MW01157083

Relational Theory
and the Practice of Psychotherapy

Other Books by Paul L. Wachtel

Psychoanalysis and Behavior Therapy: Toward an Integration

Resistance: Psychodynamic and Behavioral Approaches (editor)

The Poverty of Affluence: A Psychological Portrait of the American Way of Life

Family Dynamics in Individual Psychotherapy: A Guide to Clinical Strategies (with Ellen F. Wachtel)

Action and Insight

Therapeutic Communication: Knowing What to Say When

Psychoanalysis, Behavior Therapy, and the Relational World

Theories of Psychotherapy: Issues and Prospects (coeditor with Stanley Messer)

Race in the Mind of America: Breaking the Vicious Circle between Blacks and Whites

Relational Theory and the Practice of Psychotherapy

■ ■ ■ ■ ■

Paul L. Wachtel

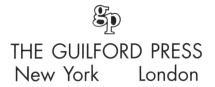

THE GUILFORD PRESS
New York   London

© 2008 The Guilford Press
A Division of Guilford Publications, Inc.
72 Spring Street, New York, NY 10012
www.guilford.com

All rights reserved

No part of this book may be reproduced, translated, stored in a retrieval
system, or transmitted, in any form or by any means, electronic, mechanical,
photocopying, microfilming, recording, or otherwise, without written
permission from the Publisher.

Printed in the United States of America

This book is printed on acid-free paper.

Last digit is print number: 9 8 7 6 5 4 3 2

Library of Congress Cataloging-in-Publication Data

Wachtel, Paul L., 1940–
   Relational theory and the practice of psychotherapy / Paul L. Wachtel.
     p. ; cm.
   Includes bibliographical references and index.
   ISBN-13: 978-1-59385-614-4 (cloth : alk. paper)
   ISBN-10: 1-59385-614-8 (cloth : alk. paper)
   1. Interpersonal psychotherapy. 2. Interpersonal relations.
3. Psychotherapist and patient. 4. Psychoanalysis. I. Title.
   [DNLM: 1. Psychoanalytic Theory. 2. Interpersonal Relations.
3. Psychoanalytic Therapy—methods. WM 460 W114r 2007]
   RC489.I55W33 2008
   616.89'14—dc22

                           2007028829

For Rajen and Tej

About the Author

Paul L. Wachtel, PhD, is CUNY Distinguished Professor in the doctoral program in clinical psychology at City College and the Graduate Center of the City University of New York. He completed his undergraduate studies at Columbia University, received his doctorate in clinical psychology at Yale University, and is a graduate of the post-doctoral program in psychoanalysis and psychotherapy at New York University, where he is also a faculty member. Dr. Wachtel has lectured and given workshops throughout the world on psychotherapy, personality theory, and the applications of psychological theory and research to the major social issues of our time. He has been a leading voice for integrative thinking in the human sciences and was a cofounder of the Society for the Exploration of Psychotherapy Integration.

Preface

A new wind is blowing in psychoanalysis. What has come to be called relational theory has introduced fresh ideas and important challenges to long-accepted views that have constrained psychoanalytic thought and kept it isolated from developments in other fields of knowledge. Relational writers have asked probing questions about how we observe and get to know another person and have redirected psychoanalytic inquiry toward the actual experiences with other people that create the foundations of personality development and constitute the texture of human life. At the same time, they have retained—and further developed—the interest in deep subjectivity that has always been the hallmark of the psychoanalytic point of view.

These new developments are of import not just for psychoanalysts. Many nonpsychoanalytic therapists have wished to extend and deepen their work, but they have been disinclined to turn to psychoanalysis for that depth because the versions of psychoanalysis they were taught (in many cases just briefly and in passing) have seemed to them alien, unscientific, or out of date. The new mode of psychoanalytic theorizing that is the topic of this book offers multiple handholds for thinkers outside the psychoanalytic realm to take hold of the discoveries and observations that have accrued from psychoanalytic investigation. Relational thinkers have already explored the interface between psychoanalytic formulations and such realms as attachment research, the broader field of mother–infant research, dynamic systems theory, and trauma research. Multiple further points of potential intersection exist in relation to family therapy and social learning theory, both of which, like relational psychoanalysis, are powerfully contextual in nature.

In this book, I aim to spell out in some detail the implications for daily clinical practice of this new development in psychoanalytic thought. In doing so, I will closely examine the main currents in relational theorizing, both to explicate the seminal contributions that have emerged and to consider where relational writings have fallen short of carrying through on their own most progressive insights. Relational theory is, in fact, not a single theory, but a set of theories, related in certain ways, differing in others. Some features of relational writing constitute a powerful critique of traditional Freudian thought and point to a radical restructuring of psychoanalytic theorizing. Other facets of the relational literature reflect still unexamined carryovers from the very assumptions and perspectives that the relational movement arose to challenge.

One of the key threads that unites these diverse theoretical efforts, giving sense to the general umbrella of "relational" thinking, is attention to people's embeddedness in a matrix of relationships, past and present, that continually shape the development of personality. Although the relational theorists I am discussing here attend to the unconscious motivations and defenses that have always concerned psychoanalytic thinkers, they generally see the structuring of these inclinations over time as strongly intertwined with the individual's actual experiences with others. Relational theories vary in the degree to which they conceptualize personality development and dynamics in a fully contextual way—this will, indeed, be one of the chief concerns of the first several chapters—but the general thrust of relational theorizing illuminates in powerful ways how even the most deeply unconscious processes must be understood in relation to context.

The version of relational thought that guides both the theoretical clarifications that are a central concern of the first half of this book and the detailed clinical discussions and recommendations that are a primary feature of the second half is one I call *cyclical psychodynamics.* Cyclical psychodynamic theory did not originally evolve as a contribution to relational theory. Indeed, at the time it was first formulated, the idea of a relational paradigm in psychoanalytic thought did not yet exist. *Psychoanalysis and Behavior Therapy* (Wachtel, 1977a), the first major expression of cyclical psychodynamic theory, was published six years before Greenberg and Mitchell's *Object Relations in Psychoanalytic Theory,* the work that is generally viewed as the first major articulation of the relational point of view. Rather, cyclical psychodynamic theory grew out of the effort to integrate the ideas and observations that were central to the psychoanalytic tradition—in which I had originally been trained and which remains to this day the core of my thinking about human behavior and experience—with those deriving from the behavioral and family systems traditions, which had become increasingly important elements in the overall spectrum of therapeutic approaches.

As will become apparent to the reader as she proceeds through this book, this different point of departure for cyclical psychodynamic theory has given it a somewhat different character from other relational theories. There are important phenomena and powerful influences on behavior and subjective experience that are not likely to be addressed when one's theorizing is focused exclusively, or even primarily, on what transpires within the psychoanalytic session. Cyclical psychodynamic theory, while remaining committed to the depth of exploration of personality associated with psychoanalytic thought, expands the frame of inquiry to include what had been left out or kept at the margins of psychoanalytic focus. It pays as much attention to the world of daily interaction with others, and even to the larger world of race, class, and culture (see, e.g., Wachtel, 1983, 1999, 2003b), as it does to the "inner" world to which much psychoanalytic discourse refers. Indeed, it aims to show how the very distinction between "inner" and "outer" is an artifact of the particular way that psychoanalytic observations were originally cast into theoretical form.

The evolution of cyclical psychodynamic theory has been influenced in important ways by many stimulating exchanges over the years at meetings of the Society for the Exploration of Psychotherapy Integration (SEPI). I had joined together in founding SEPI with a number of colleagues who were similarly deconstructing the boundaries of their original orientations, and SEPI has provided me with a valued professional home ever since. Participation in SEPI has presented me with an ever-widening web of colleagues from around the world who have repeatedly introduced me to new ideas that have required me to expand and rework the cyclical psychodynamic model. The degree to which SEPI has been a venue in which experts of quite diverse views come to genuinely listen to and learn from each other has been one of the great joys of my professional life.

My active contacts with the relational movement came a number of years later. From my base in SEPI, my professional identity had evolved as (and, indeed, remains) an *integrative* theorist and therapist. But increasingly, I found myself reading and thinking about the contributions of the writers and thinkers in the emerging relational movement in psychoanalysis and seeing striking consonances in many respects in the ways they and I thought about clinical phenomena. When Lew Aron, then the chair of the relational track in the postdoctoral program in psychoanalysis and psychotherapy at New York University (NYU), saw similar consonances, and invited me to join the relational faculty, I enthusiastically accepted the invitation.

Joining the relational faculty at NYU postdoc introduced me to a group that has perhaps been the most fertile and influential source of new ideas in the relational movement. In particular, joining the relational faculty brought me into closer contact with Steve Mitchell, a thinker and writer whose vision in many ways converges with my own. Steve and I had intermittently exchanged ideas in prior years—I had invited him to speak at SEPI and he even served on SEPI's advisory board for several years—but it was only after I joined the relational faculty that we began to meet to explore the parallels and differences in our ideas. Although our vocabularies differed in certain ways, as did aspects of our views about the relation between psychoanalysis and the larger field of psychology, we both recognized that we were tilling much the same soil and finding rather similar crops arising. Sadly, our dialogue ended with Steve's tragically early death. I still turn to his writings and continue to learn from them.

Every writer in English these days is confronted with a challenge resulting from a long history of using the male pronouns "he" and "him" to refer to people in general, as in the self-contradictory sentence "Everyone should be sure that his language usage is not sexist." Some have addressed this challenge by using plural forms, so that the gender-neutral "they" and "their" carry the weight. This serves the purpose at times, but used too regularly it seems to me to render our language too experience-distant. Others have employed the compound pronouns "he or she" and "his or her." This too can also be helpful at times, but in complex sentences it leaves English prose sounding more like German. In this book I have, therefore, chosen a different strategy. When I am referring to *the patient* in the abstract I will use "he" and "his," and when I am referring to *the therapist* in the abstract, I will use "she" and "her." (Obviously, if I am referring to a specific female patient or a specific male therapist, I will proceed differently.) This is a solution that enables me to write with the immediacy I prefer, to avoid sounding like I am writing in German, and yet to address the subtle ways in which language has shaped gender stereotypes for so many years.

This way of attributing pronouns also helps, in certain more complex sentences, to be clearer about to whom one is referring. Consider, for example, the following sequence of sentences: *Exploring the patient's transference feelings cannot proceed unless the patient has had an opportunity to test out whether it is safe to express his feelings to the therapist. He is in a potentially vulnerable position whenever he says to her something about how he is feeling about what she said.* Knowing that the "he" each time refers to the patient and the "she" refers to the therapist makes reading the second sentence considerably easier than what one would have had to deal with in the bad old days of "all he's" (and using *he or she* and "him or her" in such a sentence is a prescription for a mental hernia).

In acknowledging the enormously helpful feedback I received from friends and colleagues in the course of writing this book, I realize as well how ambitious and manifold are its aims. I seek in this book to make a contribution to critical or comparative psychoanalysis, to relational theory and practice in particular, and to the broader field and practice of psychotherapy, which extends well beyond the bounds of psychoanalytic thought altogether. I aim to be relevant to experienced practitioners who are familiar with the cutting-edge debates in the field and to beginning therapists who are looking for a clearly stated and clarifying introduction to the complexities of clinical theory and practice. And I hope to demonstrate and clarify the links between theory and practice, the ways in which sharpening and reexamining how we *think* about people, how we *conceptualize* and *formulate* our observations, can have very specific and powerful implications for how we actually practice.

This is, of course, a daunting set of aims, and it will be up to the reader to decide how well I have succeeded in each of its various elements. But broad and ambitious aims required a diverse cadre of readers to alert me to how the book might feel to readers of different theoretical orientations and different levels of experience. The individuals who gave me feedback on the manuscript varied in many respects. The one quality they all shared was a generosity of spirit and a willingness to tell me the truth about what they felt worked and what they felt needed further effort on my part. I am delighted to acknowledge Lewis Aron, Elisha Fisch, Ken Frank, Mary-Joan Gerson, Virginia Goldner, Irwin Hoffman, Libby Levitan, Lauren Levine, Judy Roth, and Marcia Sheinberg for their enormously helpful input. Some read part of the manuscript, some read all of it, but each one contributed to its improvement in important ways. I also wish to thank Libby Levitan and Becky Dell'Aglio, two outstanding students in the City University of New York doctoral program in clinical psychology, for their valuable role as research assistants.

One last acknowledgment includes much more than just reading and giving feedback. My wife, Ellen, as usual, read every chapter and offered feedback that was rooted both in her own critical intelligence and in her intimate understanding of the idiosyncrasies in my writing style. She knew when to grin and bear it and when to tell me, "No, this sentence you *have to* change." But she offered so much more than that as well. For every day of fun and depth and loving engagement I am grateful. If I understand anything about what it means to be "relational," it is due to her.

Contents

    of Subjectivity and Intersubjectivity

8. Exploration, Support, Self-Acceptance,   158
    and the "School of Suspicion"

9. Insight, Direct Experience, and the Implications   195
    of a New Understanding of Anxiety

10. Enactments, New Relational Experience,   220
    and Implicit Relational Knowing

11. Confusions about Self-Disclosure: 245
    Real Issues, Pseudo-Issues,
    and the Inevitability of Trade-Offs

12. The "Inner" World, the "Outer" World,   266
    and the Lived-In World: Mobilizing for Change
    in the Patient's Daily Life

    References   304

    Author Index   326

    Subject Index   330

Context and Relationship in Psychotherapy
AN INTRODUCTION

Human beings exist in relationships, whether those relationships be to other people with whom they have ongoing interactions, to imagoes of past important figures, to cultural traditions, values, and identifications, or to images and experiences of their own past, present, and future selves. The individual's personal life history and the relational, social, and cultural contexts in which that life history is manifested are inseparable and reciprocally determinative.

This central feature of human psychology has been addressed more fully and adequately in some therapeutic traditions than others, but it has increasingly been acknowledged across a broad spectrum of therapeutic approaches. Interest in the therapeutic alliance has increased exponentially in recent years, as has well-conducted research pointing to the central importance of the relationship in the outcome of therapeutic work (see Norcross, 2002). Family therapy, which has for some time now been a major force on the therapeutic scene, places the contextual and relational nature of human behavior and experience at the very heart of its understanding and its therapeutic approach. Behavior therapy and cognitive-behavioral therapy, though sometimes seen as quite *un*concerned with relationship, have in fact evolved from

1

a foundation (social learning theory) in which, from quite early, the responsiveness of behavior and experience to context was central, and in recent years cognitive-behavioral therapists have been paying increasing attention to the therapeutic relationship as a crucial factor in their work (see, e.g., Goldfried & Davison, 1994; Kohlenberg & Tsai, 1994; Young, Klosko, & Weishaar, 2003). Feminist approaches to psychotherapy (e.g., Miller, 1973; Miller & Stiver, 1997; Jordan, Kaplan, Stiver, & Surrey, 1991; Jordan, 1997; Simonds, 2001) have placed the relational nature of human experience at the center of their innovations in theory and practice, and the specific applications of feminist thought in the evolution of the relational psychoanalytic perspective have been very prominent (see, e.g., Aron, 1996; Benjamin, 1988, 1996, 1997; Dimen, 2003; Dimen & Goldner, 2002; Dimen & Harris, 2001; Goldner, 1991; Harris, 2005; Philipson, 1993). And, of course, psychoanalysis as a whole has been concerned with the relationship—with transference in particular—almost from the beginning.

In this book, I will especially focus on the evolution of relational thinking in psychoanalysis, but I will attempt as well to show why this development should be of interest and concern to nonpsychoanalytic practitioners and theorists as well. For the nonpsychoanalytic reader, I aim, first of all, to point to ways in which psychoanalysis has changed in recent years, and to illuminate how relational psychoanalytic approaches to exploring the individual's conflicted subjectivity can be adapted and employed within the context of a wide range of therapeutic approaches. What characterizes psychoanalytically guided work at its best is not the dogmatic application of Procrustean theories imagined by many opponents of psychoanalytic thought and practice, but, rather, careful immersion in the patient's or client's individuality and phenomenological experience. Also characteristic of psychoanalytic thought is a concern with the broader context of personality or character within which symptoms are manifested. Many therapists today, regardless of orientation, have felt the pressures from HMOs and bottom-line-oriented managed care companies that prioritize the quick fix and give short shrift to the search for greater meaning and vitality in living. Many therapists are unhappy with this turn of events and feel frustrated with the economic contingencies that impede their ability to offer their patients or clients the fullest help they are capable of offering. But in order to counter these pressures, both individual therapists and the profession as a whole need a broader and deeper understanding of personality and of mental health. In this broader and deeper understanding, psychoanalysis in general and relational psychoanalysis in particular have something vitally important to contribute.

There is, in fact, good empirical evidence that the emphasis on specific symptoms and diagnosable disorders that has been largely imposed upon the profession of psychotherapy by the weight of economic pressure by third-party payers—with some complicity by a portion of the profession itself (see Wachtel, 2006)—captures only a relatively limited portion of the larger public health challenge. In an important paper in *The American Psychologist*, Keyes (2007) has summarized much evidence that "although there is a tendency for mental health to improve as mental illness symptoms decrease, this connection is relatively modest" (p. 99). What he calls "flourishing" is a dimension that is largely orthogonal to that of diagnosable mental illness, but it is by no means a vapid luxury, the province of (as it is sometimes disparagingly put) "the worried well." Rather, as Keyes demonstrates, failure to attend to what it means to live life fully, richly, and meaningfully has in fact quite considerable consequences—even concrete economic consequences—for the nation as a whole, and it represents as well a neglect of important needs of our patients and clients.

In this, psychoanalysis is certainly not the answer in itself. Keyes himself brings an epidemiological, rather than a psychoanalytic, perspective to this research and these conclusions. But for therapists who wish to think more effectively about how to do more for the people they see than just relieve them of their symptoms, there is much to be gained from greater understanding of the contributions of psychoanalytic thought and modes of inquiry. As the dominance of psychoanalysis in the mental health professions has receded, many therapists have in fact gone through their training with little introduction to what psychoanalysis really is like or how it has changed and evolved in recent years. Or worse, they have emerged from their training with only a caricatured understanding that has enabled them to dismiss what remains a major contribution to our understanding of human behavior and experience.

I am perhaps particularly alerted to the problematic self-satisfaction that derives from holding a caricature of other orientations, because in my own graduate school training at Yale, whose clinical training at the time was largely psychoanalytic in orientation, the one departure from a very high-quality and generally quite comprehensive education was the presentation, almost as an aside, of a vision of behavior therapy that I later realized was superficial and caricatured. It was in my own later confrontation with such caricatures that I came to see the value of an approach I had prematurely dismissed and began my work on *integrating* psychoanalytic and behavioral (later cognitive-behavioral) approaches. In essence, I am now inviting therapists in the cognitive-behavioral tradition to engage in a similar journey of overcoming caricatures from the opposite direction.

This is not to suggest that psychoanalysis is without flaws or problems. Indeed, part of what is exciting about the recent contributions of relational theorists to psychoanalysis is that they address some of those very flaws and problems. They do so, however, in a way that pays intelligent and respectful attention to the phenomena on which earlier formulations were based and in a way that remains committed to understanding people comprehensively and in depth. For most of its history, psychoanalysis has been hampered by its inwardness—both in the sense of an excessive focus on the intrapsychic, without sufficient attention to how the deepest reaches of subjectivity are intertwined with the events and transactions that constitute a person's life, and in the sense that psychoanalysis has looked inward to *itself*; that is, that psychoanalytic writers have tended preponderantly to cite other psychoanalytic writers, and *not* to look to the observations and conceptualizations offered by other theories and disciplines that have also sought to understand human behavior and experience.

The relational turn in psychoanalytic thought has contributed significantly to overcoming both forms of problematic inwardness just referred to. With regard to the intrapsychic, I will argue that relational thinkers, while retaining a strong commitment to addressing the distinctive structures and regularities of personality that have traditionally been viewed as constituting the intrapsychic or the "inner world," have reconceptualized those structures and proclivities as *contextual* structures and proclivities. (I will also examine ways in which relational theories have at times fallen short of fully achieving this contextual restructuring, and will point to ways in which some prominent versions of relational thought remain unwittingly immersed in the very assumptions and viewpoints they are devoted to challenging.)

With regard to the second form of inwardness—the narrow focus on psychoanalytic contributions alone—here too relational thinking has in many instances led the way toward a transcendence of this limitation. Relational writers regularly cite the findings of infant research, attachment theory and research, elements of dynamic systems theory, and, at times, cognitive science and neuroscience. This is a natural fit, one might say, for a psychoanalytic viewpoint that is attentive to the way subjective experience is intertwined with the actual relational events that the person encounters and participates in. But here too, there are wide variations. On the one hand, not all relationalists are as receptive to the findings of other behavioral science research, and on the other, receptiveness to and interest in such findings can be found among some analysts who do not identify with the relational movement.

THE RELATIONAL SYNTHESIS, THE DEFAULT POSITION, AND THE SHADOW OF THE CLASSICAL MODEL

At the time I began working on a psychoanalytically grounded integrative model (Wachtel, 1973, 1977a), there was not yet an identified and articulated relational point of view. Although the seeds of what was later to become the relational movement could, in retrospect, be seen as already largely in place—interpersonal theory was long established, object relations thinking was a central thread in Britain and in some other parts of the world (although it had still not yet had much influence in the United States), and Heinz Kohut had already published some of the work that was the foundation of self psychology—all in all, psychoanalysis, especially American psychoanalysis, was still largely dominated by what was then called the "classical" point of view. The mainstream of American psychoanalytic thought emphasized neutrality, anonymity, caution about "gratifying" the patient's infantile needs, and the primacy of insight.

Actually, the term "classical" analysis, although by now so familiar it is difficult to excise from our vocabulary, is really a misnomer. Although it seems to suggest a fidelity to Freud's principles and practices, calling the above-noted set of rules and guidelines "classical" represents a retrospective rewriting of history that obscures the degree to which psychoanalytic practice increasingly *departed* from Freud's own way of working, which was considerably more engaged and less standoffish than the way of working that became standard psychoanalytic practice several decades later. In an interesting examination of Freud's actual practices, based on the writings of people who were his patients, Lohser and Newton (1996) argued that "classical" analysis was actually an invention of the years after World War II and is of American rather than Viennese origin (see also Lipton, 1977; Lynn & Vaillant, 1998). Hardening Freud's provisional and evolving clinical guidelines into rigid rules, these "classical" analysts advocated an approach quite different from Freud's own practices. For these highly influential postwar guardians of orthodoxy,

> silence and the absence of response [became] defined as technically correct and usually exempt from the suspicion that the analyst is acting out, a suspicion that *is* applied to talking and other more active interventions. "When in doubt, keep quiet" [became] a generally accepted prescription—yet a scrupulous analytic clinician is going to be in doubt most of the time. (Lohser & Newton, 1996, p. 178)

The further evolution of psychoanalytic technique proceeded for many years with this falsely classical view of what it meant to do psychoanalysis as its point of departure. The burden of proof fell on those who would deviate from what had become the new orthodoxy. The supposedly "classical" technique became the default position, and, ironically, innovators had to expend considerable energy justifying clinical practices whose "radical" nature largely consisted of reintroducing ways of interacting with patients that were common occurrences in Freud's own consulting room.

Today, most relational analysts and therapists—indeed, most psychoanalytically guided therapists of *all* stripes—practice quite differently in many respects from this so-called "classical" model. But the shadow of that model often falls on their practices in unrecognized ways. For relational analysts and therapists in particular, the result is that their ability to creatively follow through on their most progressive and innovative ideas can be constrained, and potentially counterproductive clinical habits are retained that, on close examination, are inconsistent with those very ideas. This may entail hesitancy about such matters as self-disclosure—a practice more common among relational analysts than among their more classical colleagues, but that nonetheless often bears a burden of proof that is not borne by the "default" position of remaining silent or purely "interpretive"—but the constraints are evident in other, sometimes more subtle ways as well. I have noticed in students and supervisees ways in which their choice of phrasing, tone of voice, facial expression, and body language reflect a close-to-the-vest caution (and consequent distancing) that has seemed not just the mark of inexperience but their unwitting imitation of the expressions of their therapists and supervisors. Hoffman (2007) describes this as "that stereotypic, stylized posture of psychoanalytic hyper-unperturbed calm."

In the following chapters, I will examine more closely the assumptions that guide psychotherapeutic work, and especially the ways in which those assumptions may be unrecognized or unarticulated or in which their impact on practice is insufficiently appreciated. I will concern myself both with older and more venerable assumptions—whether deriving from Freud, from the post-Freudian "classical" approach, or from cultural values and presuppositions widely shared by psychoanalytic and nonpsychoanalytic therapists alike—and with the newer conceptions that characterize the thinking of relationally oriented analysts, family therapists, and constructivist therapists from both psychoanalytic and cognitive perspectives (e.g., Hoffman, 1991, 1992, 1996; Guidano, 1991; Neimeyer & Mahoney, 1999). My aim is to clarify the foundations on which psychotherapy is grounded, to consider where common practices and habits are rooted in premises that are contradictory and insufficiently examined, and to spell out in some detail the implications for clinical practice of this examination.

WHAT DOES IT MEAN TO BE "RELATIONAL"?

Part of what this book aims to address is the confusion over what it means to be relational or to practice relationally. Although the two criteria I have primarily emphasized thus far—attention to context and interest in the impact of relationships in the dynamics of mental life and of the impact of the therapeutic relationship in particular in contributing to psychological change—are generally shared by relational thinkers, we will also see that different influential contributors to the relational movement offer versions of relational thinking that can differ from each other quite considerably. In part, this is one of the strengths of the relational movement. It is a loose coalition that is encouraging of diversity in viewpoint rather than seeking to impose a new orthodoxy. But this diversity of meanings also introduces confusion. Students in particular often are unclear about just what it means to be relational, and some common misconceptions are potentially problematic both theoretically and clinically. Some, for example, (mis)understand being relational as being almost relentlessly self-disclosing or as self-referentially interpreting everything that transpires as being about the therapist (Gillman, 2006).

In part, the problem lies with the very success of the relational movement. As the term "relational" has come into broader and broader use in recent years, there has been a corresponding decrease in the degree to which it communicates a clear and unambiguous meaning. This is perhaps an inevitable cost of success; relational perspectives have become increasingly prominent in the field of psychotherapy, and we have reached a point where many people want to jump onto the bandwagon. As more and more people use the term, sometimes more as a token of membership in a movement to which they wish to belong than as a substantive reference to a clearly specified set of theoretical premises and practices, the ripple of meanings makes a phrase like *relational psychotherapy* less than ideally precise.

Labels like *relational, object relational, classical,* or *contemporary Freudian* (to use examples from the psychoanalytic realm) often serve less as a medium of illuminating discourse than as a functional activity of boundary making, akin to the way our animal cousins leave their scent to mark off the boundaries of their territory. "I belong here, *you* belong *there,*" may be a sentence; but it is a sentence whose message is not very different from what is conveyed by the glands of our mammalian kin. The term *relational* has not infrequently been employed in essentially "glandular" sentences, marking a boundary in disputed conceptual territory more than promoting a process of conversation.

In a real conversation (at least in the kind of conversation I value) words are employed not just to *maintain* boundaries but to alter and complicate them. I do intend in this book to articulate the boundaries that demarcate relational approaches from others both similar and obviously dissimilar. It will become apparent, however, that the boundaries are rather permeable and shifting. There is no one meaning of *relational* that identifies all who fall on one side of the boundary and excludes all who fall on the other. Rather, we will find, the term refers to a loosely coupled *set* of ideas and set of distinctions, each element of which is shared by some relationalists and ignored or even explicitly rejected by others.

In exploring the complexities of this conceptual terrain, then, my aim is to engage in a *conversation* about the relational point of view rather than just to leave my scent and mark the boundaries. I aim, that is, to engage in that uniquely human activity in which the very process of stating what we know can contribute to *changing* what we know or how we see things. Such a description, of course, could as readily be applied to the process of psychotherapy as to conversation. And indeed, my implicitly drawing a parallel between conversation and psychotherapy is no accident. One way of thinking about the relational view of therapy is that relational therapy is an approach to psychotherapy in which the fact that it *is* a conversation—rather than a one-sided examination of one person by another—is at the very heart of how the therapist understands what she is up to.

Now, to describe psychotherapy as a conversation is at once a bland commonplace and a radical departure from the early roots of modern thinking about the therapeutic process. What went on between Freud and his patients was, of course, a kind of conversation, but one that departed so strikingly from most conversations we have in our lives that it deservedly assumed a new name—psychoanalysis. Psychoanalysis was, for many years, a therapeutic approach so thoroughly rooted in this new (and strangely different) kind of conversation that its virtual denial of the conversational heart of the enterprise was almost a defining feature of what it meant to be psychoanalytic at all. That is, within what has come to be called in recent years the "one-person" approach to psychoanalysis or psychoanalytic psychotherapy, the therapist or analyst was largely conceived of as an *observer* of what "emerged" or "unfolded" from deep within the patient (Wachtel, 1982a). And although the analyst too spoke at times, her participation was basically understood not as engaging in a dialogue, a bidirectional conversation between two people, but as offering interpretations of an inner *monologue,* emerging (often in confusing fashion) from the unconscious of the patient.

To be sure, it was often a *conflicted* monologue, one in which not only were different affectively powerful inclinations vying for expression but also in which, especially with the advent of object relations theories, different *voices* could be said to be expressing themselves. One might perhaps say that the patient's associations, reflecting these different voices, were themselves a manifestation of a kind of dialogue. But that dialogue, if one were to call it that, was not between the patient and the analyst; it was conceived of as a strictly intrapsychic phenomenon which the analyst could observe and interpret from a perspective *outside* the dialogue, as an observer rather than a participant-observer.[1]

One key element in the contemporary "relational turn" in psychoanalysis—especially as it bears on therapeutic technique rather than on

---

[1] In later chapters, I will be considering a number of different ways in which this "inner dialogue" has been conceptualized. Relational theorists, for example, have brought back into the psychoanalytic mainstream the concept of dissociation—once the dividing line between psychoanalytic conceptualizations and those of Pierre Janet. In these accounts, multiple voices and self-states are central to the story (e.g., Bromberg, 1998a).

more abstract theoretical matters—entails, in essence, an appreciation of the conversational nature of the enterprise. But like the Freudian conversation out of which it grew, it is a conversation unlike most others, a concertedly transformative activity which, while bearing more resemblances to the more "ordinary" conversations of our lives than had previously been appreciated—this is one of the key relational insights—is simultaneously unique. It is a conversation with a special capacity to be both unsettling and reassuring, and often to be both at once.

"ONE-PERSON" AND "TWO-PERSON" APPROACHES[2]

Perhaps the most common way in which relational approaches are characterized in the literature employs the distinction between "one-person" and "two-person" models. This is a conceptual distinction that bears very centrally on understanding the relational approach and its implications for clinical practice, and I will devote considerable attention to it as I proceed. But it can also be a somewhat confusing distinction, because different writers can have in mind rather different dimensions of theory or practice when they characterize an approach as one-person or two-person in nature. In the next few chapters, therefore, I will examine the various definitions and uses of these terms, attempting to clarify, critique, and sort out the various meanings and where they do and do not serve us well as guides to understanding.

When the distinction between one-person and two-person models is made, clear consensus does exist in at least one realm. There is rarely any confusion as to which term is intended to refer to more traditional psychoanalytic models and which to the newer relational models. The former are depicted as one-person models and the latter as two-person. In at least a rough way, this distinction makes a good deal of sense and does point us to a number of differences between modes of working and theorizing that are both important and real. I myself refer to one-person and two-person models quite frequently as a shorthand when I teach, and it is a useful rubric for capturing in a single phrase what is, in fact, a rather multifaceted and complicated set of differences in both assumptions and practices. The problem is that it *is* just a single phrase,

---

[2] Issues very closely related to the concept of a two-person model are also discussed widely in the relational literature in terms of the concept of intersubjectivity. I will discuss intersubjectivity in Chapter 7.

and as such it is inadequate to capture the multidimensional complexity of the actual differences among currently influential approaches. As a label or starting point it is fine. As a serious conceptualization of the issues, it is potentially confusing and misleading.

To begin with, it is worth noting that the distinction is almost always employed by putative *two-person* thinkers, as a critique of one-person modes of thought. There are rather few writers who defiantly proclaim, "I am a one-person theorist and proud of it," although there *are*, of course, many writers who declare themselves to be proponents of the models that are *called* one-person models by two-person theorists. Writing as someone who, if the dichotomy is usable at all, would without question fall on the "two-person" side of the divide, I must say I find it disquieting to be characterizing competing theorists in a way they do not acknowledge as the basis of their own thinking.

This lack of acknowledgment on the part of "one-person" theorists, of course, does not in itself invalidate the critiques. It is certainly possible that critics of one-person models are recognizing something about the theories they are criticizing that their advocates do not. Indeed, in certain respects I myself believe this to be the case. It does, however, raise a question as to whether there might be a way to frame the critique that would be more illuminating and experienced as less of a straw man by more traditional theorists.

I have suggested, only partly in jest, that in fact it comes closer to the truth to characterize the competing perspectives as one-and-a-quarter-person theories and one-and-three-quarter-person theories (Wachtel, 2002). What I mean by this is that most one-person theorists, especially *contemporary* one-person theorists, do not ignore the context or the influence of the observer as much as the label "one-person" implies and that two-person theorists are not so lost in the relational matrix that the singular properties of individuals disappear. But of course, a cosmetic refinement via fractions or decimals will not do the trick. There are much more fundamental difficulties with the one-person–two-person distinction, and I will address them beginning in the next chapter.

HOW TO READ THIS BOOK

Before immersing us in the intricate details of one-person and two-person conceptualizations, however, I wish to clarify, in this introductory chapter, some aspects of the book's structure and of its intent. This book was written with several aims and several audiences in mind. It aims, to begin with, to make a contribution to the literature of relational theory, critically examining the assumptions that have underlain some of the key contributions to the relational literature and offering alternatives and new possibilities for the application of relational thought. It aims as well to introduce students of psychotherapy to an important body of new developments and new ideas and to spell out how these new ways of looking at things can be usefully applied in their clinical work. Finally, the book aims, as has much of my previous writing, to provide a bridge between different theoretical approaches and to enable experienced therapists, clinical researchers, and teachers of psychotherapy of varying orientations to see commonalities that may be obscured by different vocabularies and emphases. In this particular book, my primary focus is on the contribution of the new relational approach to psychoanalysis. I believe, however, that readers from other orientations will find, upon close inspection, that this form of psychoanalytic theorizing and psychoanalytic practice—especially in the version I present in this book—is far more congenial to the modes of thought that have guided their work than they might have expected.

But students new to the relational literature, as well as more experienced readers who have little familiarity with relational writing, may find that their initial encounter with the key ideas of this emerging tradition is not easy going, and may not readily see at first take the consonances that I hope to make clear in this book. The vocabulary of relational theory has gradually accumulated its own jargon, and in addition relational writing retains much of the general terminology of psychoanalytic thought that has contributed to the perception by non-psychoanalytic therapists that psychoanalysis is a world apart. For readers who are not familiar with this vocabulary, I hope to clear a path and make the implications more transparent.

It may be noted that my focus on reexamining the terminology and clarifying the discourse of relational writing also has the aim of helping those who *are* familiar with the terminology to see afresh what the relational revolution has been about and to discern more clearly the new directions to which it points. The largely political aim of establishing connection and continuity with the larger psychoanalytic community has, at times, led many relational writers to use language that gives their writing a reassuringly psychoanalytic ring. The familiarly psychoanalytic vocabulary of objects and internalizations, oedipal and preoedipal, transference and countertransference, interpretation and resistance serves as a kind of psychoanalytic "identity badge," but it can make it difficult even for relationalists to be clear about what is new in their contribution and to sense fully the new possibilities that inhere in their new theoretical insights. My aim is not to "purge" our vocabulary of these familiar terms—and certainly not to ignore the phenomena to which they point. But I will examine closely in this book where they are and are not appropriate vehicles for the expression of the new directions to which relational thinking points us. In offering, at various points in the book, newer and more transparent terminology to articulate the insights of the relational paradigm shift, I aim not just to make it easier for nonpsychoanalytic readers to understand what relational theory has to offer but to illuminate for relationalists as well where the cutting edge of relational thought might lead.

The diversity of the book's intended readership, and the different relation each segment has to the material I will be presenting, suggests that different groups of readers may find that a different order of reading the chapters will be most useful and advisable. For those who are already familiar with the nature and language of relational theory and with its vocabulary, the conventional order, moving next to Chapter 2, then to Chapter 3, and so on, is probably most appropriate and useful. For those readers, however, who are less familiar with psychoanalytic or relational discourse, it may be best not to plunge right into the cold water, but to practice a more "desensitizing" reading strategy. Chapters 2 through 5 might best be read *last* by this subgroup of readers, after they have first examined and considered the concrete clinical recommendations that are central to the rest of the book.

These early chapters, constituting about a quarter of the pages of the book, are the only ones that are not amply illustrated with clinical case material. They are more abstract, examining fundamental principles and conceptual choices and probing the meanings of the terminology in which relational theory is cast. Although they are in one sense an important foundation and prologue to the later chapters (I did not accidentally or arbitrarily place them at the beginning of the book), they are also probably the most difficult chapters for a reader unfamiliar with the relational literature. For those readers, first gaining a sense of how I work clinically and how it relates to how I think theoretically—the main focus of the second half of the book—may offer them a perspective and background that will enable them to approach the earlier chapters with a clearer sense of what is at stake.

What I hope comes through in the more clinical chapters is that approaching therapeutic practice from a relational vantage point provides important links to more general principles that underlie *all* good clinical work and highlights convergences that have been obscured by political and linguistic divisions. I hope as well that these chapters illustrate the *unique* features of relational thinking, especially the ways in which it opens a path to greater depth and breadth of clinical change for therapists who had previously eschewed psychoanalytic conceptualizations as too abstruse or inattentive to the contexts of daily living.

The two middle chapters, Chapters 6 and 7, represent a kind of transitional portion of the book. They present, in more theoretical form, the particular version of relational thought that has emerged from my own particular history as a therapist and a thinker about psychotherapy and the way my "cyclical–contextual" approach compares to other common approaches to relational thought and practice. This exploration and comparison, of course, is also, at least implicitly, the topic of the entire book, but I think the reader will find these two chapters in particular to be intermediate (and intermediating) in certain respects. Moreover, unlike the earlier chapters, they include case illustrations to clarify the key points made. Thus, a useful order for readers who are not well versed in the issues and debates that are central to the relational literature—students, for example, or those from other orientations who have the intellectual openness to explore a realm that is as yet unfamiliar—might be to read Chapters 8 through 12, then to read Chapters 6 and 7, and only then to move to Chapters 2 through 5.

In whatever order you choose to read these chapters, you will inevitably find some overlap in the topics and concepts they cover. The assumptions and axioms that guide clinical work do not form a neat set of orthogonal axes. The reader will therefore find herself going over somewhat related themes in different chapters, but from different vantage points and in the context of different clinical examples and questions. The aim is to describe a way of working clinically that is rooted in the relational point of view and to spell out the thinking behind it sufficiently so that the reader can gain a better sense not only of how to practice but how to *think about* clinical practice, how to feel oriented to the patient and to the task. Put differently, the goal is to enable the reader to feel more confident in translating theory into practice, in having sufficient clarity about the aims and assumptions of the work that she can feel she *knows what she is doing.*

Obviously, this does not mean eliminating all sense of uncertainty or confusion. It is a regular feature of therapeutic work that our immersion in the conflicts and anxieties of another person inevitably means that there are times in the work—often times in *every session* even—in which we are not clear what is happening or where to go. But it is my hope that the considerations offered in this book will at least make that experience somewhat less frequent, and that even when such experiences of confusion inevitably do arise, the clarifications offered here will aid in the task—a task central to psychotherapeutic work—of using that confusion productively to understand the patient better and help him to proceed less conflictedly in the pursuit of his deepest aims.

2

■ ■ ■ ■ ■

How Do We Understand
Another Person?

ONE-PERSON AND TWO-PERSON
PERSPECTIVES

One important source of confusion surrounding the distinction
between one-person and two-person approaches is that the distinction has been brought to bear in at least three different ways—to
refer to issues of epistemology, of personality theory, and of practice.[1]
These are certainly not unrelated contexts; each in part influences and
is influenced by the others, and certain key ideas and assumptions tend
to show up in all three realms. Nonetheless, they are by no means
totally equivalent, nor do they always map onto each other in easy one-
to-one fashion.

In this chapter, I will primarily focus on the epistemological realm,
on how two-person or intersubjective theorists present an alternative
vision of what it is possible to know about another person and of what
getting to know him entails. In Chapters 3 and 4, I will turn more to

---

[1] For a different perspective on the varied meanings of one- and two-person thinking that
partially overlaps the differentiations I am pointing to here, see Spezzano (1996).

the differences between one- and two-person conceptions of personality. In all three chapters, I will consider the implications of these differing views for day-to-day clinical practice.

In the epistemological realm, two-person theorists emphasize the strong and inevitable influence of the therapist's behavior, personal characteristics, and even mere presence on what we may observe about the patient. From the two-person perspective, it is pursuing an illusion for the therapist to attempt to get a "true" or "uncontaminated" picture of the patient's inner world by diminishing her own input. "Keeping out of the way" or being "nonintrusive" in order not to distort the transference or influence what emerges or unfolds from the depths of the patient's unconscious (Wachtel, 1982a) will simply provide access to what the patient experiences or reveals *in relation to* the therapist's "keeping out of the way," since keeping out of the way is itself a way of being with another person—and one that is no less real, specific, or even evocative than any other.

From the vantage point of a two-person epistemology, the impact of the observer is so pervasive, continuous, and inevitable—so intrinsic a part of the field of observation—that to attempt to eliminate that impact is not only to engage in self-deception but actually to generate a *less* accurate or reliable picture. In part, the decrease in accuracy is due to the self-deception itself. If the therapist is not alert to her influence on what is being observed, if she denies or minimizes it, then it is difficult to take it into account, to understand that she is not really observing "the patient," but the patient *in relation to a particular kind of interpersonal relationship with a particular individual who has particular qualities and is responding to the patient's own qualities in particular ways.* The therapist who does not appreciate this tries to solve the wrong equations, so to speak; she works with equations that do not include the factor of her own influence, and hence yield misleading solutions.

A two-person epistemology does not completely eliminate the problem, of course. Knowing that one is influencing the observations does not abrogate that influence. It does, however, enable the therapist to at least ask or consider how she enters into the equation, to employ multiple perspectives to gain a better understanding of what, on the one hand, is pervasive in the patient's makeup and manifested in a very wide range of relationships and contexts and what, on the other, is more specific to the circumstances of observation that the therapy itself offers. This entails comparing how the patient feels, behaves, fantasizes, and desires in relation to the therapist in the consulting room and how he does so in the other arenas of his life.[2]

The gain in accuracy achieved in this fashion is, of course, only relative. Which events in his daily life the patient recalls or chooses to talk about in the session is itself influenced by the therapist's presence and by her characteristics and behavior. Quite different events from the patient's daily life might occur to him in the context of a different interaction with a different therapist, and these different selections from the huge menu of life experiences can give a quite different picture of what the patient's life outside the consulting room is like.

In similar fashion, *how* the patient talks about these events (whether, for example, he presents them in dry "he said, she said" terms or includes a rich account of his accompanying feelings, fantasies, and desires) also depends on the relational context in which the events are described. Consider, for example, how different your way of relating "the same" event can be when talking with someone with whom you feel very loose and comfortable and when relating the event to someone with whom you feel constricted or self-conscious.

Thus the therapist's perceptions and judgments about the patient's relationships and the affective quality of his engagements with others, even when seemingly based on the patient's accounts of the experiences of his life *outside* the office, are always also pervasively influenced by what is transpiring *within* the office. Both the actual life experiences remembered and the affective quality with which they are related might well be different with a different therapist (or with the same therapist when the therapist's own mood or affective tenor is different, or even if the therapist were operating under a different set of technical–theoretical premises).

These considerations do *not* imply, it is important to be clear, that

---

[2] A logical requirement of this position, it should be noted, is that the therapist must *pay a good deal of attention* to the patient's daily experiences with others outside the consulting room. Although this seems rather obvious, in fact much relational writing suggests that in practice many relationally oriented therapists and analysts rely rather heavily—sometimes almost exclusively—on the transference as the focus of the work. When this is the case, the ability to sort out what is a response to the therapist in particular and what is a more generalized characterological tendency for the patient is significantly impaired. I shall discuss this issue further from the perspective of therapeutic technique in later chapters.

the effort to understand the patient is futile or that the understanding arrived at is spurious. Our understanding of other people is always infused with and mediated by our own subjectivity, but we could not have survived as a social species if it were completely arbitrary. Even if imperfect, our understanding is often quite capable, to borrow from Winnicott (1953), of being "good enough." The aim of a two-person epistemology is not epistemological nihilism but a more sophisticated understanding of the ways in which we can potentially mislead ourselves in order to increase the odds that our understanding *will* be "good enough."

TWO-PERSON EPISTEMOLOGY AND ITS IMPLICATIONS FOR CLINICAL PRACTICE

Although the discussion thus far has been focused on the *epistemological* aspects of the one-person–two-person distinction, rather than on one- and two-person views regarding personality dynamics or clinical practice, it is important to be clear that the epistemological critique that is the focus of this chapter has significant implications for how—and how well—the therapeutic task itself is pursued. When the therapist believes that what she is observing is what spontaneously "emerges" or "unfolds" from the patient's unconscious (see Wachtel, 1982a), she is motivated to minimize what she views as the "distortion" introduced by her own presence and her own participation.[3] Under such rubrics as "neutrality," "anonymity," or avoiding "gratifying infantile needs" (so that those needs will build up and emerge more strongly and clearly), therapists guided by a one-person epistemology have tended to restrict their own behavior in the session, attempting, in effect, to bracket out their own influence so that what is observed comes exclusively, or at least preponderantly, from the patient.

In a variety of ways, this restriction on how the therapist may interact with the patient places unnecessary—and clinically counterproductive—

---

[3] As I discuss later in this chapter, there *is* a way in which it is useful and accurate to think of what transpires in the session as "emerging" or "unfolding," in the sense that something spontaneous and unpredictable occurs as the *two* people interact with each other. What is misleading is the view that the "true" transference or the "real" internal structure is just "there," ready to be seen in singular, undistorted accuracy if only the analyst gets out of the way and lets it "emerge."

limits on the therapist's options for helping the patient overcome his conflicts. These restrictions include not only specific interventions that considerable evidence demonstrates can be helpful (Wachtel, 1997), but limitations on the degree to which the therapist can participate in the *relationship* in ways that facilitate change. Increasingly accumulating evidence, both from clinical observation and systematic research, indicates that—over and above whatever insights are achieved in the work—the therapeutic relationship is one of the most powerful sources of therapeutic change (Norcross, 2002; Lambert, 2004; Wampold, 2001). The restrictions on that relationship deriving from the assumptions of a one-person epistemology not only hinder the establishment of a fully therapeutic engagement with the patient, they even impede the therapist from appreciating how pivotal the relationship *is* in the work, not simply as a background precondition for the "real work" of promoting insight but as a central curative agent in its own right. One of the clearest and most widely cited articulations of the rationale for attempting to restrict the therapist's behavior was offered by Merton Gill (1954). He wrote that "the clearest transference manifestations are those which recur when the analyst's behavior is constant, since under these circumstances changing manifestations in the transference cannot be attributed to an external situation, to some changed factor in the interpersonal relationship, but the analysand must accept responsibility himself" (Gill, 1954, p. 781). In this statement, Gill is specifically addressing the patient's transference manifestations, but his point clearly is intended to address the larger issue of understanding virtually *all* of the material that emerges in the course of the analysis. It is a statement of how the real insides of the patient, so to speak, are best revealed by minimizing the distorting effects of the therapist's behavior. By remaining constant, in this view, the analyst's influence is essentially removed as a variable in the equation of understanding.

Interestingly, Gill himself later became one of the sharpest critics of this one-person point of view.[4] In a series of influential books and papers, Gill (e.g., 1979, 1982, 1983, 1984, 1994; Gill & Hoffman, 1982) emphasized that the patient's transference reactions are *always* a response to something real in the analyst and in what she is doing—

---

[4] For a more detailed account of the transition in Gill's views, from a colleague who worked very closely with Gill for many years, see Hoffman (1996). See also Silverman and Wolitzky (2000).

and, simultaneously, that this in no way limits our ability to utilize the patient's transference to illuminate his psychological life or probe the depths of his character. Transference, Gill argued in these later publications, is best understood not as a "distortion," much less something made up out of whole cloth, but as the patient's particular way of making sense of and emotionally reacting to what is happening. What the patient must learn is not that he is "wrong," but that he is selective, and that that selection may be motivated and rooted in past experiences in ways he has not understood. Transference, in Gill's later view, is a matter of *perspective*, and the question to be pursued, in essence, is "Why *this* perspective, why *this* way of seeing things?" (as well as such related, and clinically important, questions as "How *else* could you see it?", "What *other* perspective might you bring to bear?", or "What keeps you from considering *that* possibility?").

Gill (1984) notes that, for reasons closely related to those he outlined in his 1954 paper, many analysts are reluctant to interact very much with their patients, fearing that they will distort the transference by doing so. But, he now argues, "the notion of an 'uncontaminated' transference is a myth," and it is a myth that fosters an unfortunate restraint on the analyst's part. This restraint may lead to emotional deprivation for the patient, but it does *not* provide a superior pipeline to the patient's emotional truth. Rather, it points to the analyst's

> failure to be fully aware that because analysis takes place in an interpersonal context there is no such thing as non-interaction. Silence is of course a behaviour too. Nor can one maintain that silence is preferable for the purpose of analysis because it is neutral in reality. It may be intended to be neutral but silence too can be plausibly experienced as anything ranging from cruel inhumanity to tender concern. It is not possible to say that any of these attitudes is necessarily a distortion. (Gill, 1984, p. 168)

Elsewhere, in a comment that again challenges the conservative position represented by his 1954 paper and still maintained by a significant portion of the psychoanalytic mainstream, Gill notes that

> if the analyst remains under the illusion that the current cues he provides to the patient can be reduced to the vanishing point, he may be led into a silent withdrawal, which is not too distant from the caricature of an analyst as someone who does indeed refuse to have any personal relationship with the patient. What happens then is that

silence has become a technique rather than merely an indication that the analyst is listening. *The patient's responses under such conditions can be mistaken for uncontaminated transference when they are in fact transference adaptations to the actuality of silence.* (1979, p. 277, italics in original)[5]

Gill's emphasis centers on two key themes—that this mistaken, epistemologically naive position can lead to unnecessary, and clinically counterproductive harshness and withdrawal, and, further in contrast to his earlier position, that it can actually render the analyst's interpretations *less* persuasive. Attempting to prove to the patient that his experience of the analyst has little or nothing to do with what she is really like or how she is really behaving is actually a formula for creating resistance. There is more likelihood of common ground, of the patient feeling seen and heard and taken seriously, and hence of the patient being in a position *really* to consider the alternative view that the analyst is putting forth, if the message takes the form of "I understand that what I did/what I said/ what I failed to say felt to you that I. . . . Is there any other way it could *also* be seen?"

ADDRESSING INDIVIDUALITY AND THE UNCONSCIOUS: ONE- AND TWO-PERSON VIEWS

More sophisticated "one-person" theorists, it should be noted, acknowledge many of these considerations, but view quite differently their implications for how best to go about understanding the patient or building theory. They recognize that the influence of the analyst on what is observed is inevitable, but they attempt to at least *reduce* that influence as much as possible, and they believe they can do so effectively enough to gain a reasonably accurate and reasonably undistorted picture of what the patient's personality and dynamics are "really" like apart from that influence. In one discussion of this issue, in a psychoanalytic group to which I belong, a proponent of the traditional rules of neutrality and anonymity remarked that although the "contaminating" influence of the analyst can never be completely eliminated from our observations, this no more implies that we should not attempt to

---

[5] For an interesting discussion of similar issues that usefully complements Gill's discussion and offers a wealth of clinical examples, see Ehrenberg (1992).

minimize that influence than the fact that the operating room too can never be a completely sterile field implies that we should do surgery in a cesspool.

At the heart of the one-person view, both epistemologically and technically, is the conviction that there *is* something "inside" the patient that exists independently of the observer and her influence and that can be seen by the observer (or at least inferred by the observer, or interpreted by the observer) even if the understanding achieved is less than absolutely perfect. This conviction includes as well that the inclinations and characteristics that come to light in the course of the therapeutic work have been long-standing in the patient's psyche, that they existed before the therapist's observation and (unless change is successfully initiated by the therapeutic process) will continue to exist long after the therapist's observations. We may not be able to exclude our influence perfectly or completely, but the effort to do so *as much as we can* will be rewarded by a more accurate and complete understanding.

In contrast, those operating from the vantage point of a two-person epistemology argue that *in principle* we cannot observe the reality of another person's psychological structures or experiences in an "objective" fashion that is divorced from the relational context within which we gain access to them.[6] Moreover, this is not just a matter of observer bias or incorrect *interpretation* of the observations. It is more intrinsic than that. What actually *is* changes as a function of the particular observer and his or her behavior and characteristics (see, e.g., Aron, 1996; Hoffman, 1998; Mitchell, 1988a; Stern, 1996). As Ogden has pithily put it, playfully tweaking Winnicott's (1975) famous phrase about mothers and babies, "there is no such thing as an analysand apart from the relationship with the analyst, and no such thing as an analyst apart from the relationship with the analysand" (Ogden, 1994, p. 4).

It is important to be clear what such a position does and does not

---

[6] This position is often likened to Heisenberg's uncertainty principle or to the ideas in relativity theory about the way such fundamental dimensions as time or distance, once thought to simply "exist" independently of the conditions of observation, are dependent on the position and relative motion of the observer. No doubt, the ways in which both quantum theory and relativity theory shook to its core our very notion of reality had a profound effect on thinkers in all realms, including the psychological. But the resemblances to these two highly mathematical conceptualizations—addressed to phenomena occurring at close to the speed of light or in the realm of the almost unimaginably small—are at best very loosely analogical. Ideas about "uncertainty" or "relativity" in the psychological realm must stand on their own feet, without the borrowed prestige of these quite different kinds of theories.

imply. Critics of two-person theorizing sometimes argue that the two-person position entails denial of the very existence of enduring psychological structures or of the possibility of understanding another person as more than a mere product of his interaction with us in the present moment. Although it is possible to find writings by two-person theorists that seem to lend themselves to such an interpretation, mostly this is an exaggeration or caricature of the two-person point of view. In my own work, notwithstanding my clearly falling on the two-person side of the divide, I comfortably assume that there is a "there" there—that however constrained our perceptions may be by our personal biases or by our relation to what is being observed (whether in the realm of perceiving the physical world or the psychological), there *is* something there to perceive. We may not be able to perceive the other "objectively," but neither are our perceptions simply arbitrary. They are meaningful, useful, and usually refer to something "real," even if they are *also* infused with our own subjectivity and particular point of view—that is, even if they are also partial, in both senses of the word (i.e., *incomplete* and *biased*).

Similarly, although it is illuminating to understand the degree to which our perceptions or memories are always *constructions*—advances in recent decades in the understanding both of perception and of memory make it clear that we do not directly "see" anything (i.e., that perception is always a creative act of putting together a picture from bits and pieces of information) nor do we ever simply remember by calling up "memory traces" that function like pictures to be pulled out of a file (Schachter, 1996, 2001; Schimek, 1975b)—this does not mean that there is no real thing or event that we are seeing or remembering or that there is not a meaningful distinction between more and less accurate memories (though of course determining which are which is not always a simple matter). We may *construct* our memories and perceptions, but we do not usually construct them out of whole cloth.

Where does this leave our understanding of the unconscious? Implicit, it seems to me, in the relational or intersubjective critique of the one-person model is a critique of "The Unconscious" as something residing inside the person, playing out its own agenda almost as a separate entity apart from the person inside of whom it is assumed to reside. "The Unconscious" is a one-person conception par excellence, something inside waiting to be *discovered.* In contrast, concern with *unconscious processes,* with the way in which so much of what constitutes psychological life proceeds without awareness, is perfectly compatible with the two-person critique. We do not "discover" or uncover what has been there all along. Rather, we engage in processes of *construction* (and co-construction) which bring forth and help articulate experiences in a dynamic, constantly evolving fashion. What emerges from the therapeutic process is not something that was previously buried and is now brought to light (see Chapter 6 for further discussion of this theme), but something that is at least in part new, something that emerges in a different sense—in the sense of an "emergent" phenomenon that cannot be reduced solely to its origins or its components.

But in conceiving of what emerges in the course of the therapeutic process as new, it is important to be clear, one is *not* engaging in the fictional caricature of relational thinking that portrays relationalists as denying that the patient had a personality or specific characteristics or inclinations before he walked into the consulting room. What is constructed in the session, we might say, is built with already existing raw materials. What changes is that experiences that were previously unformulated, to use Stern's (1997) generative and perspicacious term, achieve a greater degree not just of focal awareness but also of structure and articulation.

I shall have a good deal more to say about Stern's important concept, and its implications for therapeutic practice, in Chapter 8 in particular, but it is highly relevant to the present discussion as well. In the process of articulating previously unformulated experiences, these experiences and the psychological inclinations associated with them *inevitably* change. An articulated version of an experience is, by its very nature, different from an unarticulated or unformulated version. And, moreover, once that articulation is achieved, it almost inevitably leads to still further changes. These changes may be small and unstable; that is why psychotherapy that aims at deep and comprehensive change can take so long. But they are the daily bread of the therapeutic endeavor, the way the process continually proceeds. Change is not the product of a prior process of discovery, something that must wait until the digging is completed and the treasure unearthed from the layers in which it was buried. Change *is* the process, and what is discovered is not simply something that was there all along but something that emerges from the process of exploration and interaction itself. *Something* would have been there, in the sense (again) that the person *does* have a personality before he enters the consulting room. But what was there before is *different* from what is "discovered." We can never discover what was lying buried before we entered the scene because our entering the scene inevitably changes the person's experience of the world. The change (alas) may not always be positive, and (also alas) it may not always be large. But it is the foundation on which further change is constructed, and an understanding of the process in this fashion opens up a host of new possibilities for engaging the patient in a helpful fashion.

THE DEFAULT POSITION
AND "EPISTEMOLOGICAL ANXIETIES"

Concerns about epistemology, I have begun to suggest, are far less removed from the conduct of daily clinical practice than one might initially imagine. Indeed, in good measure, epistemological concerns were responsible for how the practice of psychotherapy evolved in its crucial early years and for the emergence of what I referred to in Chapter 1 as the "default position," the almost automatic stance that therapists assume almost without noticing and regarding which the burden of proof has fallen disproportionately upon those who would challenge or depart from it.

In principle, there were—and are—an enormous range of ways in which a therapeutic relationship might be structured. But once a particular way of working begins to be accepted as standard procedure, it is not long before habit, the wish to belong and to feel "professional," and the disinclination to reinvent the wheel all conspire, as it were, to restrict our vision and our imaginations. Certain features of the psychotherapist's stance that were to some degree historical accidents (and were certainly not the only way that one could productively or appropriately construct a therapeutic relationship) have, over the years, become "standard" in such a way that they may appear to be simply "how things are." As a consequence, these assumptions and habits of practice have persisted, little noticed or reflected upon, in the work of many contemporary therapists. The epistemological assumptions that have characterized the "one-person" point of view were the foundation on which the modern profession of psychotherapy was constructed, and although that point of view has come under increasing scrutiny and challenge over the years, many of the habits and assumptions about clinical practice that evolved in relation to this foundation have persisted. Indeed, if one looks closely, they are often evident in the work of therapists who explicitly identify with a two-person position and even of therapists whose identifications lie outside the psychoanalytic realm altogether. This is the case because much of what we learn about actual clinical practice we learn not from reading or course work but from identification with our supervisors or the direct experience of our own personal therapy. And since our profession is still relatively young, only a few generations separate the period of psychoanalytic hegemony from the current state of multiple and competing orientations and viewpoints. This means that even if one's personal therapist or one's most recent supervisors were not themselves Freudians, *their* supervisors, or their supervisors' supervisors, were. And since aspects of the basic *stance* toward the patient—the emotional tone, the readiness to answer particular kinds of questions, the degree to which one spontaneously expresses aspects of one's own views and reactions or even shares one's sense of humor—are learned largely through identification and less explicit or conscious *procedural* learning (Lyons-Ruth, 1999; Stern et al., 1998), these dimensions of the work change much more slowly than explicit theoretical positions and conscious strategies. As a consequence, the "deep structure" of many therapists' work may reflect ideas that have persisted largely unchanged and unexamined from an earlier era.

These considerations suggest that it behooves us to look more closely at the assumptions that guided therapeutic work in its early years because significant traces of those assumptions (and the practices associated with them) may be evident among therapists who do not consciously identify with the original point of view or who even explicitly challenge it.

Much of what the relational movement in psychoanalysis has been about has been, in essence, a challenge to what I am calling the default position. As we shall see in the next few chapters, however, the challenge has not always been as sharp or as thorough as it might have been. Greater understanding of how and why the default position arose in the first place—including the way in which it was shaped by concerns about potential challenges to the evidential base of psychoanalytic formulations—may facilitate a more probing reexamination that can enable us to better sort out what is and is not still valid and useful.

To a degree that is rarely discussed or appreciated, the origins of the default position lay in a set of epistemological concerns on Freud's part that it would not be an exaggeration to call his *epistemological anxieties,* concerns that the entire corpus of his work would be dismissed as merely the product of suggestion. Freud has been fairly consistently described by his biographers as a man whose primary identity and primary investment was as a discoverer rather than a healer. He shifted from a career in research to one in clinical practice only reluctantly and under the financial pressures associated with getting married and establishing a family (Jones, 1953), and he stated quite clearly that he lacked therapeutic zeal. If the judgment of the scientific community, whose respect he greatly sought, were to have been that his method "worked," but that it worked by *suggestion* and not because his "discoveries" were valid, that would have been, for him, a bitter pill to swallow.

Although Freud soon turned away from the directly suggestive treatments he had utilized very early in his career, he struggled with the recognition that nonetheless suggestion was never really fully left behind. It remained a continuing feature of the psychoanalytic relationship, threatening to corrode the very foundations of his claims to scientific discovery. Freud repeatedly alternated between, on the one hand, acknowledging how pervasive—and even therapeutically essential—the role of suggestion actually was in the psychoanalytic process and, on the other, attempting to banish, deny, or transcend its influence. As I have discussed in a more detailed examination of Freud's writings on suggestion and their clinical implications (Wachtel, 1993, Ch. 9), often these conflicting acknowledgments and claims could be found in the same paper, sometimes even on the same page.

In his *Introductory Lectures on Psycho-Analysis*, for example, Freud (1916) states:

> When the patient is to fight his way through the normal conflict with the resistances which we have uncovered for him in the analysis, he is in need of a powerful stimulus which will influence the decision in the sense which we desire, leading to recovery. . . . At this point what turns the scale in his struggle is not his intellectual insight—which is neither strong enough nor free enough for such an achievement—but *simply and solely* his relationship to the doctor. In so far as his transference bears a "plus" sign, it *clothes the doctor with authority and is transformed into belief in his communications and explanations.* In the absence of such a transference, or if it is a negative one, the patient would never even give a hearing to the doctor and his arguments. (p. 445, italics added)

Indeed, he goes on to say that "it must dawn on us that in our technique we have abandoned hypnosis only to rediscover suggestion in the shape of transference" (p. 446).

This quotation from Freud is remarkable for its frank confrontation with a difficult and thorny question. But it also highlights why Freud felt it necessary to continually offer counterarguments maintaining that in one way or another this suggestive influence was limited or transcended in psychoanalysis in a way that it is nowhere else in human relationships. If the suggestive influence of the transference creates a belief on the patient's part in the therapist's views, if the analyst is "clothed with authority," then what does this say about the epistemological foundations of the *findings* of psychoanalysis? Are they validated by the patient's assent, or even by his cure, or do both just reflect the patient's *compliance*, his readiness to believe—even to believe deeply—what the analyst has told him or what the analyst has suggested in more subtle and implicit ways? This was Freud's great nightmare, and it is what has led me to use the term "epistemological anxiety" to describe the frame of mind that so fatefully shaped psychoanalytic history.

In one of the most direct and explicit statements of these concerns, Freud stated that "whether we call the motive force of our analysis transference or suggestion, there is a risk that the influencing of our patient may make the objective certainty of our findings doubtful and that what is advantageous to our therapy is damaging to our researches"[7] (p. 452). Plunging further into the heart of darkness, he acknowledges that if this account of what transpires in analysis were valid, "psychoanalysis would be nothing more than a particularly well-disguised and particularly effective form of suggestive treatment; and we should have to attach little weight to all that it tells us about what influences our lives, the dynamics of the mind or the unconscious" (p. 452).

Freud had two major strategies for dealing with this threat to his reputation as a scientist and discoverer. One was stated in an encyclopedia article on psychoanalysis that he wrote in 1922. Its aim was to *differentiate* the role of suggestion in psychoanalysis from how suggestion is used in other therapeutic approaches:

Psycho-analytic procedure differs from all methods making use of suggestion, persuasion, etc., in that it does not seek to suppress by means of authority any mental phenomenon that may occur in the patient. It endeavors to trace the causation of the phenomenon

---

[7] Implicit in this statement, it is important to notice, is an acknowledgment that the element of suggestion *is* advantageous to the *therapeutic* aims of analysis.

and to remove it by bringing about a permanent modification in the conditions that led to it. In psycho-analysis the suggestive influence which is inevitably exercised by the physician is diverted on to the task assigned to the patient of overcoming his resistances, that is, of carrying forward the curative process. (Freud, 1923, pp. 250–251)

This strategy for addressing the impact of suggestion essentially attempts to tame the troublesome beast by harnessing it to the core psychoanalytic aims of exploration and discovery. It *acknowledges* the role of suggestion but does so in a way that interprets it as an aid to the exploratory process itself. In this view, suggestion is employed not to put new ideas into the patient's head but to discover those that were already there. Had this been Freud's only way of attempting to put to rest the threat that suggestion carried for the credibility of his discoveries, psychoanalytic technique might have evolved very differently. In Chapter 9, for example, I explore the momentous implications for therapeutic practice of a theoretical revision Freud published only a few years later (Freud, 1926), in which he radically revised his understanding of the role of anxiety in the evolution and dynamics of psychopathology. One key implication of this theoretical revision, we will see, is that it makes more central than had previously been the case the therapist's efforts to *help the patient become less afraid* of his feelings and wishes. From this vantage point, the employment of suggestion to help the patient with "the task assigned to [him] of overcoming his resistances" can best be understood as one of creating an atmosphere of safety for the patient and encouraging him to face, little by little, the very experiences from which he has previously retreated in helpless terror. As the analysis in Chapter 9 aims to make clear, *this* way of putting the demon of suggestion to rest points to a much more supportive approach to therapy and highlights why such an approach can be more, not less, effective in promoting meaningful exploration as well.

But the argument that suggestion is used in analysis, but used differently, was not Freud's only line of defense. Indeed, it was not really even his *primary* line of defense. Perhaps because the threat posed by suggestion was so great, Freud employed another strategy as well, designed not just to reinterpret the role of suggestion but, ultimately, to eliminate it. Suggestion, Freud claimed, could be used for the purposes of the work for a while, but eventually it had to be "dissolved."[8] Thus in his *Introductory Lectures*, just a few pages after the passages quoted earlier acknowledging that the transference "clothes the doctor with authority and is transformed into belief in his communications and explanations" and that "we have abandoned hypnosis only to rediscover suggestion in the shape of transference," Freud goes on to say, "In every other kind of suggestive treatment, the transference is carefully preserved and left untouched; in analysis it is itself subjected to treatment and is dissected in all the shapes in which it appears. At the end of an analytic treatment the transference must itself be cleared away" (1916, p. 453).

We may note to begin with that the phrase "in every *other* kind of suggestive treatment" clearly implies that psychoanalysis too is a suggestive treatment.[9] But even if we were to take it as meaning that it is a suggestive treatment in which, uniquely, that element of suggestion is later dissolved, we must confront a further challenge: what it *means* to "clear away," or even to "analyze," the transference, is far less clear than Freud's deft rhetorical trope seems to imply. One may, of course, *point out* to the patient the element of authority or suggestion that has been carrying the therapy thus far. And in that sense, one is "interpreting" the transference dimension, and, perhaps, *attempting* to dissolve it. The problem with this line of argument, however, is that in the attempt to "interpret away" the transference influence, the very same structure of authority and of potential suggestion exists. Why does the patient now accept *this* interpretation? Can we reassure ourselves that *this time* we have stepped outside the structure that Freud acknowledges both in the quotations above and in numerous other places throughout his writings?[10] The attempt to wriggle out of this dilemma requires us, essentially, to posit an epistemological skyhook. It also, as I will discuss next, led to the

---

[8] "Dissolved" is the word used in the English translation that appears in the edition published by Basic Books as the *Collected Papers*. In the *Standard Edition* translation the term used is "cleared away."

[9] We may perhaps wish to amuse ourselves here by noting, apropos this revealing phrase, Freud's own comment, in another context, "no mortal can keep a secret. If his lips are silent, he chatters with his fingertips; betrayal oozes out of him at every pore" (Freud, 1905, pp. 77–78).

[10] See Wachtel (1993, Ch. 9) for a more detailed account of these acknowledgments of the suggestive influence in psychoanalysis and of Freud's struggle with their implications.

enshrinement of a one-person approach to the therapeutic relationship from which psychoanalysis (and in certain ways much of the
entire field of psychotherapy) is still struggling to emerge.

THE FEAR OF SUGGESTION AND THE MINIMIZING
OF THE RELATIONSHIP

Freud's comment (quoted above) that "what is advantageous to our
therapy is damaging to our researches" holds in the opposite direction
as well. The research aim of psychoanalysis, its focus on *discovery* of
unconscious contents and the construction of the therapy around the
need to protect the findings of the research from the charge of suggestion, placed constraints on the *therapeutic* efforts of psychoanalysis,
constraints that are still being struggled with today. In particular, the
concerns about suggestion and the commitment to the idea that exploration and discovery were the heart of the therapeutic process led to a
downplaying of the *relationship* as a crucial and powerful therapeutic
influence in its own right. Rather, the relationship was seen more as a
medium through which the decisive therapeutic processes of discovery
of unconscious contents and promotion of insight could be most effectively and persuasively pursued. Transference analysis was, first and
foremost, a form of *analysis*, a way of *understanding* and *discovering*.
The role of the therapeutic relationship as a powerfully transformative
emotional experience quite apart from whatever insights it generates
was, in the foundational years of psychoanalytic work, decidedly
played down
    In later years, psychoanalytic writers such as Alexander (1956;
Alexander & French, 1946) in the United States and Winnicott (1971,
1975) and Fairbairn (1958) in England began to place the relationship
and its potential for therapeutic impact in its own right much closer to
the heart of the process, picking up a thread that had been earlier introduced by Ferenczi (e.g., Ferenczi, 1926; Ferenczi & Rank, 1925), who
encountered fierce criticism and even character assassination for his
efforts (Aron & Harris, 1993).[11] As we will see especially in Chapter
10, in recent years this appreciation of the central role of the relationship per se has increasingly become the cutting edge of psychoanalytic

---

[11] In a much more conservative fashion (see Hoffman, 1983), this dimension was introduced
relatively early as well by Strachey (1934).

discourse about the therapeutic process, and this emphasis dovetails with a rapidly expanding body of findings from systematic research (see, e.g., Norcross, 2002; Lambert, 2004; Wampold, 2001). Indeed, the attitude that insight and new relational experiences are *competing* paradigms for the therapeutic process has increasingly been replaced by the view that they are in fact complementary—that the therapist's communication of her understanding of the patient's as yet unexpressed and unarticulated yearnings *is* to a very significant degree what the new relational experience consists of, and that, conversely, what enables the insight to have a deep emotional impact on the patient is that it is achieved in the context of an intimate and meaningful relationship (see, e.g., Stolorow, Brandchaft, & Atwood, 1987). We will also see, however, that the shadow of the default position nonetheless continues to be powerfully evident in many aspects of therapeutic practice to this day.

Ironically, as I noted in Chapter 1, the restrictions were less evident in Freud's own clinical work than they were in those who relied on his *writings* as a guide to practice. But Freud was nonetheless clearly the source of what is today called the one-person model. This model may not have been so evident in his actual practice, but it was strongly evident in what Freud *wrote* about the therapeutic process. There he famously used metaphors likening the analyst to a blank screen, a reflecting mirror, or an impassive surgeon—images that both placed constraints upon the therapeutic relationship and the interaction between patient and therapist and bolstered the depiction of the psychoanalytic process as one characterized by objectivity and science.

These rules and restraints in the literature on psychoanalytic technique (largely constituting what I have called the default position) had multiple sources. In part, Freud was concerned about what he viewed as misguided humanitarianism, the consequences for the therapeutic process of the analyst trying too hard to be helpful, the ways in which impulses and inclinations which in everyday life are fine and even salutary could be harmful to the progress of an analysis (Freud, 1912a). But there is much to suggest that it was his epistemological anxieties that were most responsible for the shape that he gave to the therapeutic approach we call psychoanalysis (and, indirectly, to much nonpsychoanalytic work that followed). It was most of all the effort to safeguard the discoveries, to protect them from the claim that they were merely the product of suggestion, that gave rise to such ideas as that the therapist should remain as anonymous as possible, that she should respond to a question with a question, and so forth. "What is advantageous to our therapy is damaging to our researches," Freud said, and over time he persuaded himself, and later analysts, that it must therefore ultimately be harmful to the therapy as well.

FROM EPISTEMOLOGY TO SUBSTANTIVE THEORY

Thus we may see that epistemological concerns, far from being an abstruse intellectual preoccupation, were at the very heart of how the psychoanalytic approach to therapeutic practice was constructed and, as discussed above, in certain respects shaped the course of a still wider range of therapeutic approaches in unappreciated ways. To a significant degree, the relational point of view—with its emphasis on mutual influence and co-construction—evolved from the effort to overcome the constricting epistemological assumptions with which psychoanalysis was for so long linked, assumptions that were not really intrinsic to much that constituted the contribution of psychoanalysis to human knowledge or to its capacity to help people lead more vital, self-aware, and satisfying lives. Relational writers have incisively and probingly critiqued the epistemological foundations of psychoanalytic theory, and in the process have pointed us toward new and important theoretical conceptions. But because relational thinkers have often not been as clear about the ways in which epistemological concerns shaped psychoanalytic *practice*, they have been hampered in fully developing the implications of their critique. Many extremely important innovations have emerged from the relational movement, of course—this is, after all, a book that proudly declares itself to be a part of that movement. But I hope to show that there is still greater potential for therapeutic change and innovation implicit in the ideas that have emerged from the relational critique and that part of the realization of that potential requires us to appreciate the impact of epistemological concerns in shaping the very structure of the psychoanalytic relationship and of psychoanalytic practice.

At the same time, however, it may also be said that epistemological concerns have been *too* central in the canon of relational writings and in the demarcation of the relational point of view. The "two-person" perspective that characterizes the *epistemological* stance of most relational thinkers has not always been carried forward into their framing of the *substantive theories* that guide their work—theories regarding the dynamics of personality development and the sources of psychological dysfunction. As I discuss in the next chapter, the relational versions of these theories have often been characterized by what might be called two-person content embedded in a one-person structure. It is to this topic, and to a number of other important confusions and misunderstandings regarding the two-person point of view and its implications for practice, that I now turn.

3

■ ■ ■ ■ ■

The Dynamics of
Personality

ONE-PERSON
AND TWO-PERSON VIEWS

We have seen that two-person theorists' views of how we understand another person stress the inevitable and powerful influence of our own needs, proclivities, and active participation with the
person we are trying to understand. There is no "immaculate perception" (Nietzsche, 1885; Kosslyn & Sussman, 1995) whereby we may
simply see the person as he or she "is," divorced from our own role in
the investigative process and our own point of view. This is no mere
ivory tower abstraction; it has profound implications for how we actually proceed clinically. At the very least, it implies that the transference
does not simply "unfold" or "emerge" for us to observe it in its pristine
purity, that there is no single "real" or "true" transference that will be
revealed if only we stay out of the way and do not muddy it. The transference, as well as everything else we observe about the patient, is
drenched in our participation in the events we are observing, two-
person theorists tell us, and failure to appreciate this impoverishes our
understanding and misleads us in significant and problematic ways.

It is important to recognize, however, that how fundamentally or
comprehensively any given therapist modifies the traditional stance of

the relatively "neutral," anonymous, or minimally interactive therapist is not necessarily predictable from the position she takes on the epistemological questions that have occupied us thus far. There are therapists whose endorsement of the "two-person" epistemological position described in the last chapter is associated with an approach to clinical practice that departs quite substantially from traditional models, and there are therapists whose endorsement of such a position feels to them quite consistent with a mode of daily practice that in its basic structure or stance is barely distinguishable from the way therapists proceeded 50 or 60 years ago.[1] This diversity of practice modes among therapists who identify as relational or two-person in their point of view is a source of considerable potential confusion, especially for new therapists trying to learn how to work relationally, or even to decide whether or not the relational perspective is one they wish to explore further.

A related source of confusion is the view, held by many who are unfamiliar with relational thinking, that a relational perspective *requires* the therapist to self-disclose frequently, to be active and explicitly interactional almost all the time, and in other ways to depart from the mode of practice that has characterized exploratory or depth-oriented psychotherapy almost from its inception. As we shall see, this is a misunderstanding of the therapeutic implications of a relational point of view. What is intrinsic to that point of view is simply to question the requirement that the therapist *must not* engage in these "departures." Saying that one *may* engage in any particular activity and saying that one must are quite different. It is the very elements of choice, variability, and sensitivity to the specifics of the patient and what the patient is seeking (cf. Bacal, 1998; Bacal & Herzog, 2003) that most centrally characterize relational practice, and it is a central aim of this book to explore and clarify the implications of this way of working.

TWO-PERSON EPISTEMOLOGY, ONE-PERSON THEORY?

A key reason for the perhaps surprising lack of linkage between the holding of a two-person epistemological position and the stance the

---

[1] Arnold Modell, for example, one of the psychoanalytic authors who has written most extensively about the one-person versus two-person distinction, states quite explicitly that his version of a two-person perspective "does not lead to any modification of basic technique" (1988, p. 578).

therapist takes in clinical practice lies in differences in the substantive theories of personality dynamics and development that various "two-person" theorists hold to and advocate. As I hope to make clear in this chapter, it is not uncommon for therapists who manifest a two-person perspective with regard to the epistemological questions of how and what we actually *know about* another person and how our own participation influences what we observe (and who, partly because of this, identify themselves as relational in orientation) to manifest largely *one*-person thinking in their understanding of the dynamics of personality, the nature of psychological development, or the factors contributing to and maintaining the psychological difficulties from which their patients suffer.

Gaining a clearer understanding of the ways in which some relational approaches have more of a "one-person" than a "two-person" character is perhaps best approached by looking first at the theoretical perspectives from which relational thinkers have attempted to differentiate themselves and which they have tended to label as "one-person" theories. In doing so, we can see better how some relational thinkers have incorporated key structural features of the very models they were explicitly attempting to replace and transcend.

By and large, the theorizing that is best characterized as one-person in nature is theory that stresses the "internal" structures of the personality and depicts them as being relatively uninfluenced by current experiences or by the current relational context. In Freud's theorizing, for example, one of the key characteristics of the id, in contrast to the ego, is that it is relatively impervious to new input from reality. When Freud (1923) defines the ego as the part of the personality that "starts out from perception" and that "has been modified by the direct influence of the external world" (p. 25), he is implicitly—and with clear intent—defining the id as *not* influenced by the external world, *not* linked very closely or directly with perception. The id, for Freud, functions as a kind of free agent in the psyche, influencing the ego and our actions in the real world but not in turn being *influenced by* them, except insofar as its inclinations are blocked or diverted by the actions of defenses or further aroused by new stimulation. That is, id desires and fantasies can be stirred or triggered by current experiences, can be at least partially constrained or inhibited by the dictates of reality as mediated by the ego, but they cannot be significantly *changed* by new experience, they cannot *grow up*. Only the ego can evolve and adapt in response to new experiences. The id remains infantile, primitive, archaic, and timeless.

It is not surprising that this way of thinking was continued in those later theories which followed most closely the line of development of "orthodox" psychoanalysis—the so-called "classical" approach and its further elaboration as ego psychology. More noteworthy is that it is evident as well in some threads of theory development that have contributed significantly to the contemporary *relational* point of view and that are commonly viewed as paradigmatic examples of *two-person* theory. Object relations theories and self psychology introduce many important new ideas, and their views about the wellsprings of our motivational and fantasy life differ in significant ways from Freud's original formulations.[2] But in their theoretical *structure* they do not depart as sharply. As a consequence, many of the formulations that are widely viewed as important elements of the relational synthesis, are, in the crude terminology of "one-" and "two-" person theories (a terminology I will further examine critically in the next chapter) more one-person theories than two-person theories. This is a source of considerable potential confusion in attempting to sort out the implications of these theories.

Central to what I mean by the "one-person" structure of some putatively relational theories is their reliance, either explicitly or implicitly, on concepts of fixation or developmental arrest and their tendency to view key elements in the psyche as "early" (especially "preoedipal"), "archaic," or "primitive." The concepts of fixation and arrest reflect the assumption (shared by Freud) that early experiences, fantasies, desires, or representations are preserved in the psyche in their original form (and, in most of these conceptualizations, preserved in their original intensity as well). They imply additionally that the fixated or arrested psychological structure is largely impervious to modification by new experiences— or at least by any experience other than the unique experience of psychoanalysis itself, which is seen as fostering a regression to the early fault, flaw, fixation, point of arrest, or primitive or archaic layer of the psyche.

In much theoretical writing in the object relations and self psychological traditions, no less than in earlier Freudian accounts, crucial parts of the psyche are viewed as frozen in time, unable to grow up as the more familiar and accessible reaches of the psyche do, unable to

---

[2] In contrast to the Freudian view that our need for and ties to other people are built secondarily around primary biological and reproductive needs, these theories posit that relational needs constitute fundamental building blocks of personality in their own right. As Fairbairn (1952) put it, libido is object seeking, not pleasure seeking. As I will discuss in more detail in Chapter 5, for many relationalists this is the fundamental cleavage between relational and nonrelational theories. Clearly I am suggesting that there are other distinctions that are at least as important.

adapt to new circumstances.[3] This is why writers guided by these theories so regularly refer to psychological problems and psychological structures as being "early," or "preoedipal," or as a problem rooted in experiences at age one or two or three. It is why so huge a portion of the theoretical writing in these traditions focuses on the experience of the infant. The psychological characteristics of the infant and very young child must be studied intensively because the assumption is held that the depths of the psyche very largely retain the characteristics they had in the earliest years of life. Early in life, the psyche becomes fatefully split, and its depths are cut off from the capacity to grow and change and learn from new experiences that characterizes the more consciously accessible realms of psychic life.[4]

Psychopathology, then, in many psychoanalytic accounts—including some putatively "relational" accounts—is a function of when we got stuck. The more severe the pathology, the "earlier" our point of fixation or developmental arrest must be. And hence, as we shall see in later chapters, the need for "regression" is central in some relational and object relational accounts (e.g., Balint, 1968; Winnicott, 1955, 1971; Maroda, 1999, 2004) in order for meaningful therapeutic gain to be achieved. We must go back, recreate the circumstances of the early mother–infant bond or recreate the intensity and primitive quality of our earliest affect-fused representations in order to repair the "deepest" damage and achieve the most profound change.[5]

These features of much relational theorizing also lend themselves, at least implicitly, to the imagery of "emerging" and "unfolding" (Wachtel, 1982a) that I referred to in the previous chapter, and hence to a vision of the clinical process that retains many features of a one-person approach. That is, although they view the *content* of our key

---

[3] For further amplification on this issue, see the illuminating discussion in Mitchell (1988a, Chs. 5 and 6).

[4] In Chapter 7, I discuss the concept of dissociated self-states, which represents a different way of conceptualizing accessibility and inaccessibility to conscious experience, one which is potentially more compatible with a contextual understanding of personality.

[5] It is important to note that in the hands of creative contemporary relational writers such as Maroda (2004), the meaning of regression does not seem to be as literal. What seems to be implied, rather than a going back to an earlier mode of experience, is an *opening up* to permit more intense affective experience, a letting go of defenses that, although providing access to more "primitive" modes of experience, can as readily be viewed as a *progressive* step as a regressive one. It is clear from Maroda's writings that the letting go of the defense is a step forward, an achievement, not a return to something earlier. But the imagery and associations of the concept of regression, along with its links to venerable psychoanalytic ideas, is likely subtly to move one's thinking along more traditional lines that emphasize what Mitchell (1988a) has called the "developmental tilt" and the "metaphor of the baby."

psychological structures as relational in nature, many relational think-ers continue to view those structures as part of an "inner world" that is largely sealed off from the rest of the psyche and from the impact of daily experience. There is thus a potential warrant, from the vantage point of these object relational and self psychological theories, to prac-tice much like the one-person observer of the patient's psyche that the analyst is in more classical approaches—that is, to listen, "interpret," and, for some, to attempt to remain relatively neutral and anonymous.

In contrast, where a two-person epistemology is integrated with a thoroughgoing two-person *theory* (see below), the therapist is more likely to view the contents of the patient's psyche not as simply emerg-ing or unfolding from "within," but as reflecting a continually evolving psychological organization and framework of experience that responds meaningfully at every turn not only to the specifics of what is transpir-ing in the room with the therapist but to the ongoing flow of events and circumstances in the rest of the patient's life as well. Such a per-spective does not imply a lack of interest in the patient's unique subjec-tivity or in the more deeply unconscious sources of our behavior and experience. Rather, it emphasizes an understanding of those very depths and that very subjectivity as related (both directly and symboli-cally) to the person's actual life structure. Similarly, it does not betoken a lack of interest in the enduring structures that give coherence and identity to the personality or in the ways in which our characteristic modes of experiencing can be slow to change, "sticky," or idiosyn-cratic. It approaches those continuities differently, however, from a one-person account, emphasizing the ways that personality structure and life structure continuously and reciprocally interact. It views con-sistency and continuity not as maintained in a sealed-off realm apart from the relational world of the present but *in relation to* that world. And it illuminates how, through countless daily interactions and medi-ated by countless subtle but powerful affective feedback loops, we cre-ate and recreate a world of actual experience that is perfectly suited to maintaining those very structures (Wachtel, 1987a, 1993, 1994, 1997).

WHAT SHOULD A TWO-PERSON THEORY OF PERSONALITY LOOK LIKE?

In contending that many theoretical positions that are generally viewed as part of the larger relational synthesis are more one-person theories than two, what am I suggesting a *two*-person theory should look like?

To begin with, instead of positing an intrapsychic realm or "inner" world that is sealed off from and largely uninfluenced by what happens in daily life, a satisfactory two-person account would attend to all the experiences and observations that have been highlighted by one-person accounts (including the versions of object relations theory that are largely one-person in their structure), but would contextualize them. This is what is generally evident in relational writings when they are addressing the epistemological realm or the events of the psychotherapy session. The material emerging in the session is seen not as an unmediated or uncontaminated expression of the patient's inner world, but as an experience that is co-constructed by patient and analyst, a *mutual* product that cannot be properly understood without taking into account the continuing, moment-by-moment contribution of the analyst. In similar fashion, when relational thinkers address the process of early development, the role of context and mutual shaping of experience again tends to be acknowledged (and even emphasized). The continuous mutual impact of mother and child on each other's behavior and experience is highlighted both in relational theoretical writings and in a by now quite substantial body of empirical research (see, e.g., Beebe & Lachmann, 2002; Cohen & Tronick, 1988; Jaffe, Beebe, Feldstein, Crown, & Jasnow, 2001; Stern, 1985; Tronick, 1989).

In conceptualizing the day-to-day and moment-to-moment functioning of adults, however, and where the context of concern is their daily world of work, family, and friends rather than the relationship with the analyst, the import of mutuality and the continuing ongoing impact of context tends to be far less fully taken into account. Rather, much relational theorizing is characterized by the language of "internalization," "internalized objects," "primitive and archaic representations," "developmental arrests," and "preoedipal" levels of experiencing, and the individual is described as if "underneath" he is experiencing the world in a manner that remains largely untouched by the countless new experiences he has had since his early years.

But just as the experiences and fantasies reported by the patient in the session are assumed by most relational theorists to be co-determined by the presence, characteristics, and mode of interaction of the therapist (including that particular mode of interaction constituted by sitting and silently listening), and as the psyche of the baby is widely viewed these days as reflecting real features of the mother–child interaction, so too can *all* of personality development and dynamics—*throughout* the life cycle and *outside* as well as within the therapeutic session—be viewed in relation to the ongoing relationships, interactions, and circumstances of the person's life. In a thoroughgoing two-person account, that is indeed the aim.

This position is easily misunderstood. Critics of relational theorizing have at times pointed to particular relational formulations that may seem to imply that the person is a mere slave to stimuli, a product of the environment with no personal core, no distinct personality or personal uniqueness, no subjectivity or agency (see, e.g., Masling, 2003; Eagle, Wolitzky, & Wakefield, 2001; Meissner, 1998; Silverman, 2000).[6] It is thus important to make clear that a fully two-person theory of the sort I am pointing to here in no way excludes—or even minimizes—consideration of personal uniqueness or of what is usually referred to as the intrapsychic. Rather, what a thoroughgoing two-person theoretical structure entails is an understanding that fully addresses the person's long-standing characteristics and proclivities but *contextualizes* them (see also in this regard Orange, Atwood, & Stolorow, 1997). In so doing, such a theoretical perspective is able to provide a more complete account of how those structures—of thought, fantasy, affect, motivation, identity—are linked to each other and to the ongoing experiences of the person's life. A two-person theory of intrapsychic structure is rooted both in the many observations that point to the stubborn persistence of certain modes of thought, affect, and desire *and* in the observations—also obvious and compelling if one is not constrained by theory to minimize them—that indicate how strikingly *variable* our behavior and experience are from day to day, moment to moment, situation to situation, companion to companion, mood to mood. This variability, this flux—proceeding hand in hand with the maintenance of a relatively enduring and self-coherent structure—is a quintessential feature of all living systems and especially of human personality.

There is a consistency to people's behavior and experience that enables us to "understand" the person sitting opposite us in the therapy room, to perceive him or her as a coherent—if also conflicted—personality. But that consistency cannot be accurately characterized without taking into account how it is built upon and pulls together the

---

[6] Many of the criticisms have focused particularly on the version of relational theory put forth by Mitchell and thus are not directly relevant to the positions taken in this book. But since similar criticisms are not infrequently advanced regarding relational theorizing more generally, it seems important to address their relevance to the conceptualizations offered in this book.

enormous *diversity* in the person's way of thinking, feeling, and behaving in different circumstances, mood states, and states of desire. Nor can the experience of coherence or consistency be adequately conceptualized without examining how the individual negotiates the constantly changing world of interpersonal transactions, responding differentially to the myriad shadings of tone, affect, message, and demand that characterize every moment of our lives with other people. This is an insight reflected in Sullivan's (1953) conceptualization of the boundaries of personality dynamisms as an "envelope of insignificant differences," in Erikson's (1959) discussions of identity as a sense of sameness in difference, and in Bromberg's (1998a) and Davies's (1996) discussions of alternating self-states.[7]

TWO-PERSON THEORY FOR THE EARLY YEARS OF LIFE, ONE-PERSON THEORY FOR LATER

Some of the confusion that arises in distinguishing between one-person and two-person theories arises because much theorizing in the self psychological and object relations traditions offers essentially a two-person account of the very earliest years of life, but a one-person conceptualization of what happens in all the subsequent years. That is, the depiction of how internal structures are *laid down* is very much a relational one. Early representations of self and other are viewed by most theorists in those traditions as quite significantly influenced by the actual ways the developing infant is treated by significant others.[8] But the portrayal changes rather significantly as these early interactions are presumed to be "internalized." In the years of later childhood and adulthood, these "internal" representations or internalized objects are discussed as essentially autonomous forces in the psyche, imposing themselves on experience but not themselves being modified to any

---

[7] See Chapter 7 for a fuller discussion of dissociation and multiple self-states.

[8] This was not the case for many years for Kleinians, and the strong influence of Klein's ideas in England was very largely responsible for the negative reception that greeted Bowlby's seminal work on attachment. Bowlby was no less interested in subjective experience and the deep structure of personality than were others whose work originated in the psychoanalytic tradition, but his emphasis on relating internal structures to actual experiences marked him for exclusion for many years. Bowlby has, of course, now received the respect and interest he long deserved, and many contemporary theorists who still regard themselves as Kleinian have overcome their disinterest in the powerful impact of real experiences, even (maybe especially) in the early years of childhood.

significant degree by later events or relationships. They are rooted in relational experiences, and hence relational in *content*; but ultimately they are described as functioning in very much the same way that intrapsychic contents were described prior to the advent of object relational thinking.

Further perspective on this point may be gained via a metaphor used by both Erik Erikson and David Shapiro to illuminate a potentially problematic feature of Freudian drive theory, but that we will see has relevance to significant aspects of object relations theories as well. Erikson (1963), in discussing the libido theory, cautioned that "while we must continue to study the life cycles of individuals by delineating the possible vicissitudes of their libido, we must become sensitive to the danger of forcing living persons into the role of marionettes of a mythical Eros—to the gain of neither therapy nor theory" (p. 64). Shapiro (1989), referring at several points to Erikson's marionette metaphor, further notes that "the conception of an unconscious agent of behavior, an anomalous and irrational intruder into adult attitudes, rescued neurosis for scientific understanding and the possibility of treatment. But at the same time and apparently unavoidably, it clouded the individual's responsibility for his own behavior, seeming to make him a mere passive—or even unwilling—witness of it" (p. 19). In a similar vein, Shapiro notes that the way in which the concept of unconscious forces in the psyche evolved in psychoanalytic thought "reduced the role of the individual's consciousness to that of a compliant and innocuous bystander" (p. 19).

Now, it happens that both of these writers are focusing their critique on the libido theory which shaped the classical or Freudian tradition.[9] At first blush it thus might seem that their comments would be quite congenial to object relations thinking. Object relations theories, after all, also cast a critical eye on the theory of the drives. A closer look at Erikson's and Shapiro's critiques, however, should make it clear that they pertain as much to a great swath of object relations thinking. Both Erikson and Shapiro framed their critiques in relation to the libido theory because it (and its ego psychological descendant) was the framework in which they were brought up, and it remained the frame

---

[9] Erikson, it should be noted, was not criticizing the libido theory per se; he was too loyal to Freud to do that. He framed his critique in terms of how the libido theory *could* be used, implying that such a use was a *mis*use. It remains to the reader to judge if Erikson was politely calling attention to what he believed was a more fundamental theoretical difficulty.

of reference in relation to which their work evolved and the perspective that characterized the community of colleagues who formed their reference group. Closer attention to how "internalized objects" are written about and understood by object relations theorists, however, makes it clear that in much object relations thinking too the adult patient is cast as a marionette, tossed hither and yon by libidinal and antilibidinal egos, bad internal objects, and other internal demons that are the true drivers of the psyche.

Although object relations theorists largely replaced the drive concept with an emphasis on the impact of internalized objects, what evolved was at times less a transformation than a substitution, a plugging of the "internalized object" concept into an existing theoretical structure to serve precisely the same function as the drive concept did in the earlier theory. In replacing the role of drives with the role of object relations, the marionette conception of the relation between conscious and unconscious, or between the internal world and the lived life, remained intact. As in the old joke about Soviet style communism—before communism, society was marked by the oppression of man by man; now it is just the reverse—so too in the relation of drive theory and object relations theory, the apparent reversal leaves the underlying structure the same. A new driver is driving the psyche; drives are driven out, and internalized objects rush in to fill the theoretical void. But the relation of the hidden puller of the strings to the individual as passive container for "inner" driving forces remains intact.

Consider, for example, Greenberg and Mitchell's (1983) account of Fairbairn's (1952) theory of the relation between "internal object relations" and the "outside world." Love objects, they state, "are selected for or made into withholders or deprivers *so as* to personify the exciting object, promising, but never fulfilling. Defeat is *orchestrated* again and again to perpetuate the longing and need *of the libidinal ego* for the fulfillment of the promise of the exciting object" (pp. 173–174, italics added). Here, the libidinal ego orchestrates, pulls the strings, does the real selecting of love objects for the unwitting individual, and the individual qua marionette establishes relations in the "outside" world that he *thinks* represent his own desires but actually reflect the aims of the puppet master within.

Now in part, of course, this conceptualization builds upon the *general* idea of unconscious motivation. *Whenever* unconscious processes are at work (which means all the time), it might be said that the person is pursuing something he thinks he wants but is really pursuing something else that he does not even know he is pursuing. But there are important differences in the ways that unconscious processes are conceptualized or spoken about by different theorists. As we will see in the discussions of clinical technique in the latter chapters of this book, the unconscious dimensions of what the person is pursuing are better seen—that is, both more accurately *and* more helpfully clinically—as something *additional* rather than as something *else*. What we think we are pursuing is not simply a deception, a fraud masking a deeper reality that *falsifies* the aims we think we are pursuing. A more accurate conception of unconscious processes and unconscious motivation portrays our conscious motivations as a *part* of what we are pursuing, while illuminating the ways in which we are *also* pursuing something more (and, not infrequently of course, pursuing some aims that *conflict* with the aims that we are more aware of). As I shall elaborate in Chapter 8, the difference between the therapist addressing herself to what the patient is "really" feeling, or doing, or wanting and what he is *also* experiencing or pursuing is a central key to good clinical work.

The danger in Fairbairn's account, and in much other object relations writing, is that it can seem that there is virtually another *entity* pulling the strings and that the individual's actions, in much the way that Erikson and Shapiro describe vis-à-vis the libido theory, are in the service of aims exterior not only to consciousness but to the actual person living in the world. In this sense, the "internal" in "internal object" or "internalized object relationship" is actually *external* to the self. Thus a theoretical perspective that originated in a critique of the premise that our investments in other people were merely the vehicle for the expression of libidinal drives and that aimed to highlight the crucial role of human relationships in their own right ended up in important respects a theory that once more *played down* the relevance of ongoing relations between people. It became a theory that reduced our daily transactions with others to the unwitting play of "inner" forces from the past rather than a meaningful—if inevitably individualized and idiosyncratic—participation in the relational realities of the present.[10]

This perspective has been articulated particularly strongly by

---

[10] These limitations and contradictions in Fairbairn's thinking should not lead the reader to dismiss or overlook what were also very important contributions. I will be discussing in later chapters a variety of ways in which Fairbairn and other early object relations thinkers also *opened up* clinical thinking in important ways and pointed toward a more interactional and more related mode of practice.

Stolorow, Orange, and Atwood (2001a), who point out that although Fairbairn highlighted the crucial importance of actual relational experiences *early* in life,

> in Fairbairn's theoretical vision the endopsychic world, once established, is pictured as operating as a closed system, a Cartesian container housing an array of internalized personages. The internalized object relations are seen as dynamically active structures that behave at times like drives, at times like demons—autonomously and with a life of their own. Thus, in his view of the fully structuralized psyche, Fairbairn reverted to an image of the isolated mind, a mind whose dynamisms are insulated from the constitutive impact of the surround. (p. 471)

What these considerations amount to is that many versions of object relations theory represent two-person theory in content but one-person theory in structure. Through their lens, our daily transactions with others—much as in the Freudian theory it aimed to challenge—are reduced to a mere screen upon which is played out a drama whose script was written long ago. New people may be recruited to play the role of the objects from the past, but they do not speak their own lines; they are not full, real people in the present, they are containers into whom have been deposited expectations from long ago, and their role in the drama is precast and predetermined. As Modell (1984) has put it, these theorists, even though object relational in their content, preserved the classical one-person point of view "by referring not to the actual object but to the representation of the object in the mind" (p. 17). Citing the emphasis in writers such as Fairbairn and Kernberg on "internalized" object relationships, Modell argues that "loyalty to a one-person psychology has . . . become a deforming Procrustean bed. . . . a representational psychology that attempts to portray relationships with actual objects by means of internalized analogies makes no distinction between the actual object and one that is completely created by the subject" (p. 18). As I noted in an earlier discussion of Modell's conceptualization, "Real people are their own center of agency, responding to and evaluating others' actions toward them (and even *feelings* about them, as they are revealed in actions and non-verbal behavior); internal objects, in contrast, are not people with minds of their own, but 'fantasies' that are part of people's own minds" (Wachtel, 1997, p. 334).

In a fully two-person psychology, the affective exchange between *actual people* takes center stage, and one comes to see and understand the profound ways in which the moods, fantasies, desires, perceptions, and expectations of each intersect with, create, transform, and recreate the moods, fantasies, desires, perceptions, and expectations of the other. It is not a psychology that *ignores* those "inner" states or qualities. Rather, it aims to deepen and expand our understanding of them by looking not only at how they are structured and manifest themselves in each individual's psychological economy but also at how they are dynamically and mutually elicited in the living transactions with *others'* inner lives. That is why I disagree with Modell's contention that psychoanalysis needs both a one-person *and* a two-person psychology. If a two-person psychology is adequately understood and carried through, by its very nature it includes what is commonly thought of as a one-person psychology. The premise of a thoroughgoing two-person psychology is not that "inner" processes do not matter—*of course* they matter, and matter greatly—but that those inner processes are not adequately understood unless they are understood in context, and especially in the context of continuing transactions and interactions with others.[11]

Unfortunately, superficial versions of two-person thinking do exist, versions that place all causality in the environment and do not consider how each individual develops an almost unimaginably complex, comprehensive, and idiosyncratic way of interpreting the environmental input. It is always *individual people* who give meaning to the events they encounter, who have affective experiences in relation to them, who develop specific and fairly consistent ways of responding or reacting to particular kinds of experiences, who even, ultimately, decide whether a new experience *is* a new experience or a repetition of an old and familiar one. But it does not take a "one-person" psychology to register this, and indeed, a "one-person" understanding of those processes is misleading and inadequate. It is inadequate because in every instance, the inner processes—even the fantasies one may have while walking alone down the street or the dreams one has while asleep—must also be understood in relation to the larger context in which they are manifested and in relation to which the dream or the fantasy takes on its meaning.

---

[11] As I shall discuss in Chapter 4, that context of transaction with others includes as well the context of being physically alone, including alone with one's dreams or daydreams.

THE CONSERVATIVE PULL OF RECEIVED IDEAS

Object relations theorizing originated as a response to some of the limitations of the libido theory and the one-person model that had dominated psychoanalytic thought up till that time. And clearly, these theories were a very important advance on the path toward a more fully relational or two-person theory of personality. Yet at the same time, as I have been discussing in this chapter, there are ways in which the most influential versions of object relations thinking replicated in significant ways some of the fundamental structure of the theories they were aiming at transcending. How did this ironic outcome emerge from such promising—even revolutionary—beginnings? In part what is reflected here is the immense difficulty in extricating oneself from the frame of reference in which one's efforts originate or from the assumptive world of the community of which one is a part. Psychoanalysis has been, in many respects, a psychology of buried treasures, and for many analysts the idea of unearthing what is deeply buried is virtually a defining feature of the psychoanalytic point of view (cf. Wachtel, 2003a). In Chapter 6, I will offer a critique of this "archaeological" model and will suggest an alternative. But it is important to note that for many analysts the archaeological model is virtually a *sine qua non* for psychoanalysis itself, and the transformation of the two-person conceptualizations that represented the new and innovative thrust of object relational theories into a more traditionally one-person, intrapsychic theory was probably almost automatic, as well as psychoanalytically legitimizing.

Such pulls toward canonical ways of seeing and talking about the subject matter are characteristic of all disciplines. Philosophers and historians of science have documented this conservative tendency in great detail, and some have suggested that only a revolution (Kuhn, 1962) or, as Max Planck (1936) suggested only somewhat whimsically, the death of an entire generation of scientists who have grown up with deeply held assumptions and convictions can make way for truly new ideas. Niels Bohr, another great pioneer of modern physics, has been widely quoted as saying, "Science and medicine advance funeral by funeral."

The conservative pulls, however, are particularly strong in psychoanalysis. The tradition of institutes insulated from the intellectual give and take of the university; the unusually intense influence of the older generation that inheres in close and highly personal clinical supervision and in the crucible of a painstaking training analysis; the ways in which positions which deviate from conventional ideas can be "interpreted" and in which one's *personality* can become the issue rather than one's ideas; and the sheer ambiguity of the subject matter itself, which can make familiar assumptions and terminology feel like a port in a storm even (perhaps especially) for the critic who is bold enough to challenge some of the conventional assumptions of the discipline—all these pull for an adherence to established ideas that is over and above that in most disciplines.

CONFUSING OBSERVATIONS WITH THE CONCEPTS USED TO ADDRESS THEM

One further factor that is probably even more important to take into account in understanding how a theoretical program that was initiated as an effort to center psychoanalytic inquiry on the *relationships between people* ended up as very largely a one-person psychology of internal fantasies: The *observations* that analysts made—including those by the early relational thinkers—seemed to require a vision of a frozen past internalized beyond the reach of current relational experiences. Part of what led analysts (including many relational analysts) to frame their theorizing in terms such as "primitive" and "archaic" was that much of what their patients did or felt *looked* primitive and archaic. The psychological contents and modes of thought that became apparent in the course of the psychoanalytic process often had an intensity and a quality of affect and of thought organization that seemed to compel a vision of them as remnants from the past that had little to do with what was actually going on in the present. Similarly, the ways that people seem to cling so tenaciously to old ideas, old ties, old aspirations, old ways of feeling and behaving can seem to lend themselves to the overly internalized conceptualization noted in the previous discussion of Fairbairn; it *looks like* some kind of primitive internal presence is living out its archaic agenda through the unwitting adult who is reporting his stubbornly persistent experiences in the analytic session.

Fairbairn was keenly perceptive in his account of the ways children can remain attached to parents who have been neglectful or abusive and in his appreciation of the ways that, even as adults, we may unconsciously cling to or long for ties to early sources of comfort, to the figures who, however much they may have disappointed us, even harmed us, were all that stood between us and the utter terror and devastation of aloneness. Our understanding and our clinical work are aided immensely by his illumination of the ways in which we may continue to orient ourselves in relation to those figures (or at least to our fantasies or images of those figures), seeking in vain to win their love or approval or to be the kind of person to whom they would offer support or genuine connection. The problem lay not in Fairbairn's observations, but in the way he *talked about* and *conceptualized* these observations—the baroque language of libidinal and antilibidinal egos and the closed-system, endopsychic conceptualization pointed out by Stolorow, Orange, and Atwood (2001a).

Similarly, in the writing of Melanie Klein, we may see a variety of observations that, apart from the theoretical language in which they were expressed, attune us to dimensions of experience that are important to include in our understanding of the struggles in which our patients are engaged. Klein deserves credit for being one of the first psychoanalytic writers—perhaps *the* first—to pay serious attention to the pervasiveness and importance of envy, greed, and fears that the sheer intensity of our desires for those we love will consume and destroy them. But she also *framed* those observations in ways that it is not inappropriate to call bizarre, seeming to confuse her own fantasies with those of all human beings, attributing thought processes to infants that all evidence suggests is impossible, and imparting a concreteness and hermetic quality to object relations theorizing that continues to distort even many contemporary formulations. Most usefully, we would honor her for her observations and reconstruct our *theories* on much sounder ground. To some degree, in fact, this is precisely what has happened. Winnicott, Fairbairn, and other object relations pioneers *changed* the original Kleinian formulations in highly significant ways. And even today, when Kleinian thinking seems to be having a resurgence, the key figures in this resurgence tend to be referred to not as "Kleinian" but as "neo-Kleinian" or "contemporary Kleinian," appellations that at least to some degree derive from an appreciation that to be "Kleinian" is to hold to some rather troublesome assumptions and ways of speaking.

Analysts rightly do not want to ignore the *descriptively* primitive quality of the fantasies and urges they see in the course of their work— the unusual intensity, the voracious hungers and desperate needs, the oddly skewed, and even fantastic, ideas that become apparent in otherwise quite rational individuals in the context of the analytic process. But in addressing these phenomena, there has seemed to be an assumption that such "primitive" psychological manifestations must reflect concrete elements in the psyche that are *literally* "early," "archaic," or "preoedipal" (cf. Westen, 1989), that they are expressions of an "inner world" that is very largely cut off from everyday experience, an inner world frozen at the developmental level of early childhood. It is as if the *observation* of such seemingly primitive behaviors or experiences, in and of itself, is sufficient to validate the *theory* that has been created to explain that observation.

In one sense, my aim in what follows is to clarify how these and other key observations that have informed relational theorizing can be cast in a framework that is more thoroughly two-person in nature. In another sense, however, as the next chapter will further develop, the aim is to move *beyond* the one-person–two-person distinction altogether and to recast the essence of the relational viewpoint as a fully *contextual* psychology. Before doing so, however, it is important to examine one additional way in which the application of two-person thinking has been more limited than has generally been recognized— its restriction, in important ways, to what transpires in the consulting room.

4

■　■　■　■　■

From Two-Person
to Contextual

BEYOND INFANCY
AND THE CONSULTING ROOM

In a recent study of the views of beginning psychodynamic therapists (Gillman, 2006), an interesting finding appeared. A very large majority of these therapists strongly rejected the assumptions associated with the classical psychoanalytic approach. Yet very few explicitly associated themselves with a relational perspective either. One of the central concerns they expressed was that the relational approach, as they understood it, was too exclusively concerned with what goes on in the room between the patient and therapist and not enough about the patient's life outside the office. One of them, for example, stated, "The patient came in because she had problems *and she didn't even know you* before she came in. Too much attention to the therapist–patient relationship can veer away from problems in the patient's life." Another said, "What relational means is what's going on between you and me *in* the room . . . I think it can get overused." I believe that in certain ways, these students held a vision of what it means to work relationally that was stereotyped and exaggerated. But I also believe that they were responding to something that needs to be addressed seriously by relational thinkers. Much of this book is devoted to spelling out a relational approach in which concern with the patient's deep subjectivity is

54

not incompatible with (and is often usefully pursued through) serious attention to the details of the patient's everyday life.

THE EXCLUDED MIDDLE

A central focus of the previous chapter was the tendency of relational theorists to relegate genuine two-person thinking to the earliest years of life, with a more one-person way of thinking dominating their understanding of later childhood and adulthood. There is, of course, one major exception to this tendency. Virtually all relational thinkers, in one way or another, apply a two-person way of thinking to the psychotherapy session itself.

More often than is commonly appreciated, however, this extension of two-person thinking into adulthood stops at the consulting room door. When thinking about the interaction *between patient and analyst,* a rather consistent two-person perspective may be applied. But when other contemporary relationships and experiences in the patient's life are addressed, they are likely to be viewed in a way that reflects what I called in the last chapter "two-person theory in content but one-person theory in structure." That is, these later experiences and relationships are likely to be discussed and understood as occasions for the expression of already existing "internalized" tendencies, tendencies that are not viewed as continuing to be shaped by ongoing relational experiences, but as largely fixed and playing themselves out in a one-directional fashion. Like Freud's id, these "internalized" objects and object relationships powerfully influence our behavior and experience but are scarcely *influenced by* those experiences.

The often restricted range in which genuine two-person thinking is applied may be obscured by its anchoring in two realms that are of particularly great interest for psychoanalytically oriented therapists—the experiences of infancy and the earliest years of childhood on the one hand and the experience in the immediate setting of the session itself on the other. The particularly intense interest in these two realms is itself symptomatic of the circumscribed application of two-person thinking. As important as they clearly both are for our understanding and for therapeutic work, the degree to which these two realms are the center of relational theorizing reflects, in essence, a relative *lack* of interest in the experiences of everyday adulthood outside the session. Reams have been written by relational writers about infancy and about the therapist–patient relationship. Far less has been written about the rest of people's lives.

The applications of genuine and rigorous two-person thinking to the two realms at the center of psychoanalytic interest can make it easy to overlook the restrictions in its application elsewhere and can make it appear, without closer scrutiny, as if the two-person point of view is applied more broadly and thoroughly in the relational literature than it actually is. Consider, for example, Mitchell's comment that the most significant feature of post-Kleinian British object relations theorizing is "the importance it places on the environment—on the crucial significance of the interactions between the infant and caretakers and the crucial significance of the interactions . . . between the analysand and the analyst" (1995, p. 78). Note here that Mitchell does *not* mention the interactions between the analysand and the *other* crucial people in his life. As occurs frequently in discussions of the two-person point of view in the relational literature, Mitchell leapfrogs over the vast stretch between the mother–infant transaction and the interaction between patient and analyst. The expanse between infancy and analysis becomes a kind of "excluded middle," *seemingly* addressed by a theory that stresses relationships and "the environment," but in fact largely neglected. That is, although the experiences of everyday life are, of course, discussed and attended to by relational theorists, they are often viewed primarily as the context for *revealing* or *expressing* what is already "inside," rather than as a realm in which—just as in analysis or infancy—mutuality, co-construction, and reciprocal causation are the focus of concern.

In similar fashion, Aron (1996) states that "central to a relational, two-person model is the idea that the seemingly infantile wishes and conflicts revealed in a patient's associations are not only or mainly remnants from the past, artificially imposed on the therapeutic field, but are, rather, reflections of the actual interactions and encounters with *the unique, individual analyst,* with all of his or her idiosyncratic, particularistic features" (p. 50, italics added).

In certain ways, Aron's statement converges strikingly with my own cyclical psychodynamic point of view (see Chapter 6). In a statement that similarly addresses the "seemingly infantile," for example, I have stated:

> The key to the cyclical psychodynamic reconceptualization of the phenomena observed by earlier generations of analysts lies in examining the connection between the *seemingly* out of touch fantasies,

wishes, or images of self and other and the actuality of the person's present way of life. Through the lens of a cyclical psychodynamic analysis, the apparently archaic processes and structures are revealed as not nearly as anachronistic as they are depicted in most psychoanalytic accounts. Rather, they can be recognized as both symbolizations and consequences of the very way of life of which they are also a determinant. (Wachtel, 1993, pp. 19–20).

The difference between these two seemingly similar theoretical statements, however, is a significant one. The cyclical psychodynamic formulation refers to the patient's entire way of life. It points to how *all* of the patient's experiences must be understood in their relational context. In contrast, Aron's statement seems to limit its focus to the interaction with the analyst.

I do not mean here to suggest that relational analysts explicitly intend to reject the two-person nature of the rest of life's experiences and transactions. I know, for example, from personal conversations with both Stephen Mitchell and Lew Aron that this was by no means their intent. Mitchell, for example, having been trained first as an interpersonalist and valuing the field-theoretical dimension of Sullivan's thinking, understood very well that *all* of our experiences are contextual in nature. But at the same time, he felt that interpersonal thinking had neglected the enduring structures and attachments that serve as a keel for the personality, keeping us from being completely adrift in the prevailing winds of the particular momentary interaction. In addressing this perceived gap, Mitchell, like a number of other prominent relational theorists, was drawn to theories that described how earlier interpersonal experiences could be internalized and structuralized as internal objects and representations. I believe, however, that he failed to note sufficiently that these theories were, in the terminology I introduced above, "leapfrogging" theories, theories that jump from infancy to analysis, leaving the rest of life a vast "excluded middle." That is, although the mother–infant relationship and the relationship between patient and analyst are thoroughly probed in relational theorizing for bidirectional processes of mutual influence and mutual construction of experience, the ways in which such processes characterize *all* of life tend to be far less thoroughly explored. Concepts such as internalization, developmental level, and developmental arrest direct attention inward, to tendencies that are implicitly treated as more or less context-free properties of the single individual.

The difference between the acute attention paid to mutuality and co-construction of experience in the analytic session and the relative neglect of these same processes in considering the patient's behavior and experience outside the sessions is evident not only in the readiness to ascribe to people "preoedipal levels of personality organization" (cf. Westen, 1989), but in the contrast between the relatively sparse theorizing about the interactions of everyday life in the psychoanalytic literature and the intense focus on such interactions in the theory and practice of family therapy. For family therapists, an individual's experience— indeed, even the "developmental level" he manifests—can only be properly understood in context, in the way that the individual participates in a larger system with others, who both shape and are shaped by his behavior. This, in essence, is how relational analysts too view people when considering their participation in the analytic relationship itself or when theorizing about mother–infant interaction in the earliest years of life. It is not similarly evident, however, in much relational theorizing about what amount to rather fixed (and context-free) "internalized objects." This absence is particularly unfortunate because the psychoanalytic perspective provides a degree of sensitivity to and articulation of the conscious and unconscious dimensions of subjectivity that is usually not equaled in the family therapy literature. Combining this sensitivity with the kind of thoroughgoingly relational framework evident in much family systems theorizing provides the working clinician with an especially powerful and comprehensive vision. It is a vision, moreover, that in essence carries forth into the entirety of the patient's life the very characteristics of theorizing that relational theorists apply to the analytic session or to the mother–infant dyad—characteristics that are the essential cutting edge of the relational contribution.

THE ORIGINS OF THE TWO-PERSON POINT OF VIEW AND THE NARROW CONSTRUCTION OF TWO-PERSON THINKING

This narrow construction of the two-person point of view, with its application largely limited to the microcosm of the psychotherapy session, was, we might say, present at the creation. In a paper that is commonly viewed as the first explicit introduction into the psychoanalytic literature of the contrast between a one-person and a two-person point of view,[1] Michael Balint (1950) argued, in setting the context for his discussion, that "our true field of study is the psycho-analytical situation" (p. 120) and that the most important field of investigation for the new line of theory he was striving to develop "must be the *analyst's* behaviour in the psycho-analytic situation" (p. 121, italics in original). And indeed, as Balint develops his argument in this key foundational document of the two-person point of view, it is the events and transactions of the psychoanalytic situation that clearly occupy center stage.

Balint argued that the psychoanalytic situation, in which two people sit in the same room, is a "two-body" experience and that therefore classical psychoanalytic theory, which is a "one-body" theory, is insufficient to understand what transpires there. The concepts of classical psychoanalysis, he maintained, "were derived from studying ... the domain of the One-Body Psychology. ... That is why they can give only a clumsy, approximate description of what happens *in the psycho-analytical situation, which is essentially a Two-Body Situation*" (p. 124, italics added). Here it seems, Balint's criterion for whether a one-person or a two-person model is required comes down to counting bodies in the room. Because two people are interacting, even if one may be largely silent, a two-body psychology is required.

As a consequence, Balint, like various others over the years (e.g., Ghent, 1989; Modell, 1984) argues that psychoanalysis needs both a one-person *and* a two-person psychology. Such an argument, I believe, is linked to a limited conception of what a meaningful two-person theory might entail. If we need a one-person psychology when someone is alone, a two-person psychology when another person enters the room, a three-person psychology when still another walks in, and so forth, then we are left with an approach to theory that is both absurd and superficial. It is not because two people are in the room that a one-person psychology is insufficient to understand what transpires in the consulting room. It is because the nature of human psychology, *no*

---

[1] Although Balint's is the first *published* discussion of this contrast, it derives from a public presentation by another analyst, John Rickman. Before either Rickman's or Balint's discussions, Sullivan introduced a clear two-person perspective, but to the best of my knowledge he never put his ideas into the specific language of "one-person" and "two-person" thinking. Ferenczi, who was the analyst of both Balint and Rickman, also introduced many ideas that today we would readily label as "two-person" thinking, but again, to the best of my knowledge he did not employ that particular vocabulary.

matter how many people are in the room, is fundamentally responsive to context.

A two-person version of psychoanalytic thought, or of any psychological theory for that matter, is not about the number of people in the room but about how each of them is psychologically organized. What made classical analysis a "one-person" theory was not simply its denial of the pervasive influence of the *analyst* on what transpires in the consulting room, but its conceptualization of personality dynamics more generally—its view of the relevant factors determining our behavior and experience as residing in the "internalized" recesses of the mind, sealed off from the influence of ongoing relational events.

Elsewhere in Balint's paper, he suggests a different criterion for distinguishing between one-body and two-body[2] theories. Psychoanalytic theory, he says, evolved as a one-body psychology because it was primarily constructed around observations of only a subset of patients, those in whom "all conflicts and mental processes are internalized" (p. 119), and he contrasts them with a different set of patients, for whom "objects are of paramount importance" (p. 119). Different kinds of theories, he suggests, are needed for the two kinds of patients. This second conceptualization of the differences between one-person and two-person theories particularly highlights the problems with the way that the one-person and two-person distinction has tended to be discussed. In this second version of Balint's argument, a one-person point of view continues to be appropriate for understanding a significant portion of the patient population. In lieu of relegating two-person thinking to situations in which others are actually physically present, this version restricts it to individuals who are deemed capable of "involvement with objects." This second criterion, it turns out, is even more restrictive, for it implies that for some individuals, even when they *are* in the presence of others, they remain best understood by a one-person psychology.

In the years since Balint's paper appeared, we have learned much more about people who seem "not to relate to objects." More contemporary understandings of transference include, as one very real and very

---

[2] So that the reader will not be confused, I wish to point out that the contemporary literature uses the terms one-person and two-person as more modern equivalents of Balint's (and Rickman's) terms one-body and two-body. I will mostly use the terms one-person and two-person, even in discussing Balint, since they are the terms that are at the center of contemporary debate and discourse.

powerful transference response, the very noninvolvement "or *seeming* noninvolvement) of the patient. Noninvolvement, we now appreciate, *is* the patient's way of being involved, his way of relating to us as he relates to other significant figures in his life, and that noninvolvement is not passive and automatic but rather takes work, is resolute and painstaking, if not necessarily conscious in its effortfulness. Whether we think of Sullivan's (1953) concept of "malevolent transformation," Gill's (e.g., 1979, 1984) discussions of "resistance to the awareness of transference," Horney's (1945) concept of the moving away neurotic trend, or any of the variety of other ways in which such people can be seen as engaged in conflict and struggle, not just disinterest, the idea that they are simply "in their own world," uninfluenced by what is transpiring in the room, seems odd and quaint today.

WHAT DOES IT MEAN TO BE "ALONE"?: CONFUSIONS ABOUT THE CLINICAL AND CONCEPTUAL IMPLICATIONS OF THE RELATIONAL POINT OF VIEW

The nature of thoroughgoing two-person theorizing—and the ways in which it has been misunderstood—can be further illuminated by consideration of what it means to be *alone*. Aloneness is a topic of interest to explore for a number of reasons. To begin with, aloneness provides a kind of "one-body" test case for a two-person psychology. For aloneness, we must understand, is itself a context. Even when we are alone, we are responding to the fact that we *are* alone. In a wide variety of ways, we behave and experience things differently when we are alone than when we are with others, an indication that we *register* ourselves as being in a different context, one with different situational demands, different constraints and pulls. A variety of behaviors, often self-touching behaviors such as picking one's nose or scratching oneself in certain areas of the body, are common when people are alone but edited and inhibited when others are present. Similarly, our postures and body positions are likely to be different when we are alone from what they are when we are with others. We sit (or slouch) differently when we are alone. We may assume postures that might appear lewd or provocative if another were present but can be quite "natural" and unself-consciously comfortable when we are alone. We may engage in rhythmic self-stimulating movements such as rocking back and forth or shaking our legs, behaviors that might seem almost autistic if they were engaged in with any regularity in the presence of others. We may yawn in an undisguised or unmodulated way that we would inhibit as rude if another were present. And we are more likely when alone to engage in reverie, to daydream, to quietly "think," although at times we may engage in any of these with another person present as well. Thus, in a variety of ways, we clearly register that we are in a different psychological context, one in which "alone behavior" is appropriate.

These differences in behavior and experience are, of course, noticed by one-person theorists too. What is often *not* appreciated, however, is that behavior when we are alone is not behavior in the absence of context, behavior generated simply from "within," but is, rather, behavior that reflects our perception and appreciation that we are in a *different* context from the one in which we are with other people, a context in which different behavior is appropriate.[3] Being alone has *meaning* for each of us, whether that meaning be one of loneliness, rejection, or anxiety or whether it be relief, opportunity to think and reflect, or a welcome time out from a rewarding, if demanding, round of interactions with others. These meanings will vary from person to person, some people primarily finding aloneness a frightening or negative experience, others experiencing it as positive and welcome much of the time. They are also likely to vary for any given individual from one instance of being alone to another, and this further variability is still another example of the contextuality of experience: The meaning of the context of aloneness for any of us at any given moment itself depends on still a larger context—what has been going on, what desires or fantasies have been aroused and are operative. A formulation that states, say, that John gets anxious when he is alone or Mary enjoys being alone and feels it affords her an opportunity to listen to music and pay attention to her own thoughts is almost certain to be insufficient to capture the considerable *variability* of John's or Mary's experience of solitude, even if there are also clear and consistent differences between people in their *average* or *modal* experience of aloneness (or of anything else).

---

[3] As I have noted in a different way earlier, this emphasis on context does not mean that we are responding to the cues and demands of the situation *rather than* to our own inner promptings. Rather, whether alone *or* with others, our behavior reflects our sense (usually only very partly in consciousness) of how we can best express those very promptings *in that particular context*.

Aloneness and "Internal" Presences

The "one-body" situation of being alone is not a "one-person" situation in a theoretical sense for other reasons as well, besides the fact that aloneness is itself a context. A second major consideration is that even when alone, we are orienting ourselves with regard to other people.

Most readily acknowledged by traditional theorists is that the meanings we give to experiences, the affective tone we feel, the aims and structures that guide our behavior are rooted in our prior experiences with others and in what has been called the "internalization" of various prior figures in our lives, especially parental figures. For some writers, this dimension of our experience is central to their understanding of the two-person point of view and to what they mean when they say that human experience is pervasively relational. Mitchell's (1988a) sensitive renderings of the "internal presences" that pervade our lives and give them meaning and affective richness (though also at times a good deal of *agita*) is a good example. For other writers, however, the same phenomenon is an indication that a *one*-person viewpoint is essential to complement a two-person perspective, since the person has now "internalized" the other and is thus influenced by voices from "within."

Such a view is evident not only among "classical" thinkers but among relational and object relational thinkers as well (e.g., Ghent, 1989; Modell, 1984). It is, I think, a misunderstanding, or at the very least an underestimation, of the implications of a thoroughgoing two-person point of view. The "internal" representations, as I shall discuss further below, are not static entities stamped into the psyche and operating completely independently of what transpires in our lives. "Who" gets called up from "inside," and what qualities that representation manifests in any given instance (whether harsh, benign, accepting, directing, sharp, vague, etc.) depends on what has been happening in the person's life and what *kind* of aloneness is being experienced. That is, whether "mother," "father," "older brother," or whomever gets called up—and whether it is "harsh mother" or "loving mother," mother who cares how I am dressed or mother who cares if I have studied hard enough—is not just something that is determined from within. It depends on what the context evokes and makes relevant, and this is true even if one is alone, since aloneness can range anywhere from a momentary interim in the midst of a pleasant round of social interactions, to hard concentrated work on a project (which may be going well or poorly), to solitary confinement in a prisoner of war camp.

When there is overreliance on the concepts of "internalization" or "internal object" to theorize about the idiosyncratically private or personal dimensions of the impact of experiences with others, the two-person nature of aloneness is flattened into a one-person vision. The crucial representations of our ongoing transactions with others, both literal and imagined, are now viewed as simply "inside," and we need no longer look so closely at what is actually transpiring in the person's life.

Aloneness and the Context of Therapeutic Exploration

In the evolution of psychoanalytic technique, a key feature was the creation of a context in which the patient was, in a certain sense, both alone and with another person. It is in the contested territory between these two contradictory realities, in the simultaneous participation in the differing pulls of each, that psychoanalytic work finds its energy and its roots. On the one hand, the standard accoutrements of traditional psychoanalytic practice can be seen as attempting to leave the patient "alone" with himself and his thoughts as much as possible. Sitting behind the patient on the couch, saying relatively little, revealing little of one's personal views or one's own reactions to what the patient is saying are all ways traditional analysts have tried to make room for what is within the patient, to reduce the pulls and the distractions that ordinarily operate when we are with another person. These clinical guidelines are also designed to bring us into closer touch with who we really are, to reduce the distortions and accommodations, the "false selves" that we must put forth when we are with others.

In addition, in replicating a version of the state of aloneness, even while the patient is simultaneously in the presence of another person, the aim is to capitalize on a difference that is frequently apparent between the nature of thought and experience when we are with another person and that which is manifested when we are alone. When alone, we are more likely to engage in reverie and in thought that is more loosely associative.

The difference is only a comparative one, of course. We sometimes engage in reverie (often to our chagrin) even as we are in the midst of a conversation with others; and conversely—for the very reason that aloneness is in fact a state in which we generally remain powerfully in the presence of what is frequently called our internalized objects—the "false self" is not so easily or thoroughly left aside just because we are alone. The psychoanalytic approach, indeed, is very much centered on the *impossibility* of fully casting off the automatic defensive efforts that constrict and misrepresent our experience. Free association is never really "free," and our tailoring of our experience to the context of actual people present and unconsciously imagined parental and emotional judges is difficult to relinquish. The psychoanalytic process is based not on *free* association, but at best on free-*er* association; a crucial focus of the analyst's attention is on how the patient's associations—inevitably—fall short of genuinely free association. Nonetheless, the (inevitably only partly successful) task of free association is neither irrelevant nor, when all is said and done, a failure. The opportunity for patient and analyst to *see* the departures from really free association (and especially to discern the conflict that generates it) is at the very center of the psychoanalytic enterprise, and it is crucially dependent on the patient's associations being at least marginally freer than they are in ordinary discourse.

This alteration of the discourse—an alteration, in essence, of the balance between expression and control—is in one way or another a central feature of almost every approach to psychotherapy. In the traditional psychoanalytic version of this alteration, it is very largely the analyst's diminished presence (or, from a different vantage point, the patient's increased aloneness) that is seen as the medium that makes it possible. The analyst's relative silence, anonymity, and other features of technique that for so long characterized the mainstream of psychoanalytic practice were designed, in essence, to promote an approximation to a "one-person" situation in order to enable the necessary shift from an "outward" to an "inward" focus.

In contrast, I will suggest in the more directly clinical chapters that constitute the second half of this book that there is a much more compelling factor promoting the relative freeing of the patient's associations (and the corollary access to previously disavowed aspects of self-experience)—the *diminished anxiety* or increased sense of *safety* that a well-conducted therapy creates. This alternative perspective derives from Freud's (1926) own perceptive critique of some of the central premises of psychoanalytic thought, and it is consistent with an increased focus in the mainstream of psychoanalytic practice as well on what Schafer (1983) has called conditions of safety. As I shall try to show in those chapters, however, there are ways in which some of the standard features of traditional psychoanalytic practice can actually diminish the experience of safety and hence impede what I believe to be the most important dynamic source of the altered expression–defense balance.

Aloneness and the Pursuit of Private Experience

There is one more matter that is important to consider in further clarifying the nature of a two-person point of view. An objection that is sometimes offered to relational thinking—and especially to a thoroughgoing two-person model, in contrast to a one-person, two-person complementarity of the sort advocated by Ghent or Modell—is that it is exclusively a "social" psychology (see, e.g., Aron, 1996; Gill, 1993; Goldberg, 1986; Mitchell, 1988b). According to this critique (in which the term *social psychology* is used invidiously), such an approach lacks depth, fails to address our individuality or inner world, loses any sense of a personal core. It also, according to some critics, ignores that for many people being alone—with one's thoughts, one's creativity, one's spirituality—is an essential need. Meditation, painting, listening to music, reading, or just sitting and reflecting, the critics rightly point out, are as important a part of the full life as interacting with people.

This critique, however, is based on a significant misunderstanding of relational or two-person theory. There is nothing in the two-person viewpoint that prioritizes interaction with other people over time engaged in more solitary activities. Nor does a two-person perspective pay any less attention to the depth and subtlety of experience, the complexity of personal predisposition and identification, or any other structures of subjectivity or of conflict. Rather, what makes an account of such phenomena a two-person rather than a one-person account is the simultaneous attention to how such experiences respond to and vary with context, how they can symbolize prior and ongoing experiences with others even when we are alone, how the particulars of our experiences of the realm of fantasy, spirituality, self-reflection, or creative imagination simultaneously reflect our unique individuality and our experience of the world around us.

A two-person psychology is indeed a social psychology, in the sense that it is not an *a*social psychology. Indeed, it has been a failing of the psychoanalytic literature that it has neglected a huge body of research in social psychology that potentially has direct bearing on the questions that psychoanalysis too is concerned about (see, e.g., Westen, 1991, 1992a, 1992b, 1994). But a two-person psychoanalytic perspective is not a social psychology in any sense that implies we are mere artifacts of social forces or that when it comes to individual personality there is no there there. Rather, it is a social psychology in very much the sense implied in the following statement by Freud:

> The contrast between individual psychology and social or group psychology, which at first glance seems to be full of significance, loses a great deal of its sharpness when it is examined more closely. It is true that individual psychology is concerned with the individual man and explores the paths by which he seeks to find satisfaction for his instinctual impulses; but only rarely and under certain exceptional conditions is individual psychology in a position to disregard the relations of this individual to others. In the individual's mental life someone else is invariably involved, as a model, as an object, as a helper, as an opponent; and so from the very first, individual psychology, in this extended but entirely justifiable sense of the words, is at the same time social psychology as well. (1921, p. 69)

BEYOND "ONE-PERSON" AND "TWO-PERSON" PSYCHOLOGIES: UNDERSTANDING THE PERSON IN CONTEXT

In the last few chapters, I tried to take the widely employed distinction between a one-person and a two-person psychology as far as it will go. In many ways, it has been a valuable conceptual tool, illuminating important differences and similarities between clusters of theoretical approaches and shedding light on phenomena and dimensions of experience that had previously been overlooked or poorly understood. At the same time, however, the one-person–two-person distinction has brought its own confusions and contradictions. As we have seen, theorists who discuss one- and two-person theory often do not pay sufficient attention to the differences between epistemological concerns and developmental or dynamic considerations; in many instances they confine the applicability of the two-person point of view to the events transpiring in the consulting room; and they often leave out the crucial two-person nature of *all* human experiences, leapfrogging from the mother–infant interaction to the therapist–patient interaction without noticing that there has been an "excluded middle."

Many of the confusions associated with the one-person–two-person distinction were earlier manifested in discussions and critiques of the interpersonal point of view. Misunderstanding or rhetorically misconstruing the implications of an interpersonal viewpoint in much the same way that later critics misconceived and narrowed the meaning of a two-person perspective, many writers treated interpersonal and intrapsychic as opposing terms that referred to competing theories or to entirely different realms. Just as the claim is now frequently made that we need *both* a one-person and a two-person perspective, so too was the claim made (and indeed still is) that we need both interpersonal and intrapsychic theories. Such a way of thinking misrepresents what a two-person model or an interpersonal model *is*. That is, the two-person model is not only about what happens *between* two people, with what happens *within* each of them a separate matter altogether. The two-person model, at least as I employ it, is most fundamentally about the fact that what happens *within* each individual is itself a two-person process. Our "insides" are not a realm separate from our "outsides" or our interactions with others, and attending to the relational is not an alternative or complement to attending to the intrapsychic; it is a *different way of* attending to the intrapsychic, a way of understanding the deepest, most private, least conscious aspects of our experience but of understanding them as inseparable from the relational matrix in which we have evolved as individuals and within which we continue to evolve and express our individuality.

Consider Mitchell's (1988a) seminal articulation of the commonalities among the disparate theoretical strands from which the relational synthesis was woven:

> We are portrayed not as a conglomerate of physically based urges, but as being shaped by and inevitably embedded within a matrix of relationships with other people, struggling both to maintain our ties to others and to differentiate ourselves from them. In this vision the basic unit of study is not the individual as a separate entity whose desires clash with an external reality, but an interactional field within which the individual arises and struggles to make contact and to articulate himself. *Desire* is experienced always *in the context of relatedness,* and it is that context which defines its meaning. Mind is composed of relational configurations. The person is comprehensible only within this tapestry of relationships, past and present. (p. 3, italics in original)

This description emphasizes the embeddedness of the individual in a matrix of relationships, but it *is* the embeddedness of *individuals.* Mitchell refers not just to the relational matrix and the interactional field but also to the individual struggling to articulate himself. Desire is experienced in the context of relatedness, but it is *the individual's* desire. Such a conceptualization does not pit the interactional field against the distinctive desires and struggles toward self-definition of individuals, but rather points to the former as the *context* within which the latter evolves. Each is part and parcel of the other. They are not alternative perspectives; they are intertwined, mutually interpenetrating dimensions of a single living reality.

By now, the terminology of "one-person" and "two-person" theory is so widespread that it will be impossible to proceed with this book without falling back on it at various points to locate particular points of view within the context of the field's major divisions. But it is nonetheless sufficiently problematic that I wish to introduce a different, hopefully clarifying, term to capture what I believe to be the most important contribution of the two-person idea. What two-person theorists are most importantly pointing to, I believe, is the *contextual* nature of human psychology, and in large measure what they are criticizing in what they are calling one-person theories is the largely *acontextual* nature of those theories, the way in which they describe individuals out of context, as separate monads whose psychological driving forces are thoroughly "internalized" and hence carried around essentially unchanged from context to context. It is for this reason that such "one-person" theories do not take sufficient note of the way the therapist's qualities and her behavior in the session contribute to the experiences observed in the session. And it is for this reason that "one-person" theories also fail to appreciate (as do some purportedly "two-person" theories as well) the way in which context shapes our experience in *every* facet of our lives.

Conceptualizing the issue as contextual versus acontextual rather than one-person versus two-person helps avoid a number of potential confusions. To begin with, whereas the two-person conceptualization has at times been construed by critics as implying that we are mere reactors to the input of others, lacking core structures or enduring qualities and commitments (cf. Masling, 2003; Meissner, 1998; Eagle et al., 2001), the emphasis on contextual understanding does not so readily lend itself to such a misperception. Rather, it suggests that the very nature of those structures and commitments is contextual. It reconciles the compelling observations of how responsive we are to the events around us and the behavior of others—whether in the psychotherapy session or in any other context in our lives—with the equally compelling observations, usually stressed particularly by "one-person" theorists, of how much we experience the present through a template from the past and how tenaciously we may persist in old ways of seeing and responding that bring us continuing pain and frustration. As I shall elaborate further in the chapters that follow, appreciation of the contextual nature of the psychological structures that guide our behavior and experience does not lead us into the false dichotomies that can characterize discussions of one-person and two-person theories. It also does not call forth the facile ecumenicism—a little bit of one-person thinking, a little bit of two-person thinking—that has yielded confusion in the conceptual terrain of one-person versus two-person theory; few would suggest that in order to be comprehensive, we have to create, side by side, contextual and acontextual theories. If we appreciate what contextualism implies, we can see how it provides a foundation not only for simultaneously understanding the facts of variability and continuity or of responsiveness and apparent heedlessness, but also for understanding *when* and *why* one or the other tendency comes to the fore.

Thinking in terms of the differences between contextual and acontextual formulations introduces clarity as well into our understanding of the role of biology and of the body, realms where the one-person–two-person distinction has created particular confusion. For example, in discussing Mitchell's theorizing, Aron (1996) states the following:

> Even Mitchell acknowledges that interpersonal experience inevitably has its impact on a child, who brings to the interaction his or her own temperament and constitutional endowment, and therefore the interpersonal is always filtered through the individual's particular capacities to take in experience. *In this sense, Mitchell's two-person psychology includes within itself an implicit recognition of a one-person psychology.* (p. 60, italics added)

Here, it seems, Aron is defining as a one-person viewpoint any acknowledgment that the individual enters interactions with already formed characteristics and proclivities (whether they be genetically inherited or derived from the interaction of that initial genetic heritage with earlier experiences). Temperament and constitutional endowment, however, are not *necessarily* or *inherently* "one-person" concepts. Aron here subtly and unintendedly narrows the zone of two-person theory, creating room for a "one-person" approach as a complementary per-spective not through logical necessity but via definition. If we *define* attention to temperament or biology as a one-person point of view, then there is indeed a need for one-person thinking to complement two-person thinking unless one is willing to ignore the body alto-gether. But if instead we take as our starting point the *psychological* cri-teria for one-person or two-person theorizing that I have been stressing—particularly the issue of whether psychological structures and inclinations are understood as acontextual attributes that are essentially independent of and unmodified by the context in which they are manifested or whether they are contextual by their very nature (that is, inclinations that are real, that are indeed distinctive to and emblematic of a particular individual, but that express themselves dif-ferently and have different implications and meanings in one context or another), then one can readily conceive of temperament and consti-tutional endowment as "two-person" phenomena.

But it is also important to appreciate that in the very effort to explicate how a property such as temperament can be conceptualized in a "two-person" fashion, one is also encountering the limitations and ambiguities inherent in the one-person–two-person distinction itself. The very terminology makes it confusing to apply a "two-person" per-spective to something that seems, in a concrete perceptual sense, to reside within one person. If one approaches the issue from the vantage point of contextualism, however, the confusions and ambiguities are greatly reduced. There are *always* already existing psychological struc-tures involved in any experience or interaction. If there were not, there would not be *people* involved. But at the same time, those structures are always contextual structures, structures whose very nature entails pro-cessing and responding to events.

Each individual enters each encounter with an enormous number of interlaced and hierarchically organized structures that are part of "him" or "her." But in any particular experience or encounter, only cer-tain of those structures are elicited or brought into play; context always plays a role. Moreover, not only are different structures elicited and made relevant by particular events or contexts, the various struc-tures both change and are *changed by* those events. Mutual and recipro-cal causality is pervasive throughout. The nature of the event or con-text influences which structures are elicited, but it is equally accurate (and equally incomplete) to say that the structure or individual procliv-ity brings about the event as it is to say that the event elicits the structure. What we anticipate, how we act, how we interpret what transpires will change and influence what does transpire. But what we anticipate, how we act, and even how we interpret what happens also is *influenced by* the constantly changing context. It is not a matter of either–or, even of a simple both–and, but of constant and mutual co-construction, a co-construction in which both sides of the dialectic must be strongly acknowledged.

Put differently, recognition of structure and recognition of context are not two different points of view. They are essential components of a *single* point of view. A situation is not a *psychological* situation unless there are psychological structures to apprehend it; and those structures are not human—or even living—psychological structures if they are not structures oriented to their surrounds, capable of and inclined toward the perception of changing contingencies, demands, and opportunities, even as they seek as well to preserve themselves in the face of those changing contingencies.

Even physical properties and structures of the body, which are indeed "inside," and which, most of the time, do their thing from context to context rather reliably and consistently, are not immune from the influence of context. The heart is most obviously such an organ, which is perhaps one of the reasons it serves so often as a metaphor for the passions. Not only physical circumstances such as steep inclines, but emotional and symbolic events as well regularly alter its rate, its efficiency, its rhythms, and so forth. Other bodily organs respond similarly, if not always as obviously, to a wide range of variations in every aspect of our environment, including the social environment.

Temperament, the bodily/biological variable about which Aron (1996) explicitly states that attention to it entails "an implicit recognition of a one-person psychology," is an especially interesting case with regard to contextualism. An acontextual perspective might view the person's temperament as a property of "the individual," something more or less invariant that he brings with him from situation to situation. But temperament, as much as Freudian drives, is a borderland phenomenon between mind and body. It takes on psychological meaning and consequences only as it is perceived and experienced by self and other. Is the child's biological temperament "hyperactive" and "out of control," or is it "energetic" and "enthusiastic"? That depends quite significantly on what the mother is set to perceive, what she is comfortable with, what she nurtures, or how she defines what the child's nature is. Ultimately what the child's temperament "actually becomes" in a psychologically meaningful sense is to a significant degree co-created by the mother and other significant figures in the person's life. Temperament, we might say, is contextual down to its very core. And, it is important to note, it is contextual *at the same time* as it is, equally, a structural (and genetic) fact about the person. That is, again, a contextual view is not an antistructural view. But it conceives of structure very differently than many psychoanalytic writings in the past have seemed to.

In similar fashion, drive-related wishes or "internalized" psychological influences such as introjects or internal objects, internal working models, and the like are better understood as contextual than as fixed and simply "inside." Describing people as characterized by a particular developmental level, as preoedipal, as passive–aggressive or orally fixated fails to ask *when* they manifest whatever is being attributed to them. Implicitly, in many accounts, the times when the particular conceptualized characteristic is not manifested are treated as times when it is defended against or denied. And although it is certainly true that in many instances particular underlying inclinations *are* being defended against, in many others what we are seeing, rather, is the variability that characterizes our psychological lives, the manifestations of *other* inclinations and characteristics that emerge in different contexts and are just as real properties of the person as are the qualities that are usually emphasized in psychoanalytic accounts, which tend to highlight the "early" and the pathological. As I shall discuss in the later, clinical chapters of this book, attention to these other (and often healthier or more adaptive) ways of being—and examination of when they do and do not appear (that is, of their contextual nature)—can greatly enhance our clinical work.

After wrestling with the question of whether one-person and two-person perspectives are complementary or contradictory, Aron (1996) ultimately concludes that "the major difficulty in attempting to sort out the contradictory versus complementary nature of one- and two-person psychologies is that the referents for these terms remain unclear. . . . [They] have been used so broadly, to cover so much conceptual ground, that it is hard to know what anyone means by advocating a position that requires only one or both perspectives" (pp. 61–62). Aron further states, in a vein that strongly parallels the frame of reference that guides this book, that "dividing up the world into the innate and the experiential or the intrapsychic and the interpersonal is certainly simplistic, since each of these terms contains, organizes, and defines the other" (p. 62).

BEYOND THE SESSION:
THE CONTEXTUALITY OF HUMAN EXPERIENCE

To return to a theme discussed at the beginning of this chapter, part of the confusion at the root of the one-person and two-person distinction (and part of what contributes to its limitations) derives from its origins in addressing the specific psychological situation of the psychoanalytic session. In that realm it did offer an important corrective for a view that was once extremely prominent. The influence of the therapist or analyst on everything that "emerges" or "unfolds" in the session is palpable, and yet it had been rendered invisible by an ideological filter. But the framing of the critique of this faulty conceptualization in terms of two-person theory was an artifact of the specific circumstances of the psychoanalytic situation. In the ordinary course of psychoanalytic practice, the only *direct* observation of the impact of another person on the patient's inner experience is with the analyst. The idea of two-person theory seemed to capture that palpable experience, emphasizing the simple fact that there are indeed two people in the room and that each continually contributes to the other's experience. The seeming appropriateness of the "two-person" label was further bolstered by the light that this new conceptualization cast on traditional psychoanalytic epistemology, highlighting the way analysts had proceeded as if what was being observed in the psychoanalytic process were psychological phenomena pertaining to only *one* of the people in the room—the patient.

Family therapists, in contrast, saw the processes of mutual influence and co-construction very differently because of the observational field to which they were exposed in *their* work. They were able to directly observe mutual influences of people on each other's psychological experiences for more than just themselves and one other person. As a consequence, they did not frame the contrast between their perspective and that of earlier views as one between one-person and "two"-person theories, since "two" seemed both arbitrary and insufficient. Their critiques were more likely to take the form of linear versus circular, or individual versus systemic (see Wachtel & Wachtel, 1986), and their equivalent of the relational psychoanalytic "two-person" critique that the analyst is a coparticipant in what transpires in the room was that the therapist inevitably becomes *part of the system* that she is observing.

Put differently, a key problem with the one-person–two-person distinction is that it is largely a perspective focused on the psychoanalytic session rather than all of the patient's life. Outside the session, "one" and "two" are by no means the only possibilities. Rickman (1957), one of the originators of the two-person concept, did acknowledge this, referring as well to three-body, four-body, and multibody situations. But in the application of Rickman's ideas within psychoanalytic discourse, two usually *meant* two—the twosome together in the analyst's office. Ultimately, there is nothing magical about the number two. Although it makes a certain kind of sense to say that classical psychoanalytic theory is a "one-person" psychology, it is not really a "two-person" psychology that should replace it, but a *contextual* psychology.

5

■   ■   ■   ■   ■

Drives, Relationships, and the Foundations of the Relational Point of View

As we have already seen, there is no single criterion that definitively identifies a point of view as relational. Thinkers who identify themselves as relational characterize what they regard as the essence of relational thinking in a variety of different ways, and it is one of the characteristics of the contemporary relational movement that it takes in a broad range of positions and viewpoints. Nonetheless, there are clearly some ways of thinking and some critiques of earlier theoretical positions that are more widely shared and more strongly held among relational thinkers than others. In the last few chapters, I have explored one of those core issues—the distinction between one-person and two-person theorizing—and have found it illuminating but also potentially confusing and misleading. In this chapter, I wish to examine an equally prominent distinction in most discussions and formulations of relational thinking—personality as ultimately rooted in the vicissitudes of the drives versus personality as fundamentally derived from relationships. Here too we will find much that is clarifying and insightful but also ways in which confusions and conceptual stumbling blocks are introduced.

After examining the issues associated with the drive versus relationship distinction as the foundation of the relational point of view, I will then explore, in the next chapter, two other conceptual alternatives that I believe provide a more useful foundation for relational theory and practice—one, the distinction between contextual and acontextual thinking introduced in the last chapter; the other, the distinction between archaeological and cyclical models of personality. My aim in introducing these alternative foundations for relational thinking is not to reject the one-person–two-person distinction or the drive-relationship distinction, both of which remain valuable conceptual tools. Rather, it is to *supplement* these two perspectives and to embed them in a broader conceptual structure that enables our theory and practice to be based on a fuller range of observations, both from the clinical setting and everyday life and from the findings of systematic research.

THE MOST SIGNIFICANT TENSION
IN THE HISTORY OF PSYCHOANALYTIC IDEAS?

In the volume that might be said to have launched the relational movement in psychoanalysis, Greenberg and Mitchell (1983) state, "The most significant tension in the history of psychoanalytic ideas has been the dialectic between the original Freudian mode, which takes as its starting point the instinctual drive, and an alternative comprehensive model initiated in the work of Fairbairn and Sullivan, which evolves structure solely from the individual's relations with other people" (p. 20). This is a very strong statement: Calling any issue the most significant in the entire history of a field is no mealymouthed claim. Yet it is also very largely accurate, at least as a description of the intensity of controversy and the dominant lines of cleavage in the field.

There are, of course, other important issues and controversies as well that divide psychoanalytic thinkers, some of which have already been discussed and others of which will concern us as I proceed. But it is certainly true that few conceptual issues more centrally define the shared identification of therapists who consider themselves to be relational in orientation than the one highlighted by Greenberg and Mitchell. Skolnick and Warshaw (1992), for example, in their introduction to the book *Relational Perspectives in Psychoanalysis*, state that although there is no one single relational model or theory, all relationalists "have a common concern with the centrality of relationship in the development and structure of personality" (p. xxiv). Ghent (1992a), in the same volume, asks, "How does one recognize a relational psychoanalyst?" and answers as follows: "There is no such thing as a relational analyst; there are only analysts whose backgrounds may vary considerably, but who share a broad outlook in which human relations—specific, unique human relations—play a superordinate role in the genesis of character and of psychopathology, as well as in the practice of psychoanalytic therapeutics" (p. xviii). Aron (1996), in another influential work in the relational literature, states that "relational theory is essentially a contemporary eclectic theory anchored in the idea that it is *relationships* (internal and external, real and imagined) that are central" (p. 18, italics added). And Mitchell, in his 1988 volume *Relational Concepts in Psychoanalysis,* portrays the fundamental distinction between Freudian and relational models as one in which we are viewed in Freudian thought as "a conglomeration of asocial, physical tensions represented in the mind by urgent sexual and aggressive wishes pushing for expression" (Mitchell, 1988a, p. 2) versus the quintessential relational view that we are "fundamentally dyadic and interactive, above all else" and that "psychic organization and structures are built from the patterns which shape those interactions" (pp. 3–4).

It is worth noting, as an aside, the almost casual equation of "dyadic" with relational in this last quote from Mitchell. This emphasis on the dyadic is pervasive in the relational literature, and it reflects the influence on relational theorizing of the preponderant emphasis on the mother–infant relationship and the patient–analyst relationship described in the last two chapters. Those two *are* dyadic relationships. But as I shall further elaborate as I proceed, they by no means exhaust the relationships in people's lives that contribute to shaping and maintaining our personalities. Psychoanalytic thinkers, for example, will surely think of the triadic relationships that are central in the oedipal period. But relationships of *many* sorts have a powerful impact and shaping role *throughout* life. Our experiences in group contexts, for example, may profoundly affect our self-esteem (as anyone who has been in high school will attest), and the ways we interact with groups and the roles we assume in them have an important impact in the workplace, affecting our incomes and job prospects in significant ways. Even in the earliest years of life, when current relational theory almost exclusively directs its attention to the mother–infant dyad, there are millions of examples from around the world demonstrating that often "it takes a village."

But the issue of dyadic versus other relationships aside, what these quotations from a variety of leading relational writers indicate is that the distinction between a view of personality as built upon and organized by drives and one in which *relationships* are the central foundation is clearly of prime importance for relational thinkers, an idea that provides much of the glue that unites the rather disparate branches of the overall relational movement. It is, as well, a conceptualization that will in various ways echo throughout this book. At the same time, however, as I will explore in this chapter, the drive versus relationship distinction has also carried with it some problematic conceptual baggage that in certain respects has created a "soft foundation" for the relational movement. It is to these difficulties with the drive–relationship distinction that I now turn.

RELATIONSHIPS PAST, PRESENT, AND IMAGINED

It is difficult to imagine a "relational" point of view that was not concerned with the central role of relationships in shaping our lives and our personalities. But that does not necessarily mean that the *distinction between* a drive focus and a relationship focus needs to be at the center. Indeed, as I hope to show, there are ways in which the emphasis on the drive versus relationship *distinction* as the defining criterion for relational theorizing has actually in some instances distracted relational theorists from probing more deeply and critically into their assumptions about the exact *nature and role* of relationships in the evolution of personality, especially in the years beyond infancy. Crucial distinctions among theoretical positions on the relationship side of the drive–relationship divide may be obscured when the divide itself is taken to be so central a touchstone for defining what classifies an approach as relational.

To be sure, in directing attention to the distinction between explanations of behavior and experience that place drives at the center and those that are more rooted in the impact of relationships, relational writers have pointed to a very important issue, one that contributes significantly to our ability to transcend what could be a rather reductionistic element in classical psychoanalytic thought. As I discussed in Chapter 3, through the lens of classical drive theory, human beings may appear to be mere conduits for the expression of the drives, marionettes whose strings are pulled by biologically rooted instinctual urges that are outside of and "underneath" the aims, concerns, and perceptions that are ordinarily thought to constitute the personality or the self. But as I also discussed in that chapter, it is not uncommon for descriptions of *relational* influences to be formulated in marionette-like terms as well. The internalized representations of early object relations can similarly be viewed in reductionistic fashion, placing ongoing relations with other people in at most a supporting role or in the role of stand-in. That is, in some versions of relational thought, the new experience is largely examined as a representation of or stand-in for *early* experiences, relationships, and fantasies, and the therapist looks *under* or *behind* the present relational experience to explain the patient's behavior as a repetition and reflection of *past* (often preoedipal) relational experiences.

It is important to be clear that to question this theoretical strategy is not to dismiss the powerful impact of early experiences on later development. It is, however, to suggest a *different understanding* of that impact. Virtually all contemporary thinkers agree that we approach and perceive new experiences in terms of the expectations and schemas that have evolved from earlier experiences and earlier relationships. What is at issue, rather, is precisely *how* the earlier experience contributes to shaping later experience—whether the later experience is merely a screen upon which is projected images of "internal" object relations that have remained largely unchanged (and largely *inaccessible* to change) since early childhood, or whether the present relational matrix, the configuration of perceptions and affectively meaningful interactions with the actual key figures in one's life in the present, is taken seriously as a coequal shaper of the person's experience. Put differently, the question is whether the person is seen as genuinely responding to what is happening in the present, even if, inevitably, "in his fashion," or whether, as in some versions of both drive theory *and* relational theory, the present experience is largely bypassed in the search for the earlier and, presumably, "deeper" roots (see Wachtel, 2003a).

It is easy not to notice that these are two rather different ways of understanding the role of the "relational matrix" in generating our behavior and experience, because as we saw in Chapter 4, almost all relational theorists *do* attribute serious and consequential influence to the contemporary relational context when it is specifically the therapeutic relationship that is at issue. But (either by express intent or, often, by inadvertence) serious attention to the relational matrix within which the patient's dynamics are played out (and, so often, through which they are perpetuated) is much less common, and often tepid at best, when it comes to the *other* ongoing relationships in the patient's life.

In many versions of relational thinking, it is striking how little attention is paid to the actual nature of contemporary relationships. Attention is directed instead to the "internal" structure that is seen as almost inexorably directing the person's perceptions and leading him or her to behave in certain ways. As Mitchell puts it in discussing Guntrip (1971) and a range of related theorists whom one might describe as *proto*-relational, "*Early* mental life is conceived in terms of interaction; but once structured, the mind is perseveratively dominated by vestiges of infantile experience. . . . What is overlooked is the extent to which the analysand is involved in an interactive field" (Mitchell, 1988a, p. 162, italics added).[1] In similar fashion, addressing the developmental assumptions that lie at the heart of self psychology, another significant component in the relational synthesis, Mitchell points critically to "the assumption that there is an 'inside' to the patient which can manifest itself more or less independently of the interactive situation in which it appears," and he notes that self psychologists tend to emphasize "the importance of *past* interpersonal experience, but not the particularities of the *present* interaction with the analyst"[2] (Mitchell, 1988a, p. 298, italics in original).

With the foregoing considerations in mind, it becomes apparent that there are therapists and theorists who think of themselves as *relational* without paying a lot of attention to *relationships,* or at least to contemporary ones. They plumb the interior for the patient's *fantasies* about relationships, for the impact (especially the distorting impact) of *past* relationships on present experiences, but—again with the important exception of the therapeutic relationship—they pay little attention to the current relational matrix or interactive field that is the context for everything the patient experiences. It is with this conceptual tendency in mind that Mitchell (1988a, p. 170) cites Levenson's (1983) characterization of object relations theory as viewing the patient as an adult "stuck with an incorporated infant, like a fishbone in the craw of his maturity."

---

[1] Recall here the very similar comments about Fairbairn's theorizing by Stolorow et al. (2001a), cited in Chapter 3.

[2] Note again the way in which this last statement limits itself to the interaction with *the analyst.* There is a continuing tension in relational writings between viewing the relational matrix in which the person is embedded as significant and relevant in *every* facet of his psychological experience and the tendency to attend to the interactive context only in relation to the mother–infant relationship and the relationship with the analyst. The broader application of relationality is clearly implicit in Mitchell's overall meaning, but even he slips readily, and even frequently, into the more restrictive way of characterizing the issues.

We may thus see that there are significant and insufficiently appreciated commonalities in deep structure between the theoretical efforts of some members of the rather heterogenous group of theorists who identify with the relational paradigm and the assumptions that guide most drive theorists (for example, a highly "internal" and often rather past-oriented focus and a tendency to look "under" or "behind" what is presently going on in a way that treats present relationships largely as theoretical chaff). Knowing that a therapist places herself on the "relationship" side of the drive–relationship divide tells us relatively little about how seriously—and in what fashion—that therapist attends to the key relationships outside the consulting room that constitute the present context of the patient's life. As we have seen, some theoretical lines that are a significant part of the relational synthesis in essence minimize the significance of these relationships, viewing them very largely as the playing out of *prior* relationships that have been "internalized." Taken together, these considerations suggest that the drive–relationship distinction may *not* be "the most significant tension in the history of psychoanalytic ideas" after all, and may, indeed, at times obscure other distinctions that are at least as crucial.

COMPETING THEORIES OR COMPETING VISIONS?

How is it that theorists who pay relatively little attention to our ongoing relationships with real, present human others—whose vision of what Mitchell (1988a) has aptly called the relational matrix is largely restricted to the relational matrix of the patient's *past* or to the *imagined* or *fantasized* relational matrix, to the neglect of our immersion throughout life in *real* relationships with *real* people—can nonetheless think of themselves as "relational" analysts? Here again, our understanding can be aided by examining the centrality of the drive–relationship distinction in the emerging identity of the relational point of view. In essence, the understanding evolved (without ever quite being stated explicitly in this form) that if a theorist rejected the drive theory, if she posited that *relationships* were the basic building blocks of personality, then she was a relational thinker, regardless of whether she paid much attention to the contemporary relationships in the patient's life or not. To understand how this happened, it is useful to look at the *origins* of what has come to be called the relational turn.

Earlier writers, such as Fairbairn (1952) and Balint (1965), had introduced and highlighted the distinction between a drive theory and a theory founded on the study of relationships, but it was Greenberg and Mitchell (1983) who employed this distinction not just to distinguish their vision from Freud's but to illuminate convergences between theoretical trends that had developed largely in isolation from one another. In providing a conceptual umbrella to unite object relations, interpersonal, and self psychological theories, they not only forged an intellectual framework for bringing together theoretical tendencies whose confluences had been obscured by different language systems and professional allegiances and organizations, they also created a new *power base* in psychoanalysis. Proponents of the differing strands that they brought together had been isolated and marginalized to varying degrees. When they could be coalesced into a movement, they became a force to reckon with.

Greenberg and Mitchell's (1983) book was thus not just an intellectual contribution but, we may see in retrospect, a political one. It changed profoundly the political landscape of psychoanalysis. And perhaps as a consequence, certain problematic features of their analysis have been insufficiently examined. Because their sharp distinction between the relational and drive perspectives—the view that it is the most significant divide in the history of the field—has been the foundation for the emergence of a relational *movement* in the field, it has taken on a kind of iconic status. There are in fact *many* ways to parse the diversity of theoretical and therapeutic approaches in the field, and each one, in essence, could potentially create a different set of coalitions. The drive–relational distinction "worked"—and worked exceedingly well—on an organizational basis. It has also, however—for the very reason that it was so foundational in the emergence of the relational movement—become in a way preemptive, distracting attention from other potential distinctions among theories that, I believe, have a greater potential for illuminating "differences that make a difference" in our understanding and in our practice. These differences, which I have been discussing throughout the early chapters of this book, and will pull together in the next chapter, have to do with significant structural features of how relationships are actually taken into account, how psychological development is conceived, and (as I shall discuss in the second half of the book) how the therapeutic process is understood and carried out.

It is important to recognize that much of what made the drive versus relationship distinction seem so absolute and unbridgeable to Greenberg and Mitchell (and to many subsequent relational writers) is that they were discussing a distinction that derived not primarily from either clinical observation or systematic research but from abstract philosophical considerations. One of the strengths of their analysis, a unique feature of their book that I greatly admire, is that in contrast to most writers in psychology or psychoanalysis, they were keenly aware of the larger cultural and intellectual context of the issues they were addressing. They explicitly situate their discussion of the drive–relational debate within the larger context of two competing traditions within Western philosophical thought which, in one form or another, have contended for centuries. One school of thought, they write, "finding its fullest expression in British eighteenth-century philosophy . . . takes as its premise that human satisfactions and goals are fundamentally personal and individual. Human beings pursue their own separate aims . . . and these atomistic, discordant pursuits are likely to interfere with each other. . . . Meaning in human life resides in individual fulfillment" (Greenberg & Mitchell, 1983, pp. 400–401). The second school of thought, whose origins they locate in Aristotle and which they trace through such thinkers as Rousseau, Hegel, and Marx, "takes as its premise that human satisfactions and goals are realizable only within a community. . . . The state of nature within this approach is quite different from that envisioned by the British philosophers. . . . Human nature is felt to contain feelings of natural affiliation and mutual concern. . . . It is only in recognition by and participation with his fellows that man becomes fully human" (pp. 401–402).

Relating this debate in the larger sphere of philosophical and social thought to the specific distinction between the drive and relational models, they state, "The drive/structure model and the relational/structure model embody these two major traditions within Western philosophy in the relatively recently developing intellectual arena of psychoanalytic ideas." Like the first tradition, they argue, the drive model "takes as its fundamental premise that the individual mind, the psychic apparatus, is the most meaningful and useful unit for the study of mental functioning. That individual unit, for Freud as for Hobbes, is dominated by desires for personal pleasures and power, for private gratification" (p. 402). In contrast, the relational/structure model "takes as its fundamental premise the principle that human existence cannot be meaningfully understood on individual terms, that, as Sullivan puts it, man is not capable of 'definitive description in isolation.' . . . the very nature of being human draws the individual into relations with others, and it is only in these relations that man becomes anything like what we regard as human" (p. 403).

Drawing in particular on Isaiah Berlin's (1958) writings in political philosophy and his contention that these two contrasting visions in Western philosophical thought are "profoundly divergent and irreconcilable attitudes to the ends of life" and that "each of them makes absolute claims" (Berlin, 1958, p. 55), Greenberg and Mitchell argue that the drive and relational models in psychoanalysis occupy similar conceptual terrain. "Psychoanalytic models," they assert, "like political philosophies, are based on a 'vision by which we are consciously or unconsciously guided of what constitutes a fulfilled human life.' . . . It is neither useful nor appropriate to question whether either psychoanalytic model is 'right' or 'wrong.' Each is complex, elegant, and resilient enough to account for all phenomena" (pp. 403–404). Sixteen years later, Mitchell and Aron made a similar claim: "Each model actually *does* provide understanding of *all* the phenomena in question" (1999, p. xiv, italics in original).

In part, this way of presenting the contending claims of drive and relational theorists reflects an unfortunate anti-empirical strain that has been woven into the fabric of relational psychoanalysis from its very beginnings, and has been a continuing source of criticism of relational theorizing (see, e.g., Eagle, 2003a; Eagle et al., 2001; Mills, 2005; Masling, 2003; Silverman, 2000). Greenberg and Mitchell state quite explicitly that in their view the premises of both the drive and the relational models "are not subject to empirical verification" and that the "superordinate" criterion for evaluating these competing theories comes down to "a matter of personal choice. . . . Does the theory speak to you? Does it seem to account for your deepest needs, longings, fears?" (p. 407).

Such an attitude is by no means intrinsic to relational theorizing. Indeed, Greenberg and Mitchell themselves, in the very same chapter in which they present drive and relational perspectives as philosophical "visions" that cannot be challenged empirically, provide an indication that there *is* an empirical basis for their rejection of drive theory. For proponents of the relational model, they say, "the pervasive presence of others, real and imaginary, past and present, in every moment of our lives, demands a relational model theory and can never be adequately encompassed by a theory in which object relations are a function of primitive instinctual drives. . . . For clinicians and theorists who think in relational/structure terms, to say that pleasure seeking is at the root of all relations with others is to skew the data—it is simply too reductionistic" (p. 405).

Here it appears that, although situating their conceptualization in the context of competing philosophies, Greenberg and Mitchell are rooting it as well in what can be observed clinically. The pervasive influence of others in every moment of our lives is something that can be *observed,* and Greenberg and Mitchell tell us that these observations "demand" a relational model theory. This does not sound like a simple matter of taste. It is about whether the formulation is adequate to account for the clinical data. Those data—like the data that derive from more controlled experiments—are always to some degree theory-infused, difficult to disentangle fully from the preconceptions we bring to bear in the process of making the observations. But they are not *reducible to* those preconceptions. That idea would reflect a puerile solipsism that is certainly not Greenberg and Mitchell's understanding. To whatever degree they can trust the evidence of their senses, Greenberg and Mitchell are telling us that our behavior and experience *are* powerfully influenced by "the pervasive presence of others, real and imaginary, past and present," not that you can draw that conclusion if you're in the mood to see it that way but it's equally legitimate to say, "No thanks, I'd rather not."

When Greenberg and Mitchell claim that both drive and relational theories are "complex, elegant, and resilient" enough to "account for all phenomena," they are being excessively ecumenical and, in contrast with the overall perspicacity of their work, insufficiently incisive and substantive in their depiction of the drive model and their challenge to it. There *is* a critique to be made of the drive model that is based on more than "taste" or "feel." But Greenberg and Mitchell's primary construal of the differences between the two theoretical outlooks as philosophical rather than empirical undermines that critique. And, importantly, this emphasis on competing philosophical visions rather than on competing *observations* directs attention away from a similar critique that can be applied to some aspects of relational theorizing as well. As I have already alluded to, and will elaborate further in the next chapter, the claim that the drive theory "is simply too reductionistic" can be applied to some formulations common in relational theorizing as well.

OBSERVATIONAL TUNNEL VISION

A good part of how competing drive and relational formulations can seem each to "account for all phenomena" is not because of their inherent comprehensiveness but because their adherents engage in a form of tunnel vision, restricting their attention to observations that are consistent with or seem to confirm their theoretical assumptions. Indeed, not infrequently, they even restrict their very *opportunity* to observe to contexts in which congenial (or at least sufficiently pliable) observations will arise. One way this is accomplished was noted in the previous chapter. By directing their attention more or less exclusively to the events in the session, many analysts render their theories impervious to observations from other realms that would require modifications in their theories. Moreover, the particular way in which the events of the session are attended to in contemporary psychoanalytic practice often excludes as well (or at the very least pushes to the margins) observations that are gathered *in* the session but are not primarily *about* the session—that is, the patient's references to the events of his ongoing daily life. Serious attention to those events would virtually compel changes in the overall theoretical structure through which clinical phenomena are understood (see, e.g., Wachtel, 1993, 1997; Wachtel & Wachtel, 1986), and in tandem with the attention to the transference and the vicissitudes of subjectivity that have always been of central interest to psychoanalytic observers, would yield a more comprehensive and satisfactory grasp of the person's experience and of the clinical challenges that need to be addressed.

Neither the classical drive theory *nor* most versions of the relational paradigm explain all the data sufficiently. They each focus their attention on somewhat *different* data, and they retain their adherents not through personal choice among equally viable and fully comprehensive theoretical accounts, but through tunnel vision. They *ignore* palpable and important observations that might require them to change.

No psychological theory is viable that does not address the *empirically demonstrable* impact of context, the ways that people (and even the intrapsychic structures that may be revealed via analytic inquiry) vary—vary enormously—from situation to situation. As we will see as we proceed, theories that depict people as arrested at a particular developmental level or that characterize unconscious psychological structures and tendencies as sealed off from the influence of new experience, as "timeless" and more or less direct manifestations of early states of mind impervious to the events of later life, are not just an alternative "taste" or preference or "vision." They are *wrong*.

WHAT DO PRACTICING THERAPISTS
ACTUALLY LISTEN FOR?:
ABSTRACT THEORIZING AND CLINICAL REALITY

There is still another difficulty with conceptualizing the distinction between drive and relational perspectives as fundamental and irreconcilable and, in the process, grounding the relational approach in its opposition to drive theory. This distinction is at a level of abstraction that is actually rather far removed from the discriminations and judgments that actually guide clinical practice. There are obviously important differences among therapists in the way they listen, understand, and respond. But those differences are not well captured by the question that many relationalists view as the key issue—whether drives or relations with others constitute "the basic stuff of mental life" (Mitchell, 1988a, p. 2). That is a question of *abstract* fundamentals, of a priori philosophical assumptions about the essential nature of things. Although it is in one sense a question of origins, it is of origins in almost an ontological sense rather than a question of what earlier experiences were the forerunners or causes of the experiences the patient is now reporting. Consequently, although it is a question that may bear quite directly on therapists' theoretical *identifications*, it actually has relatively little import for the categories through which practicing clinicians make sense of the diversity of things that patients say, think, and feel during the course of the therapeutic work.

The reason I say this is that clinical work guided by drive theory—especially drive theory as it is employed by most *contemporary* analytic therapists who identify with that point of view—*also* conceives of human relations as utterly central to what is listened for when listening to patients. Analysts virtually *never* listen for "drives." Even when they employ that conceptual terminology or keep that conceptual framework in their consciousness when they are listening, they are listening for *drives as they are attached to objects*. The oedipus complex, for example, so close to the heart of Freudian theory, has at its very core that it is *not* the mere occurrence of sexual desire that is the problem, but sexual desire toward a *particular* object. When broader inhibitions or distortions in the patient's love life or sexual life are understood as a result of oedipal conflicts, it is not because sexuality per se is assumed to be threatening, but because, through this lens, there is assumed to be an unconscious confusion between the contemporary object of sexual desire and the earlier forbidden object. Similarly, "orally" biting comments or dependent behavior, "tight-assed" behavior or "anally" explosive vituperation, and so forth also tend to be understood by most analysts who use these concepts as reflecting a structure of relatedness, a particular way of experiencing and interacting with the significant others in one's life rather than an abstract exercise of a bodily function divorced from a relational context. This is especially true of those Freudian analysts who have absorbed the ego psychological formulations of writers such as Erikson (e.g., 1963), but it is evident in the daily clinical work of almost all analysts.

There are certainly real and important differences between traditional Freudian and relational points of view; indeed, much of this book is devoted to articulating and clarifying those differences. But they do not constitute the sharp dichotomy of competing "visions" except in the most abstract realms of what might be called theoretical fundamentalism. I believe that good theory is essential to good clinical practice, but I have also been struck by how often theory either remains in a realm of its own or influences practice in highly idiosyncratic ways that can make it impossible to predict from the formal premises of the theory what any given therapist will make of them as guidelines for practice. Often, what might be called *abstract* theory (the modern residue, even in relational theories, of what used to be called metapsychology) takes center stage, but is largely divorced from the theory of therapy or of change that guides the clinician's daily work.

There are indeed large and consequential differences in the ways that different therapists work, and there are almost certainly ways in which some of these differences correlate rather significantly with the self-identification as, say, Freudian or relational in orientation. But, as I will elaborate further below, the most significant foundation of differences in practice lies less in the question of whether drives or relationships are the fundamental building blocks of personality than it does in how the structuring of personality is viewed over time—whether the past is seen as preserved via "internalization," fixation, or developmental arrest or via the *continuing* influence of bidirectional transactions throughout the life cycle (cf. Zeanah, Anders, Seifer, & Stern, 1989).

When we persist over many years in perceptions and life patterns that are rigid and problematic (a phenomenon that is, of course, not a rare one to the practicing psychotherapist), it not because our inner world is hermetically sealed off from the impact of life experience, but because it is a key consequence of those very patterns, and of the psychological structures associated with them, that they tend to yield the kinds of life experiences that are likely to confirm and maintain them. The patterns and structures persist, that is, not in spite of the new realities that are encountered but precisely *because of* those realities, which are skewed in such a way that they ironically tend to bring about the very outcome the person is trying so hard to avoid (Wachtel, 1987a, 1993, 1997). Without understanding how other people are unconsciously recruited as "accomplices" (Wachtel, 1991) in the perpetuation of our life patterns and even of our "internal" structures, without understanding how the inner world is repeatedly *co*-constructed conjointly with others, our ability to understand how we may help people to *change* those patterns and psychological structures is severely limited.

BIOLOGY DOES NOT EQUAL DRIVE THEORY

Human beings are physical beings, biological organisms. No viable theory can ignore this reality, and even to minimize it is to reduce one's thinking to vapid evasions. Our genes, our hormones, the neurotransmitters that flow across our synaptic gaps—these are utterly crucial contributors to our psychological state, and any useful relational theory cannot push them aside or ignore them. The question is not relationships versus biology but what the relation *between* the two is and what the nature is of the biology that is posited.

This does not imply or require any particular position on questions of monism, dualism, psychophysical parallelism, or any of the other ways that philosophers have attempted to come to grips with what has traditionally been called the mind–body problem. Relationalists, I believe, can reasonably place their theorizing under any of these philosophical banners. However it may be conceived on the most abstract level, we are *embodied* minds and we are as well, one might say, minded bodies; that is, bodies or organisms that think, not *mere* bodies. There can be little doubt that certain kinds of perceptual experiences or thought processes cannot occur if certain parts of the brain are not intact; that imbibing alcohol or taking a serotonin uptake inhibitor will have some consequence for subsequent thoughts and feelings; that being hit or cut will, most of the time, be followed by the subjective sensation of pain. No viable relational theory can ignore biology, and indeed, because relational theory is sometimes mistakenly thought to do so, relationalists have taken pains to discuss explicitly and in detail the role of the body in relational theory (see, e.g., Fast, 1992; Aron & Anderson, 1998).

Where relational thinkers differ from drive theorists is not in the role of biology per se—which any reasonable person recognizes is enormous—but how that role is conceptualized. Freud's drive theory, it is important to understand, represents only one of many possible ways of conceiving of the biological substrate of behavior. Claims, appearing with increasing regularity in the psychoanalytic literature, that modern neuroscience research confirms the basic postulates of Freud's drive theory reflect strenuous conceptual pirouetting and highly selective citation and interpretation of findings. What contemporary research reveals is not a few simple "drives" that fit a poetic or dramaturgic aesthetic (sexual and aggressive, life and death, or ego and self-preservative) but a biological substrate of daunting complexity, with an almost unimaginably elaborate network of feedback loops, a dazzling choreography of proteins and nucleic acids, neurotransmitters and membrane receptors, hormone flows and electrical impulses.

The resemblance of this intricate set of multiply intersecting processes to the two titanic prime movers of Freud's dual instinct theory[3] is minimal at best. Yes, we are biologically programmed to want sex, and we *may* be biologically programmed to be aggressive (we certainly are biologically *ready* to be aggressive, and we most likely have some kind of "built-in" inclination to seek a certain position in the dominance hierarchy that social species tend to establish). It is certainly an important advance in knowledge to learn that sexual and aggressive inclinations can be aroused not only by ordinary life experiences but by stimulating different parts of the brain or that these desires can be facilitated or inhibited by the release of certain neurotransmitters. But such findings, while by no means inconsistent with Freud, are also consistent with virtually *every* modern thinker's views on human nature and human psychological functioning. The understanding that has emerged from modern neurobiological and neuropsychological research is not an understanding that can be rea-

---

[3] The particular names or conceptualizations of the two primary instincts or drives varied at different stages of Freud's theorizing, but the tendency to depict the psyche in terms of the contending demands of two conflicting drives remained a constant.

sonably equated to that in Freud's dual instinct theory. Indeed, the dual instinct theory per se probably is the one element in the drive–relational debate and dichotomy that comes closest to Greenberg and Mitchell's depiction of psychoanalytic ideas as expressing a philosophical "vision," a formulation at once so sweeping and so abstract that it is indeed beyond empirical inquiry and capable of "accounting for all phenomena."

Closer to substantive empirical claims was the part of the libido theory that posited a series of psychosexual stages (oral, anal, phallic, latency, genital) that the individual goes through beginning in infancy, and the corollary statements about the role of other "component instincts" such as sadism, masochism, exhibitionism, and voyeurism in the course of development and the eventual construction of adult sexual desire. Here Freud is basing his theories on observation rather than armchair philosophizing. He is pointing to aspects of the child's behavior that can be *observed,* and the power of his contribution derives from enabling us to see phenomena that social convention had conveniently ignored.

But even in this more substantive and differentiated form, the drive theory is by no means the definitive statement of how our biology contributes to our psychological lives. The seeming accuracy of Freud's hypotheses in the eyes of contemporary Freudian observers owes much to creatively Procrustean thinking in which a huge range of behaviors are ingeniously fitted to their contours. Too many objects of a certain shape lend themselves to being seen as "phallic" (precisely *why* Freud's witticism that "sometimes a cigar is just a cigar" is so widely quoted); too easily is any reference to bodily damage of any kind assumed to represent "castration anxiety"; too often do analysts (professional or amateur) assume that they know what drinking or smoking "really" are about; and so on.[4] For holders of the drive theory, its gravitational pull is such that virtually *all* data of human living are pulled into its orbit.

To some degree, of course, this is what Greenberg and Mitchell are pointing to in contending that the drive theory (along with, in their view, the overarching relational paradigm) can explain "all phenomena." But much of the problem (when it comes to the stage theory rather than the dual drive theory) resides not in the absence of substantive (and potentially adjudicable) empirical claims, but in formulations

---

[4] Karen Horney's (1939) insufficiently cited or appreciated critique explores these tendencies brilliantly.

of those claims that are insufficiently precise to make evaluation meaningful. It has been one of the weak links in the relational movement that it has often been associated with attitudes toward evidence and toward scientific inquiry that serve to render conceptual territory inviolate to empirical evaluation. This has served to protect relational territory from encroachment by potentially hostile observations (as it were), but it has also blunted the cutting edge of the critique of the drive theory. It is *difficult* to evaluate the formulations of the drive theory, to be sure. But who could have anticipated that the seemingly even more abstruse formulations of relativity theory and quantum theory would one day be subjected to multiple and meaningful empirical tests? If they had been relegated to the realm of abstract "visions," immune to confirmation or disconfirmation, our understanding of the world would be seriously impoverished. As I will discuss in the next chapter, there are already a variety of observations that strongly bear on the competing claims of drive and relational theorists, and at least in certain respects these observations favor the latter.

In particular, the accumulating body of empirical knowledge points to problems in the acontextual way in which drive theory formulations tend to posit universal sequences, forms, and meanings. A comment by Mitchell (1988a) states particularly clearly and incisively the differences between the two approaches to taking biology into account:

> The distinction between the drive model and the relational model is *not* equivalent to the distinction between biology and culture, or between the body and the social environment. Both the drive model and the relational model contain considerations of biology *and* culture, the body *and* the social environment. What is different is the way they conceive of the interaction between these factors. In the drive model, "anatomy is destiny" . . . ; social factors are shaped by inherent, underlying drive pressures. In the relational model, biology and interpersonal processes constitute perpetual cycles of mutual influence. . . . The body houses mental processes, which develop in a social context, which in turn defines the subjective meanings of body parts and processes, which further shape mental life. . . . Human biology and human relatedness both generate and are the creation of each other. (pp. 4–5, italics in original)

In contrast to the "two alternative visions" position he took just a few years earlier (Greenberg & Mitchell, 1983), this statement suggests that the drive theory, as it had been traditionally formulated, *did not* "account for all phenomena." Observations of the reciprocal influences among the biological and psychological forces that shape our behavior and experience raise serious challenges—*empirical* challenges—to the standard drive theory conceptualization (and, it must be said, to some versions of relational thought as well). In highlighting the essentially *contextual* nature of human motivation, experience, and psychological organization, this statement by Mitchell accords particularly well with the vision that guides this book. And, as Mitchell makes clear, to emphasize context is *not* to ignore that there is something there to *be* influenced by context. Psychological structure or selfhood or personality do not melt away in the crucible of relational thinking but rather are understood in a more complete and differentiated way

BEYOND THE DRIVE–RELATIONSHIP DICHOTOMY: AN *EMBODIED* RELATIONALITY

What conclusions can we draw from the foregoing discussion? Clearly, attention to relationships is a hallmark of any approach that is meaningfully labeled as relational. But if highlighting the emphasis on relationship rather than drive as a core theme in diverse theoretical efforts helped to illuminate important similarities, it also served to cover perhaps equally important differences among the theorists who were attempting to supplant drive theory. The diversity of viewpoint and conceptual emphasis among relational theorists is, in one sense, a strength of the relational movement. Employed effectively, it offers the movement a kind of hybrid vigor. But if the differing implications of different versions of relational thought are not sufficiently examined, the "pax relatiana" that has been so successful in building an intellectual movement may also end up yielding a vapid consensus signifying little more than a shared interest in "relationships" in some way, shape, or form or a shared distaste for the excesses of drive theory.

Perhaps more generative a focus than the distinction between drive and relationship models is an issue that is being increasingly appreciated by thinkers and researchers in all of the disciplines that concern themselves with human behavior and experience, from psychology and psychoanalysis to anthropology and sociology to psycholinguistics, history, economics, or neuroscience—the limits of simple linear models to capture the extraordinary complexity of human thought and feeling. What distinguishes more fundamentally what might be called "old paradigm" or "new paradigm" thinking than the drive–relationship distinction is whether there is an understanding of the remarkably variegated feedback loops and reciprocal influences that characterize our lives. What makes at least the older versions of the so-called "drive" model quite *far* from capable of "accounting for all phenomena" with any degree of success or precision is their emphasis on direct, linear cause and effect explanations; their relative lack of attention to the *continuing* way that biology both influences and *is influenced by* our experiences with other people at every single moment; the ways that our images of the past are continually being reconstructed in the present even as they also greatly influence the nature of that present; the ways in which culture, race, class, ethnicity, and history shape the very way our genes express themselves in behavior, even as our genes and our early histories in our families contribute to the ways we participate in and define ourselves as members of the various groups to which we belong (Jencks, 1987; Francis, Szegda, Campbell, Martin, & Insel, 2003; Sapolsky, 2000; Moore, 1999; Ridley, 2003; Wachtel, 1999).

By and large, relational theorists have tended to be on the "new paradigm" side of this set of distinctions, but the correspondence is by no means one to one, and there are versions of relational theorizing in which these issues are far from fully explored or realized. In going beyond the "drive versus relationship" definition of the new emerging paradigm in psychological thought, it is necessary to turn to a different way of distinguishing between new and old, a different way of conceptualizing what it means, one might say, to be fully and wholeheartedly relational. It is to this further way of honing in on the deeper implications of relationality that I now turn.

6

The Limits of the Archaeological Vision

RELATIONAL THEORY AND THE CYCLICAL–CONTEXTUAL MODEL

In a 1931 letter to the writer Stefan Zweig, Freud wrote, "I have sacrificed a great deal for my collection of Greek, Roman and Egyptian antiquities, [and] have actually read more archaeology than psychology" (E. Freud, 1960). Archaeology was a powerful and abiding interest of Freud's—an interest difficult to miss by anyone who has seen pictures of his office, filled as it was with those treasured objects from the ancient world. But archaeology was more than a hobby for Freud; it was a central metaphor in his theorizing, a source of images that not only expressed but shaped his theoretical vision. In attempting to articulate how the relational perspective I describe in this book differs from the approach to theory and practice that characterizes the more conservative or traditional versions of psychoanalytic thought (as well as in clarifying how the views described here differ in certain important respects from some versions of relational thinking as well), the distinction between the archaeological model on which much of psychoanalytic theory and practice was originally founded and what I call the *cyclical–contextual* model is crucial. Indeed, for the purpose of illuminating the essential features of the relational approach I explicate in this book, this distinction is even more pivotal than that between one-person and two-person theories or between drive conflict and relational conflict theories.[1]

What I mean by the archaeological mode of thought is the view that personality is organized in terms of more and more deeply buried layers that, by virtue of their being deeply buried, have been cut off from the influence of new experiences. In accord with this view of personality, psychotherapy is viewed very largely as a process of uncovering, recovering, or reconstructing the past and of digging through successive layers to get at the "archaic" material that lies below. Personality is seen as most fundamentally organized, most deeply influenced by the most archaic depths of the "inner" world, while the "surface" manifestations, the ways in which we seem to be responding to what is actually going on "outside," are relegated to the realm of the superficial (see Wachtel, 2003a).

One indicator of how pervasive this model is in psychoanalytic theorizing is that, for many readers, what I am describing—the structuring of personality in the form of hierarchically organized layers or "developmental levels," with "earlier" modes of psychological organization more deeply buried and fundamental—may not seem to be a *particular kind* of psychoanalytic theorizing (that is, an archaeological kind), but simply what a psychoanalytic point of view *is*. If psychoanalysis is not the study of the "depths" of personality, of the "inner world," of the infantile core that has not grown up and that remains attached to the figures and the circumstances of childhood, they may ask, then what is it?

The cyclical–contextual paradigm that I will discuss in this chapter addresses that question by presenting an alternative form of psychoanalytic theorizing, one that is *not* rooted in the archaeological model but that, nonetheless, addresses all the observations and clinical phenomena that have been of concern to proponents of that model. It is a theoretical point of view that is informed by developments in relational thought over the last two decades and at the same time is rooted in a still broader integrative effort that aims to incorporate a substantial range of phenomena that have tended to be largely ignored or minimized by psychoanalytic theorists (Wachtel, 1997). On the one hand, it

---

[1] This is not to suggest that the distinction between one- and two-person psychologies or between drive and relationship-focused theorizing is unimportant. I would not have devoted several chapters to these distinctions if I did not view them as of major significance in understanding the current landscape of clinical theory and practice. But, as I noted, they both are also in certain respects flawed distinctions, distinctions that can lead to unnecessary confusion.

Relational [handwritten annotation in left margin]

is concerned with the pervasive evidence for unconscious wishes, fantasies, and images of self and other that silently guide our behavior and color our experiences; with the many ways in which these unconscious mental structures and processes can at least *seem* to be infantile, archaic, or primitive; and with the many ways in which our experience of new circumstances and new figures in our lives seems to reflect the influence (and often, seemingly, the distorting influence) of our *earlier* experiences, including the phenomenon of transference which is so central to psychoanalytic thought. But on the other hand, it aims as well to address a whole *other* set of crucial observations that have been given short shrift by psychoanalytic theorists, especially those who operate from within the archaeological model.

Among these additional observations are particularly those bearing on the enormous variability of behavior and experience from one context to another. This variability and responsiveness to context includes not just the impact of the immediate interpersonal environment, but also the critical role of culture, class, race, ethnicity, and other broad social, economic, and historical influences which are as much a part of the essential context of our behavior and experience as is the more immediate and intimate relational matrix that has been the prime focus of relational theorists (see, e.g., Wachtel, 1983, 1999).

It is again important to be clear that in emphasizing the crucial role of the specific context in determining the individual's behavior and experience one is in no way positing an "environmental determinism." Rather, one is simply averting an equally simplistic characterological or developmental determinism, in which the answer to how the person will respond already lies "inside." There *is* a structure to personality, a unique individuality that leads each person to respond in his particular fashion to even to the most compelling and seemingly unambiguous of situations; the variance does not simply lie in the situation (Bowers, 1973; Wachtel, 1973, 1977; see also Frankl, 1959, for a more dramatic example). But, as noted in a previous chapter, that structure is a *contextual* structure. As Stolorow and Atwood (1992) have put it:

> A person enters any situation with an established set of ordering principles (the subject's contribution to the intersubjective system), but it is the context that determines which among the array of these principles will be called on to organize the experience. . . . The organization of experience can therefore be seen as codetermined both by preexisting principles and by an ongoing context that favors one or another of them over the others. (p. 24)

CRITIQUES OF THE ARCHAEOLOGICAL MODEL

Stolorow and Atwood's contextual approach to psychological structure is part of a larger intersubjective critique of the assumptions of the
archaeological model. Thus, in discussing problems and contradictions
with the concept of neutrality (cf. Wachtel, 1987c), Stolorow and
Atwood (1997) note that "the commonly held idea that interpretation
simply lifts into awareness what lies hidden within the patient is a rem-
nant of Freud's topographic theory and archaeological model for the
analytic process. . . . This model fails to take into account the contribution of the analyst's psychological organization in the framing of interpretations" (p. 436). Elsewhere (Stolorow et al., 2001b) in discussing
the fundamental assumptions of their intersubjective approach, they
state quite explicitly that "psychoanalysis, in this view, is no longer an
archaeological excavation of ever deeper layers of an isolated and
substantialized unconscious mind" (p. 47).

Other prominent psychoanalytic writers have also offered critiques of the archaeological model in recent years. Spence (1982), for
example, makes reexamination of the archaeological model a central
element in his influential book, *Narrative Truth and Historical Truth*.
Mitchell (1992a), further extending the critique, states, "The analytic
method is not archaeological, analyzing and reconstructing; it does
not simply expose what is there. The analytic method is constructive
and synthetic; it organizes whatever is there into patterns supplied by
the method itself" (p. 279). And even from a more classical or
Freudian view, Blum (1999) expresses similar concerns about the
nature of the material that comes forth in the analytic process: "The
beautiful archaeological model was oversimplified, and did not do
justice to the complexity of memory modification and validation, or
to the need to establish or restore meaningful connections and context" (p. 1131).

A key thrust of many of these critiques is epistemological, highlighting how the archaeological metaphor misleads us about what we
can actually know or discover. But the problems with the archaeological metaphor and the psychoanalytic model constructed on its basis go
beyond the epistemological. Apart from contributing to a misleading
sense of certainty about the historical accuracy of the constructed past,
it also is the foundation for serious misunderstandings about the
way that the past influences the present. The archaeological model, in
all its various manifestations—whether they be Freudian, Kleinian,
Winnicottian, Fairbairnian, Kohutian, or what have you—posits an

"inner world" that is, in significant and fateful ways, hermetically sealed off from everyday experience.

This is not to say that, from the vantage point of these theories, the inner world does not *influence* everyday experience. It is a central tenet of these theories that the impact of the inner world on our daily lives is enormous. Rather, the inner world is hermetically sealed off in the sense that it is not *changed by* our daily experiences as are the more conscious or "surface" manifestations of our personalities. It remains attached to the circumstances and fantasies of infancy, even as, outside of awareness, it drives the psyche of the adult.[2]

Within this model, in order to understand the person as he or she is now, one must dig through the successive strata that lie closer to the surface in order to get to the hidden core. In the theorizing of Freud and of later analysts in the classical tradition, that core consists of desires and fantasies that have been generated through a series of sequentially programmed phases by the vicissitudes of the drives. Some of these early desires and fantasies evolve over time in response to maturation and new experiences, but other parts of our early mental life are isolated from the reality-oriented ego and remain preserved in their original form. They do not "grow up" but rather, as Freud (1915b) described it, they "proliferate in the dark" (p. 149). They may send out derivatives that make some contact with the ego and find partial expression in more modulated and acceptable ways. But the core lies there unchanged, as sealed off from the daylight of new experience as the shards of pottery buried under layers of debris in archaeological sites. Therapy conducted from this point of view consists, to a significant degree, of digging down until the earlier layers are reached.[3]

Object relations models, of course, differ in important ways from this "drive"-focused conception. But in many ways, object relations models also frequently manifest the same fundamentally archaeological structure. It may be *internalized objects* that are buried rather than drive

---

[2] The model does posit, of course, that these "inner" experiences and structures can be modified by one particular set of circumstances—those deriving from the special experience of being in analysis. But the impact of the ordinary experiences of daily living is taken into account in far more limited fashion.

[3] In certain respects, this model might more aptly be described as geological than archaeological. That is, what is found is *not* actually like inert shards of pottery, but more like the intensely hot magma that lies beneath the surface layers of the earth, always ready to erupt. But in part reflecting Freud's especially keen interest in archaeology and in part because it has simply been the metaphor used in psychoanalytic discourse over the years, the term "archaeological" is almost always used when examining this way of looking at the psyche.

representations, and these affect-laden images may derive more from actual relational experiences than do the more endogenously generated fantasies posited in the drive model; but the *structure* of the theory (as opposed to the content) is often quite similar—successive layers that are more and more deeply buried and that, *by virtue* of being buried, persist in essentially unaltered form despite later experiences that might otherwise be expected to modulate and modify them. As with the drives of classical theory, the "primitive" or "archaic" representations of internalized objects that are depicted by object relations theorists do not grow up, do not mature and evolve as new experiences accrue in the course of living.

There are, of course, many versions both of Freudian and of object relations theorizing, and sorting out precisely where a particular model manifests the assumptions of the archaeological model and where it is organized around a different conceptual structure is not always easy. Psychoanalytic thinking has evolved, and today there are few "pure" forms of the archaeological model. More often, what appears are unexamined hybrids, in which the influence of the archaeological model remains strong, but the parameters of that influence are less easy to identify than once was the case. Considerable ambiguity is maintained by the deployment of a variety of forms of linguistic fudging that are very common in the psychoanalytic literature. These include depicting a particular pattern or problem as *having its origins* in a certain developmental period, *having its roots* or *precursors* in that period, *deriving from* that period, and so forth. Phrases such as these are so common in the literature that most readers scarcely notice their ambiguity. But there is a vast difference between the unobjectionable (but largely banal) point that everything has a beginning or origin, that something starts the ball rolling, that earlier events lead to later events, and the potentially more problematic assumption that seems often to be implied—that the "roots" are still there, that the trees and branches that are more evident to the eye are still being fed and maintained by those roots, and—to move away from the botanical and metaphorical and toward the implied literal meaning—that what the person is "really" pursuing is not what it seems to be but in fact the more infantile and "archaic" aim that, in archaeological fashion, lies beneath.[4]

---

[4] I shall have more to say later about the issue of the person not "really" pursuing what he thinks he is pursuing. At first blush, this may seem to be merely a statement of the idea that some of our aims are unconscious, or indeed, a logically necessary corollary of that idea. As I will elaborate, however, there are other ways to conceptualize unconscious processes that are sounder both theoretically and clinically.

The ambiguities are further illustrated in a passage from Mc-Williams's (1994) influential textbook on psychoanalytic diagnosis, along with a particularly clear statement of the premises of the archaeological model. In spelling out some of the key assumptions that tend to be shared by classical and relational thinkers alike, she states the following:

> Although most analytic diagnosticians now conceive the relevant stages through which young children pass in less drive-defined ways than Freud did, psychoanalysis has never seriously questioned three of his main convictions: (1) current psychological preoccupations reflect infantile precursors; (2) interactions in our earliest years set up the template for how we later assimilate experience, making that experience comprehensible unconsciously according to categories that were salient in childhood; (3) identifying a person's developmental level is a critical part of understanding him or her. (pp. 40–41)

The ambiguity is embodied in terms such as "precursors" and "template" (as well as in the meaning of "reflect" in her first proposition). But in the third proposition, we seem to be moving into a mode of thought that more pointedly affirms the archaeological model. The person's way of being does not just have *origins* or precursors in an earlier period; the person, in significant ways, *remains* in that period, stuck at a particular "developmental level."

McWilliams's characterization of the standard assumptions of psychoanalytic thought parallels May's (1990) depiction of psychoanalysis as "wedded to a notion of developmental stages and more particularly to the idea that disruptions at particular phases of infancy or childhood have effects on particular systems of motives or character traits" (p. 165). May, however, adds the noteworthy additional sentence, "It is remarkable how little evidence we have for this idea in spite of voluminous and energetic research over the last half century." Able reviews of the empirical findings in this regard by Westen (e.g., 1989, 1990) and by Zeanah et al. (1989) among others, have further documented the substantial empirical challenges to this widely held way of thinking.

In reflecting on the limitations of the archaeological model and on the substantive alternatives for conceiving of the development and dynamics of personality, Mitchell (1993b) has stated that "rather than regarding the past as the underlying, archaeological substratum of psychic reality, I regard the past as the relational context in which characterological patterns of integration were established and shaped. In this view, the past does not underlie the present but, rather, provides clues for understanding the way in which meanings in the present are generated" (p. 464). Elsewhere, he similarly argues that "disturbances in early relationships with caretakers ... seriously distort subsequent relatedness, not by freezing infantile needs in place, but by setting in motion a complex process through which the child builds an interpersonal world (a world of object relations) from what is available" (Mitchell, 1988a, p. 289).

Mitchell's comments take the critique of the archaeological model an important step further. The image evoked by Mitchell's account is not one of successively more deeply buried layers, with the original still down at the bottom causing mischief. Rather, it is one of a process that, as he puts it, is "set in motion" by early experiences; that is, a picture not of fixed layers but of constant evolution and change. To be sure, as I will elaborate further in this chapter, the *direction* of that evolution is powerfully influenced by early experiences and the *degree* of change is constrained by the very processes they set in motion. Early experience indeed has a powerful impact; but the nature of that impact, the process by which it is perpetuated, needs to be rethought.

THE CYCLICAL PSYCHODYNAMIC MODEL

The conceptual thrust embodied in Mitchell's position—early experiences affecting later experiences not by "freezing infantile needs in place," but by setting into motion a complex, ongoing process in which the consequences emerge from the kind of interpersonal world the child builds as a result—parallels very closely the model I have previously called *cyclical psychodynamics* (e.g., Wachtel, 1977a, 1977b, 1987a, 1993; Wachtel & Wachtel, 1986). That label is still an appropriate one, and I will continue to refer to cyclical psychodynamics in the discussion that follows. But I will also refer to the model in this discussion as a *cyclical–contextual* model. The original name (cyclical psychodynamics) was introduced because the model was grounded in a psychoanalytic point of view, but it organized the observations associated with such a point of view in a different manner—a manner that highlighted the central role of cyclical feedback processes in the dynamics of personality. The term "cyclical–contextual" similarly identifies the model as one that emphasizes cyclical processes, but it highlights as well the *contextual* emphasis which I believe to be one of the most distinctive and valuable contributions of the relational point of view.

The cyclical psychodynamic model was designed from the outset to take into account not only the findings and ideas of psychoanalysis but, additionally, those of therapists and researchers from outside the psychoanalytic world (Wachtel, 1997). What psychoanalysis highlighted was the ways in which we persist in thoughts, fantasies, and behaviors that seem "out of touch" with present reality and governed by the past rather than the present. In contrast, what was highlighted (in equally persuasive fashion) by influential theorists and researchers from outside the psychoanalytic tradition was that our behavior and experience are responsive to the immediate context and to changes, even subtle changes, in what is transpiring (see, e.g., Mischel, 1968, 1973; Wachtel, 1973, 1993, 1997; Wachtel & Wachtel, 1986).

Cyclical psychodynamic theory was an attempt to reconcile these two lines of thought and the phenomena associated with each. It entailed a depiction of the ways in which, on the one hand, our behavior and experience—and even the *unconscious* dimensions of our psychic life—were profoundly influenced by the events and emotional nuances of what was actually transpiring around us and, on the other hand, our response to that context was determined not by any "objective" property of what was going on but by our particular *experience* or *interpretation* of what was going on, by our unique, idiosyncratic, subjective take on those events. It is not a matter of one or the other—being governed by our inner world of deeply private and largely unconscious psychological meanings and inclinations or by the events and stimuli of everyday life. It is that *each creates and evokes the other.* Consistency is maintained both by our *perceptual* inclination to *see* the old in the new and by our *behavioral* inclination to *evoke* the old in the new.

Consider a simple example that I introduced in one of the earliest presentations of the cyclical psychodynamic point of view (Wachtel, 1977a):

> The two-year-old who has developed an engaging and playful manner is far more likely to evoke friendly interest and attention on the part of adults than is the child who is rather quiet and withdrawn. The latter will typically encounter a less rich interpersonal environment, which will further decrease the likelihood that he will drasti-

cally change. Similarly, the former is likely to continually learn that other people are fun and are eager to interact with him; and his pattern, too, is likely to become more firmly fixed as he grows. Further, not only will the two children tend to evoke different behavior from others, they will also interpret differently the same reaction from another person. Thus, the playful child may experience a silent or grumpy response from another as a kind of game and may continue to interact until perhaps he does elicit an appreciative response. The quieter child, not used to much interaction, will readily accept the initial response as a signal to back off.

If we look at the two children as adults, we may perhaps find the difference between them still evident: one outgoing, cheerful, and expecting the best of people; the other rather shy, and unsure that anyone is interested. A childhood pattern has persisted into adulthood. Yet we really don't understand the developmental process unless we see how, successively, teachers, playmates, girlfriends, and colleagues have been drawn in as "accomplices" in maintaining the persistent pattern. And, I would suggest, we don't understand the possibilities for change unless we realize that even now there are such "accomplices," and that if they stopped playing their role in the process, it would be likely eventually to alter. (p. 52)

As I noted in originally discussing this example, however, it is very difficult for the accomplices to break out of their roles. The repetitive behavior that has maintained the patient's dominant patterns over the years constitutes a powerful force field and exerts a strong pull on others. In a host of ways, many of them not easy to identify or notice, each of us repeatedly induces others to behave in ways that are very likely to *maintain* the pattern between us.[5] If the therapist understands this, then she will seek to illuminate, for herself and for the patient, the often subtle ways in which the patient induces others to act toward him in a manner that perpetuates the assumptions about the world he already holds, and she will examine in detail the repetitive *sequences* that characterize his interactions with other people. Because so much of this mutual eliciting of pattern-maintaining responses goes on outside of awareness, or is only dimly in awareness, bringing this interactive pattern more focally into awareness is as crucial a part of the therapist's task as is the more traditional task of elucidating unconscious wishes and fan-

---

[5] In Chapter 7 I discuss how this conception differs from those of projective identification and the repetition compulsion.

tasies. That is, it is not only our wishes or fantasies that must be made more conscious, but our *behavior*, the repetitive actions and interactions with others that constitute our lives and that, from another perspective, define our personalities.

Put differently, and highlighting the contrast with the archaeological model, the early pattern (not just of behavior but of affect, fantasy, self-experience, and experience of others) does not persist because it is somehow buried and sealed off from the influence of daily life but because the pattern itself creates, over and over, a *particular kind* of daily life, one that maintains that very pattern. In this sense, far from ignoring the reality of what is actually going on around us, neurotic patterns are, in important respects, *acutely responsive* to what is going on. To be sure, they depend as well on the element of active construction and interpretation that is characteristic of all of our encounters with the environment and is especially evident in the ambiguity-soaked realm of affective experience and interpersonal transactions. Every stimulus, every situation, every context, every interpersonal event is filtered through our subjectivity, given meaning through the perceptual and interpretive structures that have evolved in the course of our lives. To a significant degree, we see what we *expect* to see and, often, what we want or need to see. That is the side of the maintenance of old patterns that psychoanalytic accounts have always stressed. But, short of psychosis (and even in certain respects in psychotic states as well) the capacity for distortion has its limits. We always are *also* responding (if always "in our fashion") to what is actually going on;[6] and without understanding this dimension, without understanding how the seemingly internal structures of our psychological lives are maintained through our transactions with the "accomplices" in our relational patterns, both our theoretical understanding and our capacity to be helpful to our patients are severely diminished.

---

[6] I will not consider here the philosophical conundrums that are introduced by a term like "what is actually going on." Much fruitful and illuminating philosophical analysis has been directed to this question, as has a good deal of stance-taking sophistry. Suffice to say that in daily living (if not necessarily in the pages of philosophical journals) failure to assume that there *is* a real world out there is a sign of serious mental illness. At the same time, especially in the realm of relational and affective experiences, to assume that "what I perceive" is necessarily equivalent to what "is" is itself a formula for considerable interpersonal mischief, as well as a formula for disastrous incompetence as a psychotherapist.

THE CYCLICAL MODEL AND CONTINUITIES
IN ATTACHMENT STATUS

Much the same kind of process of mutual perpetuation and interpenetration of internal and external influences needs to be considered in understanding a wide range of other continuities in behavior and experience from early childhood. Consider, for example, the phenomenon of attachment. It has been one of the remarkable discoveries of developmental research in the last few decades that indicators of attachment status assessed very early in childhood can be seen to predict attachment status in later childhood and, to some degree, even in adulthood (Grossman, Grossman, & Waters, 2005; Sroufe, Egeland, Carlson, & Collins, 2005; Cassidy & Shaver, 1999). Here again, we seem to come upon a persistence of early modes of psychological organization and of the impact of very early experiences. But although Bowlby's (1973) concept of an "internal working model" valuably advances our understanding of the way that new experiences are inevitably perceived and filtered through psychological structures deriving from earlier experiences, an overly "internal" account of how this set of expectations about human relationships persists over time can be rather misleading.[7]

To begin with, and very germane to a contextual understanding, it is not only the child's attachment status or internal working model that remains the same; the child's *context* is likely to remain the same as well. Although there are obvious (and usually traumatic) exceptions, children generally continue to have the same mother and the same family throughout childhood. Thus, whatever characteristics of the mother and ways of interacting with the child had originally brought about the child's attachment status are also usually *continuing* in the child's life. It is thus impossible to attribute the continuity in the child's attachment status to a kind of "setting of the cement" in the personality, because an equally plausible explanation is the continuity in the child's key relationships. As Westen (2002) has put it:

> The attachment literature has given us good reason to believe that certain forms of dyadic interaction can indeed lead to insecure or

---

[7] For an analysis of our ties to early objects that parallels the examination of the persistence of attachment patterns presented here, see Wachtel (1997, pp. 56–60).

disorganized patterns of attachment and problematic ways of experiencing self-in-relation-to-others by at least 12 months of age (Fonagy, Steele, and Steele, 1991; Lyons-Ruth, Bronfman, and Parsons, 1999; Main, 1996). But the same parents who are misattuned with their infants are often misattuned with their toddlers or their teenagers, and we have precious little data that bear on the question of when the primary damage is done and when it can be undone. (p. 878)

Westen notes that the failure to sufficiently take into account the continuities in the child's context over time skews psychoanalytic thinking about other aspects of development as well. Reviewing the assumptions prevalent in psychoanalytic discourse and how they compare to the findings of careful research, he raises questions about the widespread tendency to assume that particular difficulties in adulthood are attributable to difficulties encountered at a particular stage of development. He notes, like May (1990), that there is precious little evidence for this idea. A more relevant consideration, he suggests, in understanding the relation between problems that may have been encountered at an early developmental stage and those occurring later is that the same problematic parenting that marked the preoedipal years is likely, in slightly different form, to mark the oedipal, latency, or adolescent years.

A second source of continuity also is rooted in the continuity of the developing person's context over time, but highlights the *dynamic* relation between individual and context. As Robert Merton (1948) pointed out many years ago in a classic formulation, our expectations can often become "self-fulfilling prophecies." The secure child, whose internal working model leads him to anticipate a sensitive and attentive response to his needs, is likely to behave differently toward his attachment figure than the child who has learned to fear an unpredictable or inadequate response or who has learned that it is safest to turn away and seek to minimize his attachment needs. As a consequence, the behavior of the attachment figure is likely to *continue* to be different toward the secure child than toward the child whose attachment experiences have been compromised. In response to the child who is comfortable needing the parent and gratifyingly reassured by her ministrations, further sensitive response on the parent's part is much easier than in response to a child who fights showing or experiencing those needs (the "avoidant" or "dismissing" child) or who interacts in a fitful and potentially off-putting manner (the "resistant/ambivalent" or "preoccupied" child). In this fashion, whatever potential there is for sensitive, responsive parenting in the mother is enhanced in interacting with the secure child and diminished in interacting with the insecure. In the emotional realm too, it seems, the rich get richer and the poor get poorer.

Of course, the mother is not just *responding*, not just encountering a child whose behavior has nothing to do with her or with her own inclinations. The attachment style she encounters is one that she has very largely *created* through her own prior behavior.[8] Thus her continuing with that behavior is not just a function of the child's behavior but of inclinations that characterized her even before the child was born and that were responsible for initiating this pattern of interaction in the first place. But the point is that even if, in some patterns such as this, we actually *can* decide which is the chicken and which is the egg, before very long the results become scrambled. Whatever potential there was for change (positive or negative) is diminished over time by the continuing pattern between them, which becomes self-fulfilling from both directions. With attachment as with virtually all facets of personality, the past matters greatly. But the past matters not as something simply stored, not as the ultimate frame of reference for the present, but as *what starts us on a particular path*. What we encounter on that path then becomes our destiny.

TRAUMA, BRAIN, AND BEHAVIOR: FURTHER ILLUMINATING THE CYCLICAL MODEL

Even when early experiences seem to create a change in the very structure of the brain, as seems to be the case, for example, with the occurrence of severe trauma[9] (van der Kolk, McFarlane, & Weisaeth, 1996), the process of cyclical transactions I have been depicting remains essential to understand. For whatever changes in the brain (as well as in emotional and behavioral proclivities) may occur as a result of trauma,

---

[8] It may be that there is as well a genetic or temperamental component to the attachment status and attachment behaviors of both mother and child. But this should not lead us to overlook the role of the continuing interaction between them, which is also a crucial element in maintaining the continuities that are found repeatedly in the research.

[9] Of course, because we are embodied beings, we can also say that *every* experience results in physical changes in the brain in some respect.

the person then further reacts to those very changes, and the concatenating consequences of those reactions, including the ways other people experience and react to them, begin to take on a life of their own. People who have experienced traumas, for example, manifest a variety of behaviors that have further significant impact on their relations with others. They may show considerable wariness with other people, be inclined toward intense and unpredictable emotional outbursts, have difficulty establishing intimate relationships or reliable friendships, have difficulty performing at work or holding a steady job. They may have severe sexual inhibitions or be conflicted and ambivalent in sexual situations. These problematic patterns are consequences of the trauma, but they also over time become a source of *further* life experiences that are painful in their own right and that maintain the impact of the trauma over the years.

Thus, for example, if as a result of the trauma the person has developed a deep fear and mistrust of other people, then he is likely to recoil from the possibility of closeness or intimacy and perhaps to present a face to the world that is perceived as unfriendly, unapproachable, even hostile. As a consequence, he will be less likely to elicit or encounter the "softer" side of people, and the world will *continue* to feel like a harsh and dangerous place, perpetuating his stance of mistrust (and the same consequences) once again.

Similarly, if as a consequence of the trauma, the person is prone to unpredictable or inappropriate-seeming emotional outbursts, this too is likely to keep others away or keep them wary, and the consequence once again is of making the world feel less safe or welcoming, setting the stage for still more of the same. Other common sequelae of trauma, such as impairments of attention or concentration, distraction due to anxiety, or difficulty following through, can perpetuate the state of vulnerability and traumatization in a different way. They are likely to create difficulties both in school and on the job, and these school and job failures, especially in a society such as ours which is marked by considerable economic inequality and inequality of living conditions, can generate further stresses. They may, for example, lead to depression, proneness to aggressive behavior, or a variety of other reactions that then generate further consequences, including further disruptions of work capacity or career advancement which create a vicious circle of still more of the same.

Thus, the source of the problematic sequelae of trauma does not lie simply or directly in the stored memories of the trauma in the brain.

It lies as well in the *further* experiences that occur as a result, experiences which probably would not have occurred, or would not have occurred in quite the same way, had the person not undergone the original trauma, but which now are as much a part of the problem as the original trauma was. As I put it elsewhere in discussing this topic, "a way of life that may have originated in trauma can become itself a continuing source of traumatization that, in turn, further perpetuates that same problematic way of life" (Wachtel, 2002).

Even if some patients are indeed helped by recovering access to the early experience so that they can work it through, without understanding how the problem has evolved into a *way of life*, and without attending to the ongoing, and very real, consequences of that way of life in the present, the therapeutic effort is likely to be insufficient to the task. Here too, the causes of the patient's difficulties do not lie simply in the past. They lie in the way of life that ensues and in the cyclical patterns that, over and over, create and recreate the same situation.

CYCLICAL PSYCHODYNAMICS: A CASE ILLUSTRATION

In further elaborating on the cyclical psychodynamic model, it may be useful to present at this point some material related to a concrete clinical case. The patient's difficulties (I will call him Richard) could readily be understood in terms of his earlier experiences with a mother who was severely limited in her capacity to empathize with his experience or to value him for who he was rather than for what she needed him to be. In important respects, Richard did persist in a way of experiencing the world that was traceable to his early experiences with his mother and that represented a striking continuation of the early patterns in his life. But rather than understanding this persistence as a result of the wishes, fears, fantasies, and representations that dominated his earliest years being sealed off from influence by the ongoing events of his life, the cyclical–contextual understanding highlights how those very events are crucial in maintaining the pattern.

Richard was, in certain ways, a rather gregarious man, capable of being charming and outgoing. But it soon became apparent that these social skills were in large measure being used in a way that warded off more intimate relationships, and that on those occasions when the possibility of intimacy did begin to emerge, it was associated with quite considerable anxiety. Richard had many friends, many dates, and a hectic social calendar. But he was lonely, sometimes to the point of quite considerable depression. He rarely permitted himself to expose his deeper feelings to a woman, or even to a close male friend. He was, one might say, relentlessly superficial.

But it was not easy for him—or even for others—to be clear about this. For his superficiality, as it were, was *sophisticated* superficiality. He was a very bright, very well educated, very funny and interesting person. He could tell a good story and keep people engaged. At the same time, there was a sense that his friendships were not really very close, and that the people he regarded as his good friends did not regard him in similar fashion.

As noted earlier, there were many elements in Richard's childhood and in his upbringing that could help explain these tendencies. One could, that is, easily find the "roots" or "origins" of the pattern. *Both* his parents were preoccupied with appearances to a quite unusual degree. Multiple cosmetic surgeries, at all stages of the life cycle for all members of the family, were a part of the picture. So too were expensive clothes, continuing redecoration of the house, and conversations about other people that, to a striking degree, centered on whether they looked good or not. I have the image that Richard received more "air kisses" in his childhood than genuine embraces. And although much of what his parents had to say about him was positive, there was a very strong sense that he was valued for how he could enhance the image of the family, not out of any genuine appreciation of his own unique qualities or with any real understanding of his subjective experience.

In a certain sense, then, it is rather easy to "explain" Richard's present pattern in terms of his past. And indeed, without knowing about how his life patterns constituted an understandable adaptation to the experience of growing up in his particular family, our understanding of Richard would certainly be deficient. But understanding of Richard's difficulties is also deficient if it does not include the way in which he reproduces those dynamics over and over in the course of living, in large measure through the very way he tries to defend himself against their consequences. This pattern may have *started* (had its "origins," "precursors," "roots," "template") in his response to the emotional circumstances of his early relations with mother and father; but it continues not just because it became part of his "inner world," but because his entire *way of life* now is organized around it. The unconscious anxieties, conflicts, fantasies, and identifications that originated in his childhood can be seen as the cause of this way of life. But it is equally true that this way of life is what keeps those anxieties, conflicts, fantasies, and identifications alive. Because he is so adept at keeping people away from the more intimate (and hence more vulnerable) core of his affective life, day after day he has the *actual experience* (not always consciously registered, but registered powerfully nonetheless) that others are not interested in his deeper feelings, that they respond to his social skills and self-presentation but keep a certain distance. Even as, with little awareness, Richard worked hard to keep a moat around his deeper feelings, he also (again with little conscious awareness) *yearned* for deeper contact. Consequently, the distance that others maintained in response to cues from him could feel, at some level, like a confirmation of the unacceptability of the more private, vulnerable, and deeply personal side of him—an experience that, in turn, led him still again to retreat behind the very wall that kept him from deeply meaningful contact with others. In this fashion, over and over, his "inner" state produced predictable "outward" consequences, and those consequences served to sustain the "inner" state. Neither the inner state nor the outward events were more basic or fundamental. They were part and parcel of each other, inseparable and insufficiently understood without reference to the other.

In our sessions, in parallel fashion, what frequently ensued was that Richard would lead me away from the emotional core of what he was experiencing, until I actually did begin to lose interest and start to drift. That would then confirm for him that I, like everyone else, wasn't really interested in him, and even though the apparent disinterest actually resulted from his *not* revealing his deeper feelings, the implicit (if usually not conscious) conclusion that he would reach from this experience was that he had *better not* reveal those feelings. This would then set the stage for still another round of "you don't really care so I won't take the risk of revealing myself to you."

This could happen in a variety of ways. At times, for example, he would tell a story in great detail—sometimes even in *interesting* detail—but in a way that made it extremely difficult to see what it had to do with the work we were doing together or to keep track of the emotional thread. Other times he would use (really use up) much of the session in efforts to entertain me,[10] but his efforts to keep me inter-

---

[10] Interestingly, Richard did not particularly try to *impress* me. Although he was proud of his skills as a raconteur, and did want to impress me with *that*, the overall sense was much less of his trying to impress me than to please me and to make me "safe" to be with by keeping things light and pleasant. In the conceptual framework of Horney, (1945) the dynamic was much more one of "moving toward" than of "moving against," though there were obviously elements of the "moving away" dynamic as well.

ested in this way would have the opposite effect. I would grow bored and restless, even at times almost hopeless that anything "therapeutic" would ensue. The content of his conversation was of a sort that in another setting I might well have found quite engaging. But *because* our relationship was a therapeutic one, in which disclosure of his more private and vulnerable side was part of the expectation, the ways in which Richard's almost relentless "socializing" became an impediment to intimacy were particularly salient.

Other cyclical patterns related to Richard's conflicts over intimacy were evident as well. Richard was a successful information technology entrepreneur, and so he had enough money to initially attract women with the lavish amounts he spent on them. He would almost instantly, as soon as even the beginnings of a relationship looked in the offing, buy the woman very expensive clothing and jewelry or take her on extravagant vacations, with first-class flights and five-star hotels. The sense of "buying" these women's attention was quite palpable, but disappointment followed quite regularly. The healthier of the women began to feel used, felt *bought* in some way, sensed that they were being given money and clothes and jewelry *instead of* intimacy with Richard. Others were the kind of women—those, after all, more likely to be drawn to someone like Richard—whose own dynamics pulled more for wanting material displays than for wanting genuine intimacy. In the first case, the woman would eventually withdraw, often with a sense of disgust and disappointment. This would leave Richard feeling devastated, and confirm for him (again not always with clear awareness) that he had *better* "buy" women because he sure as hell couldn't really interest them in him. In the second kind of relationship, his view that women were not interested in him as a person, but only in what he could provide them, was confirmed in a different way, but equally persuasively.

It is particularly important to understand that unless the daily dynamic that characterizes his life in the present is taken into account, it becomes virtually impossible to liberate someone like Richard from the endless round of repetitions of the same pattern again and again. For the perpetuation of this pattern is *not* just a function of an "inner" fantasy or fear. His vision, though in many ways *continuous* with that of his childhood self, is not just an irrational holdover from years before. In an important way, it is a relatively *realistic* response to the particular life experiences that he encounters again and again. At the same time, the very fact that he does encounter those experiences over and over is a product of the "internalized" assumptions that he holds and the highly individual reaction patterns associated with them. Having learned to be mistrustful and despairing of the prospect of real intimacy, he lives in such a way that intimacy becomes impossible, and then has confirmed again and again that that mistrust is justified.

In the work with Richard, as in all work guided by the cyclical psychodynamic point of view, the "internal" dynamics are by no means disregarded. In the course of the work, the fantasies, memories, fears, and shameful desires that are the central focus of standard psychoanalytic work were addressed in good measure. But those internal dynamics were understood not just as residing in an "internal world" apart from the events and circumstances of his life but as *Richard's particular way of experiencing and responding to* those circumstances.

Put differently, rather than the events of daily life being treated as a mere *reflection* of "deeper" processes, as a *product* of those processes but not a cause, the cyclical–contextual perspective views the influence of early experiences and the psychological structures that evolved as a consequence through a different lens. The influence of those psychological structures is indeed powerful, but it is manifested through (and inseparable from) the *later* life experiences that they contribute to bringing about; and, in reciprocal fashion, those later life experiences are what maintain some version of those early-arising structures of thought, affect, and action over the person's lifetime. The person is seen to persist in old patterns not in spite of new experiences which would change them if they were only accessible to influence, but *precisely because of* the ongoing experiences those patterns repeatedly bring about. No one, in fact, lives in an "average expectable environment." Rather, if the clinician looks closely and sensitively enough, it becomes readily apparent that we each live in a relationally and emotionally *unique* context, a context that is generated by the often subtle distinctive characteristics of our particular way of interacting with others and that both reflects and maintains our ongoing psychic structures.

IRONY AND INTENTIONALITY

The ends we regularly bring about are not necessarily the ends we seek. A common feature of the life patterns that bring people to a psychotherapist is irony. Sometimes, to be sure, the repetitive nature of the pattern does reflect a direct intention, even if an unconscious one; the person may not be *aware* of what he is seeking, may not be *aware* of the hidden intentionality, but it is difficult to make sense of the patterns that may be observed clinically without assuming that precisely such an intention is operating beneath the surface. But viewed through the lens of cyclical psychodynamic theory, a different configuration often becomes evident, one in which unconscious thoughts, meanings, and intentions are no less a matter of concern, but in which irony rather than straightforward intention takes center stage.[11]

As is almost always the case, the ironic consequences in the case just discussed were intermixed with consequences that were indeed intended, even if not conscious. Although Richard craved intimacy he also feared it, and a good part of the pattern of his life seemed to reflect unconscious efforts to ensure that the danger that intimacy represented would be averted. In that sense, the absence of intimacy in his life, though genuinely painful, was also unconsciously sought by him in the pursuit of safety. At the same time, though, many of the ways that Richard attempted to prevent rejection and the accompanying feelings of inadequacy and undesirability ended up making rejection more likely. In that sense, ironic (and *un*intended) consequences were also central to his dynamics.

In many other cases, the role of irony is even more evident and more central. In these cases, the primary consequences of the problematic patterns in the patient's life are *not* really intended, even unconsciously. They are *ironic* consequences, the result of efforts to prevent the very thing that ends up happening. Consider, for example, the case of a patient I will call Edward. Edward was plagued by a painful feeling of insubstantiality, a sense of being "a straw in the wind." Here again, as in most cases, the factors that contributed to this troubling experience of himself included a complex web of conscious and unconscious representations and of repeated experiences that began fairly early in childhood. But in order to understand how this troublingly fragile sense of self was perpetuated over time. it is necessary to understand how Edward *responded* to this disturbing feeling and what the *consequences* for him were.

Whatever the origins of this experience of insubstantiality, much of what the experience reflected and symbolized—and what contrib-

---

[11] Irony figures especially prominently in the writings of Karen Horney (e.g., 1939, 1945, 1950). I have drawn on Horney's thinking in a wide range of my own formulations throughout my career and have explicitly drawn attention to the dimension of irony in her work in Wachtel (1979).

uted to perpetuating it—was Edward's inclination, over and over, to accommodate or accede to others, to fit in in a way that led him to lose touch with his own views and desires and his own vital center. Whether it be what restaurant to go to, what movie to see, what political opinion to express, or, more profoundly and significantly, what emotions to experience and express, Edward found himself under the sway of other people's wishes and feelings. This would usually begin as an almost automatic response, not initially noticed or experienced by Edward as ignoring his own inclination. But usually, before very long, Edward would begin to sense that something felt vaguely uncomfortable, not quite right. This experience was often associated with a feeling of "hollowness" that would emerge for him in a conversation in which he realized he had been feigning enthusiasm. Whether this was about the food, the movie, the direction of the conversation, what have you, there would be a discernable subjective experience of falseness and lack of vitality, the result of his taking on *others'* views, and so having little to support what he was saying from within his own vital experience.

Some of the origins of this kind of self-experience have been insightfully discussed by Winnicott (e.g., 1965) in his classic discussions of the "false self." But understanding the perpetuation of the experience for Edward requires attention to the ironic processes whereby the very efforts he makes to deal with this distressing experience end up recreating it over and over again. Once established, the sense of weakness and emptiness that plagued Edward made it difficult for him to feel safe or justified in asserting his own views. Not feeling whole or "real," not feeling an inner sense of integrity, he felt little sense that he even knew or could count on what his own views were. Thus, feeling lost and without grounding, he looked to others for direction as to what he should do or even feel. Moreover, as a consequence of feeling like a straw in the wind, maintaining his own boundaries was a task for which he did not feel he had the requisite strength. Thus, feeling unable to reach or to value or trust his own views or preferences, he would once more conform to the preferences and expectations of others, and, as a consequence, once more feel like a straw in the wind, once more feel he lacked an internal compass. Not very much of this process was articulated or conscious for Edward at the time he began therapy, and what was was limited to fragments that provided little if any illumination of the sequence of events and experiences or its repetitive nature. Nonetheless, Edward repeated the pattern in one form or another over and over. Feeling weak and uncertain of his own real desires and perceptions, he would look to others for direction; looking constantly to others, he would feel ungenuine and insubstantial, "like a straw in the wind"; feeling like an insubstantial straw in the wind, he felt compelled to look to others for direction. The circle turned again and again, with each turn justifying the next.

For whatever reason, in the case of Edward, the experience of suppressed anger never emerged as a central feature of this pattern in his life.[12] For Marina, on the other hand, this did seem to be the case. Manifestly, Marina's life pattern was a lot like Edward's. She too had difficulty asserting her own views and often accommodated to others. But for Marina, the driving experience that led to the repetition of this pattern was not a feeling of insubstantiality and hollowness as it was for Edward, but rather a fear of the *anger* that might be released if she dared to let her own natural inclinations be expressed. She was constantly holding herself in check, as if putting her finger in the dike to prevent everyone (her *and* her potential victim/rejecter) from being flooded and drowned. I say victim/rejecter because Marina had *two* fears, equal and opposite from one vantage point but cumulative and additive from another (that is, from hers). She feared, on the one hand, that she would destroy the other, that her rage would lead her to be overwhelmingly hurtful. On the other hand, she feared that her anger would drive people away, that she would be left alone and vulnerable.

When the latter aspect of her anxieties was in the forefront, she often feared her anger would be laughable and dismissible, that she would at most be perceived as an annoying gnat. This part of her fears was, of course, inconsistent with her fear that her anger was so powerful it would destroy those she loved. It was somewhat more accessible to consciousness than the fear of her anger's destructiveness, but the two states of mind were largely dissociated from each other, and thus the "logical" inconsistency between these two visions of her anger was unable to diminish the impact of either.

To keep these fears of her anger in check, Marina behaved in a manner that was rather strikingly "nice," conforming to others' wishes and going along to a degree that hurt her own interests quite considerably. This was not, however, the product of a conscious strategy.

---

[12] Obviously this brief vignette, which describes only one specific element in the complex dynamics that characterize any case, is not intended as a *comprehensive* account of the dynamics even of this one pattern in Edward's life. It does illustrate, however, some of how the dynamics of irony contribute to perpetuating patients' difficulties.

Marina was only dimly aware of this pattern at the time she entered therapy. It took a good deal of work to illuminate even the degree to which she did go out of her way to be "nice," much less the anger she thereby hoped to keep at bay.

Marina's life story is representative of a sizable subgroup of patients who seek help from psychotherapists. They present as strikingly meek, or cooperative, or helpful, or "nice." They suffer from a variety of symptoms—perhaps headaches, or depression, or low self-esteem, or a frustrated and sometimes mystifying sense that life feels empty and unsatisfying. Before long, it becomes apparent that they have great difficulty in asserting themselves as well as in expressing anger. Indeed, the two are confused for them. They are hesitant to make their needs or preferences known or to express their views or ask for their due; to do so makes them feel too "pushy" or aggressive. They also have a hard time not just in *expressing* anger but even in letting themselves *feel* angry, even if they have been badly treated. They try hard to smooth things over or they "understand the other person's point of view" to such an extent that *their* point of view virtually disappears. If they do feel anger—and, as I shall discuss in a moment, the occurrence of anger is actually not inconsistent with this clinical picture—they feel guilty, apologetic, maybe even humiliated. In attempting to make amends, they may go out of their way to an extreme degree (and sometimes to the considerable detriment of their own interests) to get back in the good graces of the other person.

In Marina's case, for example, as afraid of anger as she was, she would periodically erupt in intense angry outbursts. These outbursts, however, hardly ever were accepted by her as appropriate to the situation that elicited them. They felt to her "crazy," incomprehensible, and shameful, and the main way she dealt with them consciously was to ask, "What's wrong with me?" or "What happened? *That's not like me!*" She would, through such a response, reassert her sense of herself as a *non*-angry person for whom being angry is "not like her," but would thus also prevent herself from ever *standing behind* her anger, and thereby rectifying what had angered her in the first place.

Not uncommonly, people caught in this kind of pattern may withdraw altogether from the person who has made them (consciously or unconsciously) angry, finding the tension intolerable or finding it impossible to integrate the normal occurrence of anger into any relationship that means something to them. Such withdrawal, of course, is often as well *an expression* of the anger, an aggressive rejection, even if not necessarily acknowledged as such. At times—and here we get deeper into the tangled knot of the patient's way of life—a good part of the patient's anger at the other person may include anger at him for *being someone he gets angry at*; that is, for contributing to the breaching of the patient's *defenses against* anger. In essence, the feeling is: "How *dare you* make me angry! Don't you know how uncomfortable that makes me?" This, more than what the person actually did may be the most significant offense.

From the vantage point of classical psychoanalytic theory, such patients are commonly described as manifesting a reaction formation against anger that has been there since childhood. The excessive nice-ness is a way of keeping away angry feelings that are constantly in dan-ger of breaking loose. This vision, more a product of the drive theory than of relational accounts because it focuses on the defense against the impulse rather than on the relational configuration that gives rise to it or that it represents, views the anger as primary, as something that arose in childhood and that is stored "within." Put differently, the anger is the independent variable, and the reaction formation is the dependent variable. The cyclical psychodynamic point of view leads us to expand our field of vision. What becomes evident when one does so is that, however the pattern began (and such patterns very frequently do start in childhood), once it gets going it has certain consequences. The person who is inhibited in this way from pursuing his aims and interests is much more likely than most people to feel thwarted, deprived, even cheated. Marina, for example, was bypassed for promo-tions at work, was somewhat of a wallflower socially, and even in her family was the caretaker adult child who seemed to get less love and appreciation than her more "selfish" sister. Such experiences are very likely to lead to the kind of frustration that has made the hypothesized connection between frustration and aggression (Dollard, Doob, Miller, Mowrer, & Sears, 1939) such a psychological mainstay.

But there was little room in Marina's makeup for much aggression, at least of the overt kind. When angry or aggressive feelings were stirred, they were experienced by Marina as dangerous and toxic, and the result was that she redoubled her efforts to be "nice," to be cooper-ative, pleasing, unthreatening. And in doing so—exaggeratedly, com-pulsively, and largely unconsciously; not as a reasoned and tempered product of a religious or moral philosophy—she once again set the stage for *further* experiences of being dismissed, frustrated ... and angry. And then, since this anger too had to be immediately buried and repudiated, she laid the ground for still another turn of the circle in which she was caught.

The problem for patients such as Marina is often exacerbated further by their not knowing very well how to *express* anger in an effective and socially acceptable way. The very tendency to suppress their anger deprives them of the cumulative experiences that enable most of us, over time, to learn how and when to express anger—how, that is, to express anger so that it serves the purposes of changing the situation that has *made us* angry.[13] As a consequence, the alternatives feel to such patients like either "bury it" or explode, and neither alternative gets them what they want or need. Moreover, because they do not know how to be angry *effectively,* they feel less able to *back up* any aggression that is stirred in them, and so they back off. And, of course, the result is *still more anger,* because they continue to be deprived of their fair share.

People like Marina lead a way of life designed to stifle anger, and that very way of life, instead, *generates* it. They may talk about their childhood in the therapy, and in doing so may even express some degree of anger about things that happened then (an indulgence made safe by the therapist's encouragement and the distance of the consulting room from the time and place when the anger was most hot and dangerous). But the anger that they struggle with is no longer the anger from childhood, and going back to its "origins" or "roots" may miss the key point—the patient's *whole way of life* has become an anger generator, and *that* is what is most essential to understand. The anger the patient struggles with now is not the anger from the distant past but from experiences today and yesterday, and their cause is very largely the *suppression* of anger the day before that

Similar patterns of internal state generating action in the world that ends up maintaining or strengthening that same internal state can be seen in virtually every clinical case. The deeper one probes into the person's history, experience, and unconscious wishes, fears, and fantasies, the more it becomes evident how powerfully they are all linked to the *ongoing* patterns between people in the patient's life today (for further examples, see Wachtel, 1993, 1997).

---

[13] I will discuss later in this book the important work of the Boston Process of Change Study Group (e.g., Stern et al., 1998; Lyons-Ruth, 1998), which has introduced to the literature of psychotherapy attention to processes of "implicit relational knowing." Knowing *how to be* angry in an effective and socially and personally acceptable way is an important dimension of implicit relational knowing.

VARIABILITY AND CONTEXTUALITY

It is important to be clear that rarely are any of these patterns utterly pervasive. To begin with, as I have already alluded to, it is not uncommon, say, for people like Marina to quite regularly become overtly angry or resentful, notwithstanding their prodigious efforts to prevent this from happening. But in addition, there are often pockets—sometimes very important and extensive realms—in which the pattern is not evident, in which they are able to be assertive, effective, even to stand up for themselves quite directly and forcefully. This might be at work but not with friends, or vice versa. It might be in *certain aspects* of their work and not others (say, in getting a project under way but not in salary negotiations). It might be in a particular relationship (say, with a spouse or a sibling) and the relationship might be highly valued—perhaps overly so—for this very reason.

This variability is frequently omitted from clinical case reports and formulations, which often tend to focus on the patient's dominant patterns and to relate them to particular developmental experiences. But it is an essential feature of clinical descriptions deriving from a contextual point of view. In order really to understand another person, we must understand the impressive variability in both behavior and subjective experience that is almost certain to be evident if one pays attention to it. Almost everyone, from the sickest to the most healthy, feels good or does well in some settings and not others, with some people and not others, in some activities and not others, on some days and not others, and so forth. It is essential that we understand—or at least attempt to understand—the ways in which these variations are related to their context. We must know, that is, *when* the person feels depressed, confident, outgoing, inhibited, sexually aroused, sexually inhibited, and so forth. For only when we know how the person's experience is related to the setting do we really know sufficiently what the experience is "about."

CYCLICAL PSYCHODYNAMICS, REPETITION COMPULSION, AND PROJECTIVE IDENTIFICATION

The conceptualization I have outlined in this chapter has certain similarities with two other concepts that have been prominent in psychoanalytic discourse—repetition compulsion and projective identification.

The concept of repetition compulsion, a concept Freud introduced in *Beyond the Pleasure Principle* (Freud, 1920), also depicts the person as bringing about the same pattern over and over again. Where the concept of repetition compulsion differs from the conceptualization described in this chapter is in its presumptions about motivation. There are actually two versions of the motivation to repeat. In one, what is at issue is a biologically innate tendency to repeat that is closely related to Freud's philosophical speculations about the death instinct. In the second, the person repeats the same scenario over and over because he is attempting to recreate the old situation in order to make it *come out differently* this time. This effort at coping is usually futile, however, in large measure because it is engaged in unconsciously and hence in a way that is unlikely to be flexible or nuanced enough to actually make things happen differently.

The cyclical psychodynamic conception is certainly not lacking in ideas of motivation, including unconscious motivation. But it is more agnostic with regard to precisely what the motivation is or what the engine is that powers the repetitive set of occurrences over and over. As noted above, in many instances the result that is repetitively achieved is *not* sought, but is an ironic consequence of the very effort to *avoid* that result. The burden of proof, we might say, is more even-handed. There are certainly instances where we do unconsciously recreate the same situation over and over for the purpose of mastery, of coping better the next time around, even of just having "better luck" this time. There are instances as well when the person unconsciously *seeks* punishment or failure, *aims* to bring this about, just as proponents of the concept of repetition compulsion and certain closely related ideas assume. But there are many instances as well where the aim (even the *unconscious* aim) is *not* to bring about the same problematic set of events again and again, but rather, as I described above, where the repetition derives from the ironic consequences of trying to *prevent* the very events that keep occurring. In this, what transpires from the cyclical psychodynamic vantage point includes patterns that are quite different from what is depicted in the theory of the repetition compulsion.

The role of irony is what distinguishes the conception described here from that of projective identification as well. The concept of projective identification has undergone considerable change over the years, from its origins in Klein's drive-dominated, preponderantly intrapsychic proto-object-relations theorizing, through the modifications introduced by theorists such as Bion (e.g., 1959a, 1959b, 1970) and its further elaboration by Ogden (1979, 1982) and by contemporary relational theorists. But it remains very largely a concept in which what the other person is feeling and how the other person responds is assumed to be what the patient unconsciously *intended* her to feel and do. Gabbard (1995) has noted that it is not uncommon in references to projective identification to portray the analyst as "virtually empty and . . . simply a receptacle or container for what the patient is projecting" (p. 479). And Eagle (2000), after describing an interaction with a supervisee who was convinced that she was having headaches during sessions with a particular patient because the patient was "putting the headaches into her" via projective identification, states:

> I have read references to projective identification in the literature that are not essentially different from the account I have just given. There is frequent talk of the patient putting something into the analyst without any seeming awareness of the need to at least try to specify the interpersonal process (e. g., cues emitted by one person) by which one person gets another person to feel certain feelings—or without any seeming awareness that such ordinary, nonmagical processes must exist. . . . I am not maintaining that there are no actual phenomena that people who use the term projective identification are trying to capture. What I am trying to highlight is the fuzzy and muddleheaded nature of much discussion of and thinking about concepts such as projective identification . . . in contemporary psychoanalysis. (pp. 34–35)

In contrast to this very concretistic concept, the cyclical psychodynamic account of the way that people evoke feelings in others is concerned precisely with what Eagle notes that proponents of the concept of projective identification so largely ignore—the particular behaviors and cues that evoke the feeling (see the discussion of the important role of *actions* in cyclical psychodynamic theory in the chapters that follow). Moreover, the cyclical psychodynamic conception of how feelings are evoked in the other again considers irony and *un*intended consequences to be a real and not infrequent possibility.

Today, the concept of projective identification is widely viewed as a bridge between the "internal" world and the world of everyday experience. But closer examination of how the concept is often employed reveals it to be one of those bridges on which the tolls are collected only in one direction. Although the posited phenomena of "putting feelings into" others and then having them "put back into" one's own psyche after appropriate "metabolization" may seem to imply a two-way flow (putting aside for the moment the conceptual incoherence that conflates moving the feeling to a different *representation* in the person's head and putting the feeling into an actual other person), the focus in discussions of projective identification is usually preponderantly on what *the patient* is doing, with, as Gabbard notes, the other person essentially just a vessel for the patient's projections to be poured into (see also Slavin, 1996, p. 622).

It is interesting to note in this regard that Bion (1970), who is often credited with "interpersonalizing" the concept of projective identification, directs the therapist to enter the session "without memory or desire," an idea that is utterly and quintessentially a one-person conception. The therapist is empty, has no motives or expectations of her own, and is simply an external receiver (a "container") for the projections that come from inside the patient. It is thus surprising and disappointing that so many relational writers discuss Bion's conceptualizations so positively and uncritically. It is precisely such a view of the therapist as not bringing *her own* contribution to the interaction, but merely observing and responding to the patient's, that the entire relational movement was created to challenge. As Renik (1999a) notes in discussing a somewhat related conceptualization of projective identification by Bollas (1987):

> From this point of view, the analyst, the analyst's subjectivity is rendered essentially inconsequential. Such is the patient's power to determine the analyst's experience by projectively identifying that the analyst's individual psychology is, in effect, overridden. Now, instead of the analyst looking at the patient *out there* and observing him or her objectively, the analyst is looking at the patient *within* and observing him or her objectively. The familiar positivist conception of the analyst as objective observer is preserved. (p. 518, italics in original)

If one instead approaches the phenomena that have been addressed through the concept of projective identification in a more fully two-person way, what becomes apparent is that the patient evokes whatever he evokes in a *particular* therapist and hence, what he "puts into" the therapist is not just a product of the patient's insides but of the therapist's sensitivities and readiness to perceive. What to one therapist might be evidence of the patient's masochism (because it evokes the therapist's sadism) to another might be evidence of the patient being bravely forthcoming about his frailties (because in that analyst the patient's vulnerability evokes *respect* rather than sadism). As a consequence, not only are the two therapists' *perceptions* different, but—à la cyclical psychodynamics (see also the discussion of schemas, assimilation, and accommodation in the next chapter)—what the patient's feeling "is" becomes different, because over time the way the patient feels and construes his experience is powerfully influenced by how the other person responds to it and by the quite different ensuing sequence of events that *continues* to shape the experiences and perceptions of both parties.

Now, in saying that what the feeling actually becomes is changed by the perceptions and the response of the particular therapist, I am not implying that the patient's experience is arbitrary or simply "determined" by the therapist. There are significant and meaningful constraints or boundaries in at least two ways. First, where *the patient* goes with the experience is not completely arbitrary. It has to be in some way a version of what was there to begin with, a path consistent with where he was going. The patient's experience may be somewhat malleable, but it is not *infinitely* malleable. Second, similar constraints exist on how the therapist will *perceive* the patient's experience. Her perception is not completely malleable or arbitrary either. The therapist too is responding and perceiving to what is actually transpiring, even if she too is doing so selectively and "in her fashion." In that sense, the therapist's response *is* a function of what the patient is feeling or doing, and so the responsibility for what the patient evokes in her does partly belong to the patient, but in a very different (more transactional and mutual) way than in the objectivist fashion that Renik calls to our attention.

It is true that the concept of projective identification and the ways that it is employed in clinical formulations have continued to evolve. Maroda (2002), for example, has stated that "the analytic literature is replete with examples of projective identification, moving from the old view that the patient uses it to 'dump' unwanted feelings on the analyst and force her to feel bad, to a more constructive view of projective identification as an attempt to communicate disavowed affect to the analyst" (p. 107). But in "moving from the old view" to the newer view, which Maroda employs with great sensitivity and skill, the meaning has been *radically* altered. Yes, in both cases it's about how we pick up feelings from the patient; but the conceptualization is so fundamentally—and importantly—different that it is confusing to use the same term.

NEW WINE IN OLD BOTTLES?

The standard complaint about proffered conceptual innovations is that they are just old wine in new bottles, ideas that are tired and familiar that are simply given a new name. This has certainly often been the case in psychoanalysis as it has in other realms; jargon can provide impressive, technical-sounding wrapping for ideas one's grandmother was familiar with. But, as the above discussion illustrates, in psychoanalytic discourse, there is often what might be described as an equal and opposite problem—*new* wine in *old* bottles; that is, genuinely new and useful ideas whose implications are obscured and constrained by a tendency among psychoanalytic writers to be overly reverent toward (one might even say, to fetishize) older, widely used terms that have come to be almost membership shibboleths. Psychoanalytic writers often seem to sprinkle their writings with such terminology in order to be perceived as still members in good standing of the psychoanalytic community—*especially* if they are introducing innovations.

As we have just seen, "projective identification" is one of those terms, an old bottle into which have been poured a variety of new and genuinely important ideas and observations. But the distinctiveness and specificity of these innovations are somewhat obscured—and even limited—by the older connotations and associations that are called up by continuing to use the older terminology. As I proceed, it will be apparent that this is by no means an isolated instance. In various ways, terms like neutrality, interpretation, transference, and countertransference have all been stretched well beyond their original meanings as new ideas have been formulated in familiar terms, obscuring the full import of the new conceptualizations that have been inserted into comfortingly familiar containers.

To be sure, in *all* disciplines, the meanings of terms are constantly evolving and building metaphorically on older conceptualizations (Lakoff & Johnson, 1980; Wachtel, 2003a). *Some* allusive ambiguity and ties to older ideas can be helpful and enable connections that are lost if we are too obsessionally precise or literal. But the process is considerably more extreme, I believe, in psychoanalysis, which, we might say, is a "transference-based" discipline in more ways than one. (See the discussion in Chapter 3 of the influence on psychoanalytic thought of the model of training that for so long predominated in the psychoanalytic world.) There is always considerable difficulty in extricating oneself from the frame of reference in which one's ideas were originally shaped. Lifting one's leg out of quicksand often drives the other leg in more deeply. Many of the issues I have been discussing in this book derive from the ways in which the critiques and new ideas of psychoanalytic innovators were often expressed in language forms that subtly perpetuated the very assumptions that were being challenged. The chapters that follow will be devoted to spelling out the implications for clinical practice of a more thoroughgoing adaptation of relational thinking in general and of the cyclical psychodynamic point of view in particular.

7

■　■　■　■　■

Self-States, Dissociation, and the Schemas of Subjectivity and Intersubjectivity

In an increasingly prominent line of relational theorizing (e.g., Bromberg, 1998a; Davies, 1996; Harris, 1996; Mitchell, 1993a; Pizer, 1996; Slavin, 1996) some of the phenomena that were of central concern in the previous chapter—for example the substantial variability that is evident in all people's behavior and experience and the responsiveness of even "deep" psychological dynamics to the constantly shifting intersubjective context—are discussed in the language of dissociation and multiple self-states. Of particular import in the conceptualization of multiple self-states is the fact that not only can we behave differently and feel differently from moment to moment, but even our sense of self, our understanding of *the kind of person we are*, is far from constant. Just a moment's reflection makes it clear that this fluctuation of self-experience is an everyday occurrence, overlapping in part with the familiar concept of mood. It is problematic or pathogenic only when, while immersed in one state of mind or sense of ourselves, the others become so thoroughly alien that we have no access to them. When such a wall exists, when we cannot "stand in the spaces" between them

as Bromberg (1996a) puts it, then we suffer from the kinds of dissociation that have problematic implications for our mental health and well-
being.

There are many points of convergence between the recent theorizing about dissociation and multiple self-states in the relational literature and the cyclical psychodynamic perspective presented in the previous chapter. Davies's (1996) discussion of multiplicity, for example,
like the cyclical psychodynamic model (see below), draws on Piaget's
concepts of schemas, assimilation, and accommodation to illuminate
the ways in which already established psychological structures and the
new experiences that we encounter at every moment of our lives continuously and reciprocally shape each other. Noting similarities in the
theories of Piaget and his teacher, Pierre Janet, Davies points out that
for both thinkers, "schemas affect the way in which each individual
views reality, *and* reality affects the ongoing structural nuances of
schemas" (1996, p. 557, italics added). In calling attention to this latter
half of the bidirectional process of personal evolution, Davies thus
offers—in a fashion quite parallel to the arguments presented in this
book and in previous presentations of the cyclical psychodynamic
point of view (e.g., Wachtel, 1981, 1987a, 1997)—a corrective to the
vision of the past as buried like archaeological remains and of psychological structures as sealed off from the influence of new relational
experience. Moreover, in a convergence with the integrative aim of
cyclical psychodynamic theory, Davies states that she favors a schema
model not only because she views it as more consonant with a relational point of view but also because it is "more conducive to an integration of psychoanalytic theory with other branches of academic psychology" (1996, p. 561).

ASSIMILATION, ACCOMMODATION, AND THE INTERPLAY OF STRUCTURE AND NEW EXPERIENCE

In the course of development, two different things tend to happen that
jointly shape the nature of the personality and of the person's individuality: (1) an expansion and *consolidation* of the cyclically self-
perpetuating patterns described in the previous chapter, in which the
pattern (whether problematic or a source of pleasure and satisfaction)
becomes more and more deeply entrenched; (2) a *differentiation*, in
which, in relation to different contexts and cues, the dominant patterns

are manifested much of the time, but variations and contradictions are evident in certain contexts with some regularity. It is the first trend that is preponderantly highlighted in most clinical theories, and for obvious reasons. People come to us to address the persistent patterns that seem to dominate their lives, patterns they have tried to change and found they could not. But the second dimension of personality dynamics, the ways in which behavior and experience *do* keep evolving and changing in response to new contexts, is equally crucial for the clinician to attend to. For change to occur, at least the kernels of a different way of life must be there to begin with. Much of the skill of the effective psychotherapist entails noticing those kernels, however rare or submerged they may be, and working to amplify and build upon them (Wachtel, 1993; see also Chapter 12, this volume).

It is in bringing together these two seemingly contradictory tendencies in psychological life that I have found Piaget's concepts of assimilation and accommodation particularly helpful.[1] No psychological theory is viable that does not pay careful attention to the enormously powerful role of the psychological structures and motivational and perceptual inclinations that begin their evolution very early in life and shape our experience of the present at every moment. But no theory is viable as well that is not equally attentive to the exquisite responsiveness to context that is *also* a hallmark of human experience (and indeed, without which our species—endowed neither with great speed nor sharp claws or teeth—never would have survived). The challenge is to reconcile and integrate these tendencies toward consolidation and differentiation in a way that does justice to the pervasive presence of both and, as well, to the full range of phenomena and observations that present themselves for theoretical understanding.

I first turned to Piaget's ideas in coming to terms with certain problematic features of the way that the phenomenon of transference was conceptualized by psychoanalytic theorists (Wachtel, 1977a, 1981), but I wish here to extend that analysis to a consideration of personality development and dynamics more generally. Transference was for many

---

[1] Harris (1996) notes that Piagetian ideas can be problematic when they are taken to posit a single core organizing structure as characterizing the entire individual. It should be clear that the aspects of Piagetian thought emphasized here represent instead the conflict-based model of change that Harris notes is also a key feature of Piaget's model. Indeed, Harris's critique of certain features of contemporary Piagetian-inspired developmental research is highly consonant with the critiques offered in this book of the tendency in psychoanalytic writing to depict people as characterized by a singular underlying "developmental level."

years a phenomenon in which psychoanalytic writers tended to think almost exclusively in terms of the patient's *distortions* of reality, his seeing the present in terms of the past to such a degree that he seemed virtually *not to see* the present, not to experience the "reality" of the analyst. This is not to say that Freud completely ignored the role of what is really transpiring in the room. As Schafer (1977) put it in discussing Freud's conception of transference, "On the one hand, transference love is sheerly repetitive, merely a new edition of the old, artificial and regressive . . . and to be dealt with chiefly by translating it back into its infantile terms. . . . On the other hand, transference is a piece of real life that is adapted to the analytic purpose, a transitional state of a provisional character that is a means to a rational end and as genuine as normal love" (p. 340). We may note as well that one important element in Freud's legacy includes a wide-ranging literature on the therapist's role as *both* old and new object (e.g., Aron, 1991a; Greenberg, 1986; Loewald, 1960). Nonetheless, it is accurate to depict the classical tradition in psychoanalysis as one that emphasized to a preponderant degree the transference as a *distortion.* Greenson (1967), for example, who in one way liberalized the understanding of the therapeutic relationship through his influential introduction of the concept of the therapeutic alliance and the "real" relationship (Greenson, 1965, 1971), nonetheless states unequivocally that "transference reactions are always inappropriate" (p. 152). Similarly, Langs (1973) contended that "to identify a fantasy about, or reaction to, the therapist as primarily transference . . . we must be able to refute with certainty *any* appropriate level of truth to the patient's unconscious or conscious claim that she correctly perceives the therapist in the manner spelled out through her associations" (p. 415, italics added).

In this traditional conception, the analyst's real qualities were seen as at most an arbitrary "hook" or "peg" on which the patient, driven by the virtually inexorable inner need to see the present in terms of the past, hung the ready-made outfit that had already been purchased to dress the analyst in. One of the signal contributions of the relational point of view has been its insistence that the portrayal of the patient's "distortions" be replaced by a more dynamic and dialectical account in which the patient's long-standing inclinations are seen as in constant tension and interaction with the impact of the actual qualities and behavior of the other person in the room (e.g., Hoffman, 1983; Aron, 1991b).

In understanding the dynamic tension between these two facets of the patient's transferential experience, Piaget's conceptualization of the interplay between assimilation and accommodation is an invaluable tool. From the vantage point of this conceptualization we may see that, in essence, the traditional conception of transference (with its emphasis on the patient's "distortions") posited a process of assimilation virtually without accompanying accommodation. But as Piaget's analysis illuminates, in every encounter with the world, we *both* assimilate the new experience into our already existing schemas and, as part of the very same process, accommodate those schemas to the ways in which the new experience *differs* from the previous experiences from which the schemas were constructed (Flavell, 1963; Wachtel, 1981)[2] We need not choose between a conceptualization that emphasizes the sometimes remarkable tenacity people show in maintaining old ways of experiencing themselves and other people, even in the face of seemingly dramatic disconfirmation,[3] and one that highlights our continuing responsiveness to the events of our lives. We are *always* experiencing the world in terms of the structures that evolved in the past and *always* modifying those structures to accommodate to the present. To understand why this is the case, let us begin with an illustration I have previously offered (Wachtel, 2005a) of one of the simplest instances of this process, the way a young child develops his understanding of what a "dog" is:

> Consider, for example, what happens when a child who has developed an initial schema of dog comes into contact with a kind of dog that he has not seen before, say a Chihuahua or a Great Dane. When the child learns to include either of these new experiences in his schema of dog, he is clearly assimilating them to that schema. But in the very effort to do this, the child is also *accommodating* the schema to take them in. It is no longer the same schema, simply because it is now a schema that includes these new outliers that previously were not part of the child's vision of what the category dog included. It is the very act of assimilation that produces the accommodation and

---

[2] Flavell (1977) has argued that "schema" is a mistranslation of the Piagetian French original, "scheme." However, because of the particular connotations of the word "scheme" in English (think of detective stories or insurance scams), and because the term "schema" more readily facilitates comparison between Piaget's ideas and those of a variety of other approaches to cognition and cognitive development, I prefer the term "schema," the term that has more and more become the standard English translation.

[3] For an interesting perspective on this phenomenon from the vantage point of systematic research, see Swann (1997).

the very act of accommodation that enables the assimilation. Neither could proceed without the other. (p. 244)

Much the same thing happens in the processing of experiences more closely related to our emotional life and our relations to other people Consider for example what happens when we encounter someone whom we experience as being critical or insulting. As with every other experience, we do not passively register what is happening as a camera registers the light falling on it, but rather we actively *construct* the event, making sense of it on the basis of the psychological structures that have evolved for us up to that point (Schimek, 1975b; Neisser, 1976; Schacter, 1996). In this process, the schemas we already hold for making sense of the world are applied to the new experience, and because each of us has had somewhat different experiences in our lives and has developed a different set of psychological structures for encountering the world, each of us interprets the experience somewhat differently. Where one person might register a particular interaction as one of criticism and hurtful intent (or put differently, might assimilate the experience to the schema for processing and dealing with criticism), someone else, with a different personality and different life experiences, might assimilate the very same interaction to his schema for friendly banter.

What is particularly important to understand—and what particularly characterizes our schemas for emotional and relational experiences (that is, for interactions with others whose own schemas are simultaneously interpreting and reacting to *our* behavior)—is that almost from the very first moment, the perceptions that each person has *will change what happens next.* Perceiving the other person's comment as criticism will likely lead to behavior toward him (whether hostile, or tense, or inhibited, or withholding) that is less likely to elicit a warm or positive response in return. Perceiving the behavior instead as friendly banter will lead to quite different behavior and hence to a likely somewhat different response in return. And so the experience that evolves over time is in very large measure a function of how the experience was perceived (by both parties) in its very early stages. That is, an initial *mis*perception (if we can call it that for now) can, in the fashion of the self-fulfilling prophecy, eventually turn out to have been an "accurate" perception—but it will be accurate only because the perception itself brought about its confirmation by eliciting behavior from the other that seems to confirm it.

What transpires, I have previously suggested (Wachtel, 1981), is a kind of race (often with the quality of "a race against time," as that phrase is used to convey an effort to head off a crisis or disaster). If the person one is "misperceiving" (say as hostile) can continue to behave benignly, the element of accommodation that is an essential feature of every perceptual act will eventually lead to the registration of this difference from initial expectations. But the process of coming to terms with the differences between one's expectations, rooted in past experiences, and what one is presently encountering does not occur instantaneously or totalistically. For a time, the initial perception of the situation is likely to continue to guide the person's behavior to a significant degree. This is the "stickiness" (as we may call it) that has been observed countless times by psychoanalysts and other clinicians, often leading them to posit a sealed off or split off part of the psyche that is no longer responsive to the events transpiring in the present. But that *apparently* almost inexorable persistence, the *apparent* unresponsiveness to new contingencies and new possibilities, is actually an artifact of the way that the other person's response is itself a part of the process. Because the schema evolves and accommodates only slowly and gradually, and because we initially perceive matters as we are *set* to perceive them and begin to respond to them accordingly, there is a considerable likelihood that before the accommodation can proceed very far, the *other* person's behavior will have responded to the way he is being perceived and responded to by the first. In that case, the first person's expectations *do not* change very much. Rather, his view of the world continues to reflect his earlier expectations and assumptions because the world *comes to look like them.*[4]

Notice here that this is very much a two-person or intersubjective process, a reflection of life patterns that are mutually created between people over and over again. Notice as well that this two-person or intersubjective or interpersonal process is *not* in contrast with or antithetical to an "intrapsychic" process. Rather, the intrapsychic processes of each party are crucial to and embedded in the transactional process, just as the transactional processes are an essential element in the operation and the maintenance of the intrapsychic state of affairs for each individual. Each is part and parcel of the other.

---

[4] A similar phenomenon occurs in the realm of race relations and ethnic misunderstandings, where mutual stereotypes receive "pseudo-confirmations" (Wachtel, 1999) that keep the stereotypes alive to create the same mischief the next time. Pseudo-confirmation is a central process in the maintenance of problematic personality patterns as well.

MULTIPLICITY AND ACCEPTANCE

I wish to return now to the conceptualization of multiple self-states that I referred to earlier in this chapter as a way that a prominent line of relational thought has addressed many of the same phenomena that I have just been pointing to. This emphasis on multiplicity has been associated with a way of thinking and of working clinically that is in important ways both more creative and more humane than the conventional linear and hierarchical approach to personality associated with more traditional versions of psychoanalytic thought. Bromberg, for example, in discussing one of Freud's earliest cases, states, "What Freud was unable to see at that time was that his failure was not a lack of patience with Emmy's symptoms as symptoms, but a lack of patience with her symptoms as representing her perceptual *reality* and in this sense more than 'pieces of pathology' that should or could be 'taken away' " (Bromberg, 1996b, p. 64). This emphasis on *acceptance* of the patient's various modes of experience rather than attempting to "correct" them is evident throughout Bromberg's writings on dissociation and multiple self-states. Viewing *multiple* modes of experience as real and valid points him toward a kind of "equal opportunity" exploration rather than engaging in what Aron, adding further meaning to a term introduced by Kohut (1979), has called "maturity morality," a view in which certain of the patient's experiences are immature, infantile, archaic, or primitive, and hence must be *renounced* when they are uncovered in the course of the work (Aron, 1991a).[5]

Central to the therapeutic strategy that is repeatedly expressed in Bromberg's writings is an emphasis not only on acceptance, but on a measure of restraint regarding what is usually depicted in the analytic literature as "interpretation." Bromberg (1993) emphasizes that interpretation can often feel to the patient like the therapist's imposing *her* views on the patient as if she is the arbiter of what is "real" and what is illusory. Citing also Ghent (1992b) and Pizer (1992), he regards the determination of what is real or valid in the patient's experience as "a relational process of consensual negotiation" (p. 152). The aim, he suggests, is not one of showing the patient where he is distorting or misrepresenting, but the "pleasurable construction of a more inclusive reality." Citing Winnicott (1951, 1960, 1971), but emphasizing a differ-

---

[5] The issues of renunciation and acceptance, and their implications for clinical practice, are further considered in Chapter 8.

ent perspective on Winnicott's work than is often evident in the literature, Bromberg argues that a prerequisite for meaningful therapeutic
change is that the patient not be "pressured to choose between which
reality is more 'objective' . . . and which self is more 'true' " (1996a,
p. 525).[6]

This emphasis on *acceptance* of the patient's experience, it is
important to understand, can only be part of an effective therapeutic
strategy if it is understood to be in continuing tension with an equal
and opposite dimension of the therapeutic process, working to help the
patient to *change.* Thus Bromberg notes, "The ability of an individual
to allow his self-truth to be altered by the impact of an 'other' . . .
depends on the existence of a relationship in which the other can be
experienced as someone who, paradoxically, both *accepts the validity* of
the patient's inner reality and participates in the here-and-now act of
constructing a negotiated reality discrepant with it" (1993, p. 160).
From an integrative perspective, it is worth noting that this view of the
therapeutic process is very similar to that emphasized in dialectical
behavior therapy (Robins, Schmidt, & Linehan, 2004). It resembles as
well a point that has been a key feature of my own approach to clinical
work (Wachtel, 1993—see especially Ch. 8, "Affirmation and
Change").

Davies similarly (e.g., 1996) utilizes the concept of multiple self-
states in a way that highlights both acceptance and playfulness. In contrast to the critical and demeaning tone that is often unwittingly a characteristic of psychoanalytic interpretations (for further discussion of
this tendency, see Wile, 1984; Weiss & Sampson, 1986; Aron, 1991a;
Wachtel, 1980,1993), Davies conceives of the good interpretation as
"an *invitation* we make to the unconscious to enter the future along
with us, to give its potential for fantasy full reign, in order to witness
together different aspects of what it might become if allowed to flower
uninhibited by other, more practical concerns" (1996, p. 571).[7] This is
nicely illustrated in an exchange she reports with a patient, Helen, who
had reacted in an unsympathetic and even hostile way to Davies feeling
ill during a session. In the next session, Helen clearly felt embarrassed

---

[6] In this respect, Bromberg's conclusions parallel those of Mitchell (1993a), who, in also
advocating a view of multiple selves and examining Winnicott's ideas about true and false self,
notes that "deciding what is true and what is false when it comes to self is a tricky business"
(p. 130).

[7] See Wachtel (1993) and the remaining chapters of this book for further applications of and
variations on this theme.

at how she had behaved and was eager to apologize and move on to another topic. Davies, however, stayed with the experience of the previous session:

> I told Helen that I believed I had seen a new and different part of her—someone I had not quite met before. "I'd like to know her better," I said. "I think she's got quite a different perspective . . . I bet she's been there all along."
> The patient smiled, "Oh she's very bad, you don't want to know her, she's very very bad."
> "How bad could she be?" I asked.
> "The worst a person could ever imagine," Helen replied.
> "What if we let ourselves imagine," I said. "What if we invite her in." (1996, pp. 570–571)

One of the noteworthy qualities in this exchange is its playfulness. Very much in the spirit of Winnicott's (1968) emphasis on play as a crucial component of the therapeutic process, both Davies and Bromberg exhibit a noteworthy playfulness in their interventions, a form of playfulness that is at once profoundly serious and encouraging of forbidden pleasures and loosening of scleroticized boundaries. One might indeed say of Davies in particular that—in the service of enhancing the patient's growth and vitality—she works to replace the scleroticized with the eroticized (Davies, 1994, 1998).

MULTIPLE SELF-STATES OR MULTIPLE SELVES

One potential pitfall of theorizing in terms of multiple self-states is that the idea of multiple self-states, each with its own individuality or "personality," can lend itself to reification. Bromberg, for example, whose use of this way of conceptualizing leads to clinical interventions that converge quite considerably with the clinical approach described in this book, nonetheless at times depicts what he does in a way that can create ambiguity for the reader regarding the boundary between misplaced concreteness and creative and generative metaphor. For example, in emphasizing the importance of the analyst "allowing himself to become immersed in the here-and-now intersubjective field as it exists at that moment" (a position I resonate to and highly endorse), he adds, "He must *form authentic relationships with each of the patient's self-states* as it exists in the moment and engage with it in its own terms without surrendering his own vision of the present moment as also a way station linking the patient as he used to be (the past) to what he ultimately might become (the future)" (1998b, p. 228, italics added).

This passage can be read in two different ways. On the one hand, it seems almost to imply that the analyst or therapist must treat each mood of the patient, each facet of his complex personality as a separate being with whom a separate relationship must be established and maintained. On the other, the emphasis on the *way station* and the *linking* of the various moments of being to an *ongoing* being suggests something rather different. To some extent, this apparent contradiction reflects Bromberg's creative embrace of the paradoxes of human experience, a viewpoint similar to Harris's (1996) emphasis on "polarities" and on the value of "determinacy remain[ing] unresolved" (p. 548). But although life is indeed full of ambiguities and paradoxes, and too hasty and linear an attempt at resolution may yield a neat but insufficiently deep and complex appreciation of nuances, there is an equal danger of too easy and fashionable an embrace of paradox and indeterminacy in this "postmodern" era. We are best off, I believe, *trying* to achieve resolution, while being prepared for limits to our capacity to do so at any given point and taking care not to do so in a way that achieves only *pseudo*-resolution, by which I mean a merely *apparent* resolution that is achieved only by ignoring the complexities and contradictions in favor of a misleadingly tidy formulation. For myself, I am more comfortable with the idea of multiplicity as a *transitional* phenomenon, a playful stretching beyond the familiar but not a substitute for continuing with the hard intellectual work of attempting to integrate the competing perspectives and observations into a coherent new synthesis.

In further considering how best to employ the concept of multiplicity, I would suggest that there is an important difference between referring to multiple self-states or multiple self-experiences on the one hand and multiple *selves* on the other (see in this regard the exchange between Lachmann, 1996a, 1996b, and Slavin, 1996). The literature at times uses these terms interchangeably, but to my mind their implications are different. This difference seems to be recognized in a clinically astute way by Davies (1996) in the following further exchange with Helen, in which Davies shifts from a third-person discourse in which she refers to Helen as "she" (that little girl we are talking about) to a more direct form of address in which she refers to Helen as "you," a single person and the person being spoken to:

At my invitation to "let this part of her in," Helen's smile faded and she remained quiet for quite some time. "What are you seeing?" I asked her. I was aware that her face was scrunched up into a tight little pinch, and still she remained quiet.

"She [Helen's still referring to herself in the third person, rather than as "I"] walked right over her grandmother when her grandmother was sick and lying on the floor one day. That's how bad she is . . . that's what I thought of when you were choking and I walked right out of here! I haven't thought about that in so many years. I walked right over her frail little body." (1996, p. 571)

In response to this, Davies says, "I guess you were tired of people being sick. Maybe you got scared and frightened that day when my cold wouldn't go away."[8] Notice that Davies does *not* say at this point, maybe *she* got tired of people being sick, or maybe *she* got scared and frightened. Here Davies instead works to integrate the experience into, essentially, the patient's singular integrated, first-person self, the center of self-experience and agency. Earlier in the exchange, the little girl who walked over her grandmother's body ("she") or the "very bad" little girl who responded with hostility to the therapist's bad cold and choking cough are *strategically* looked at as quasi-separate beings. (I say *quasi*-separate because both parties—I presume—maintained a background awareness of the playful and metaphorical dimension of this way of speaking.) But, in a temporal version of Winnicott's spatial metaphor of transitional space,[9] this way of speaking is *transitional*: at just a slightly later moment, when the fruits of that playful moment have ripened, the structure of the conversation shifts in a highly important way to a more direct conversation between two *persons* rather than fragmentary self-states or self-parts.

One cue to proceed in this way was the patient's own shift of pronouns. *The patient* shifts from "*she*" (that little girl) walked right over her grandmother to "*I*" walked right out of here. But even if the patient had not made the shift first, the kind of transition introduced by Davies would be called for, either at that moment or at a later one. At some point

---

[8] A crucial element in Helen's history, and a crucial part of the background both for the recollection that occurs to her regarding her grandmother and for her reaction to Davies's severe cough in the previous session, is that Helen's mother tragically died from cancer when she was a child, and on top of it her father's response was a guilt-inducing rather than a helpful one. Thus, the meaning of her caretaker being sick was a very loaded one for her.

[9] See Mitchell's (1993a) insightful discussion of the differences between spatial and temporal metaphors (pp. 99–102) and its applications to Winnicott (pp. 125–134).

the patient needs to be able to fully "own" the experience, even if, at an earlier point, the very ambiguity about who owns it is what enables it to enter the room at all. The earlier, transitional stage is a frequent one in good psychotherapy, and it is part of what makes Davies's term *therapeutic dissociation* (1996, p. 567) so apt. By first enabling the patient to talk about what "she" (that girl over there) did instead of what "I" (Helen) did, the material is made safer to explore and reexamine. Only when it is experienced as less dangerous and more acceptable, less subject to the preemptive foreclosure that comes with self-condemnation, can the temporary therapeutic dissociation be relinquished.

THE RESURGENCE OF INTEREST IN DISSOCIATION

As is already evident from the discussion thus far, the conceptualization of multiple self-states by relational theorists has proceeded hand in hand with an emphasis on dissociation. Dissociation is a concept that, with the exception of the Sullivanian branch of psychoanalytic thought (e.g., Sullivan, 1953), was for many years very largely ignored in psychoanalytic discourse (Berman, 1981; Bromberg, 1996b; Loewenstein & Ross, 1992) In recent years, however, the concept of dissociation has had a remarkable resurgence (see, e.g., Bromberg, 1998a; Davies & Frawley, 1994; Howell, 2006). A number of factors have contributed to this revival of interest. The first has been the recognition in the last two decades or so that psychoanalysis had vastly overreacted in its movement from an emphasis on trauma to one on fantasy. The reconceptualization by Freud that led him to conclude that his patients' memories were the result of wish-driven fantasies rather than actual traumatic occurrences was, at the time, a stimulus for very important advances. Much of the structure of psychoanalytic thought derived from it, as did a much enhanced understanding both of the nature of our unacknowledged feelings and desires and the extent to which we reconstruct our memories and subjective experience to accord with the imperatives of inner promptings and the structures through which our experience of the world is filtered. But the reframing went much too far, leading analysts for many decades to underestimate the impact of real experiences in ways that seriously compromised the foundations of psychoanalytic theory and practice.

Some early analysts recognized clearly that understanding of the powerful role of unconscious wishes and fantasies was not incompatible with attention to the actual events and realities of the child's life. Particularly noteworthy in this regard were Ferenczi (1926, 1952, 1955) and Horney (e.g., 1939, 1945). Ferenczi's influence and prescience has increasingly been recognized by relational thinkers (see, e.g., Aron & Harris, 1993). Horney's equally powerful contribution to a conceptual synthesis between the impact of actual events and their unconscious elaboration has, in contrast, still not been sufficiently acknowledged.

Several other developments over the years have also contributed importantly to the redress of the imbalance introduced by Freud's overemphasis on fantasy. Certainly to be included must be the evolution of ego psychology, with its concern with how to integrate the impact of actual life events into a theory that had seemed at times virtually to imply that the basic psychological equipment with which we were born was limited to the capacity to fantasize the occurrence of what we wished for (e.g., Hartmann, 1939; Rapaport, 1951, 1959; Erikson, 1963). More directly impacting on the evolution of relational thought was the increasing influence of object relations theories, especially the theoretical contributions of Winnicott (e.g., 1965, 1971) and Fairbairn (1952), who highlighted much more than Freud the impact of the actual occurrences between parent and child. In related fashion, Kohut's (1971, 1977) development of self psychology similarly highlighted the impact of the parent's actual empathic attunement or lack thereof on the child's development, placing these actual experiences on a co-equal basis with the internal fantasies that had been the almost exclusive concern of "official" psychoanalytic theory.[10] Finally, as an additional spur to what might be called the rapprochement with reality, psychoanalysts began to pay much more attention to research studies concerned with mother–infant interaction (e.g., Cohen & Tronick, 1988; Jaffe et al., 2001; Beebe & Lachmann, 2002; Tronick, 1989; Stern, 1985), with attachment (Ainsworth, Blehar, Waters, & Wall, 1978; Cassidy & Shaver, 1999; Main, 1995; Main, Kaplan, & Cassidy, 1985; Slade, 2000), and with the relational events that contribute to the development of mentalization and reflective function (Fonagy, Gergely, Jurist, & Target, 2002; Fonagy, 2002; Fonagy, Target, Gergely, Allen, & Bateman, 2003).

---

[10] I refer to "official" psychoanalytic theory because *no* intelligent or observant psychoanalyst could ignore the actual events of the patient's life, but there was for many years a gap between what was addressed in the everyday exchanges in analysts' consulting rooms and what was highlighted in the writing of theory.

But the "return to reality" that most affected the upsurge of interest in dissociation was surely the increasing concern with the impact of trauma, both in the course of early development and in later years (e.g., Herman, 1997; van der Kolk et al., 1996; Davies & Frawley, 1994; Howell, 2006). Sparked especially by the attention directed by feminist thinkers to the victimization of girls and women, but then extended to include other kinds of traumatization, the new appreciation that early formulations attributing psychopathology to the consequences of trauma had much more validity than had been appreciated—and should be regarded more as incomplete than wrong—led to a renewed *study* of trauma and to interest in the dissociation that is so often one of its major consequences.

VARIETIES OF DISSOCIATION

In reflecting on the concept of dissociation in contemporary theorizing it is useful to notice that the term dissociation in fact refers not to a single phenomenon but to an only partially overlapping *set* of phenomena which have different implications both for theory and for clinical practice. Much of the recent resurgence of interest in dissociation has been largely focused on the *massive* dissociations arising from severe trauma. But once one begins to think in terms of dissociation, it becomes clear that dissociation is a concept that helps us to understand as well the more subtle nuances of everyday experience and to extend and deepen our understanding of the *wide variety* of alterations of experience that constitute the realm of "defenses." The evolution of psychoanalytic thought from as early as 1920 to the present is an evolution of the increasing appreciation that *not being conscious* is not the be-all and end-all it was originally thought to be. What psychoanalysis and dynamic psychotherapy are most of all about is the restricting, foreshortening, and fragmenting (that is, dissociating) of experience that results from the pressures of anxiety, guilt, shame, or the need to retain important relational ties. Put differently, what is crucial in the work is most often not what we *don't know* about ourselves, but what we *both* know *and* don't know, the ways in which certain things we "know" do not really influence very much what we do or what we feel.

Let me illustrate this way of viewing dissociation with an example (see Wachtel, 2005b, for more details about the case and its theoretical implications). One of the very first patients I was assigned as a beginning therapist was a woman in her twenties whose primary complaint was what seemed to be a "hysterical" tendency to gag severely when eating solid food. Doctors could find no physical basis for her difficulties, but eating solid food was extremely difficult for her. Other than liquids, virtually the only food she could swallow without great distress and difficulty was M&M's, which she ate a great deal of.

Only after many months of treatment did she mention that struggles over food were a central feature of her childhood, that her mother was morbidly obese, and that the mother's preoccupation with her daughter not eating candy in particular led the patient, as a young girl, to hide candy under her pillow and indulge in this secret pleasure at night under the covers. It will certainly not surprise a sophisticated readership to learn that the food most often smuggled into bed in this fashion was M&M's.

I wondered then—as I do still today—whether my not hearing anything at all about this before quite a few months had gone by was due to my inexperience at the time. But I also was struck at the time by what seemed to be the dramatic confirmation of the theory of repression provided by this turn of events. As a graduate student, I had learned that significant childhood experiences could be cast into the unconscious, able to be recovered only by extensive psychotherapeutic work. This case seemed to offer an example par excellence. What else but the theory of repression could account for the disappearance of a memory so strikingly relevant to her difficulties and its reappearance only after months of therapeutic work?

My patient's experience of these events, however, was quite different. When I commented (in the overly stilted and restrained fashion that was taught to young therapists in those days) that it was "interesting" that such a powerfully relevant memory had taken so many months to emerge, she did not find it very interesting at all. My aim was to initiate a process of her recognizing that she had been actively keeping certain thoughts and memories out of her awareness. But the patient's response to my comment took me aback. Rather than being struck by her having "forgotten" something so obviously relevant, she stated matter-of-factly, "I could have told you all along. I hadn't forgotten it, it just didn't occur to me as relevant when we were talking earlier."

As I stated in my previous discussion of this case, I do not think she was lying. But I do not think she was telling the full truth either. She was telling as much of the truth as she had access to. Had I asked her, "Did you and your mother struggle over food when you were a child, and were M&M's a central part of that struggle?", I have no doubt she would have answered yes, and could have told me about at least the general outlines of what transpired. Thus it was *not* something that she "could not remember." Rather, what she could not do was *have that memory occur to her spontaneously.* What was repressed, one might say, was not the content per se but the associational network.

In considering this experience, it is worth recalling a passage from Freud's (1914a) important paper "Remembering, Repeating, and Working Through":

> Forgetting impressions, scenes or experiences nearly always reduces itself to shutting them off [translated in the *Collected Papers*, where I first read the passage, as "*dissociation*" of them]. When the patient talks about these "forgotten" things he seldom fails to add: "As a matter of fact I've always known it; only I've never thought of it." He often expresses disappointment at the fact that not enough things come into his head that he can call "forgotten"—that he has never thought of since they happened. (p. 148)

This passage is a striking one to find in Freud, because it seems to contradict the idea, so central in much of his thinking and writing, of the unconscious as a bounded, inaccessible realm apart from consciousness. But if one shifts from the theory of repression as the cornerstone of psychoanalytic thought (Freud, 1914b) and the archaeological model of uncovering buried material as the key aim, Freud's comment is not so surprising. If one takes a closer look at the actual observations that characterize most psychoanalytic sessions, they point to far greater complexity than is captured by a vision of two overarching systems (whether conscious/preconscious versus unconscious or ego versus id) or by a sharp distinction between more or less permanently *accessible* material and more or less permanently *unconscious* material.[11] Actual session material usually looks more like Davies's (1996) account, in which "we deal not with one unconscious, but with multiple levels of consciousness and unconsciousness—a mul-

---

[11] It may be noted that Freud (e.g., 1915b) too depicted repression as a process that is "variable," "specific," and "mobile." But he was referring primarily to a shifting of the edge or boundary between two fairly discrete systems, enabling material that is generally part of the unconscious to occasionally find its way into consciousness, not to a multifaceted organization of multiple parallel processes, interconnections, and disconnections.

tiply organized, associationally linked network of meaning attribution and understanding" (p. 562). Mental contents are not simply "conscious" or "unconscious"; they are capable of being experienced and of being articulated and elaborated to *varying degrees*, depending on one's particular state of mind and on the situational, relational, and cultural context.

This way of thinking does not mean that the concept of the unconscious is adulterated or abandoned, though it requires that it be modified and understood in a more complex fashion. There *are* certain thoughts and experiences that are very hard for the person to notice, acknowledge, or accept as part of him, and some that are scarcely *ever* acknowledged or admitted to awareness at all. Freud's distinction between mental contents that are simply out of awareness at the moment (the preconscious) and those actively being defended against and avoided (the dynamic unconscious) remains of crucial importance. But the range of ways that potentially disturbing experiences are warded off and the many different forms and degrees of awareness and articulation goes well beyond any simple dichotomy between conscious (or preconscious) on the one hand and unconscious or dynamically unconscious on the other. The overall picture of what is actually observed clinically resembles much more closely the account of unformulated experience offered by Stern (1997), the phenomenologically articulated version of psychoanalysis introduced by Stolorow, Atwood, and Orange (e.g., Atwood & Stolorow, 1984; Stolorow & Atwood, 1984, 1992; Orange et al., 1997), and the depictions by Shapiro (e.g., 1965, 1981, 1989, 2000) of consciousness itself as having so many varied qualities and gradations of articulation that it virtually subsumes the classical view of conscious and unconscious (Wachtel, 1982b).

Overall, much as Freud acknowledged in the passage quoted above from "Remembering, Repeating, and Working Through," in psychoanalytic or psychotherapeutic work, we do not so much dig up material that has never been consciously experienced before, or that has been thoroughly banned from consciousness since the day it was buried, as we enable material that has, up till now, been but dimly or occasionally grasped or experienced to be more readily and thoroughly acknowledged, elaborated, and accepted. Moreover, apropos the expanded understanding of dissociation I am discussing in this section, not only does the work aim to further the *articulation* of the experience but to enhance the *connections* between that articulation and *other* experiences that have been heretofore mysterious, misunderstood, or difficult to modify. Overcoming dissociation means restoring, or enhancing, the capacity to be *moved* by what one sees or understands, both in the sense of being moved emotionally and in the sense of being moved to action.

Freud's original concept of defense, which was so centered on the particular defense of repression, was a product of the archaeological model and of his aspirations as a discoverer. Something was buried and hidden and had to be unearthed. Over time, Freud himself began to modify this view. With further experience of how patients responded to his interpretations, the dichotomous distinction between what is accessible to consciousness and what is dammed up, walled off, sealed away, began to shift to a more detailed understanding of the complex phenomenology of defenses, the ways in which people keep things from disturbing them, not just by keeping them out of consciousness, but by *muting* them, keeping them from having their full *emotional meaning* registered, acting without noticing or noticing without acting, reexplaining and rationalizing, and so on. Freud showed some recognition of these phenomena almost from the very beginning of psychoanalysis, but much in the very fashion being discussed here with regard to our patients, his appreciation of their implications was fluctuating and dependent on context (in this case very largely on the context of what theoretical point Freud was focused on making). It was with *The Ego and the Id* (Freud, 1923), and then with Anna Freud's (1936) *The Ego and the Mechanisms of Defense,* that the figure and ground between the older more dichotomous account of conscious and unconscious and the newer, more differentiated account began noticeably to shift. Ego psychology became a new foundation from which further departures from the older simple dichotomy between conscious and unconscious could build.

But ego psychology continued to emphasize "mechanisms" of defense, and it continued, in large measure, to assume that the "real" representations and memories were "down there," disguised but recoverable. It remained for later theorists, mostly from the emerging relational point of view, to take the next step of converting psychoanalysis from a mechanistic account to a phenomenological one. In this, a central feature was the more differentiated understanding of *dissociation* and of the ways in which, depending on the particular context and particular state of the relational or intersubjective field, different configurations of thought, feeling, and self and object representation will be placed in the foreground or the background and will be articulated to varying degrees.

DISSOCIATION, PHENOMENOLOGY, AND SUBJECTIVITY

What the foregoing considerations point to is that, in contrast to much of the rhetoric that long dominated psychoanalytic discourse, psychoanalytically oriented clinical work is most aptly characterized as a particular and distinctive form of phenomenological inquiry (see in this regard Atwood & Stolorow, 1984; Basescu, 1972; Orange, Stolorow, & Atwood, 1998; Stolorow & Atwood, 1984, 1992; Stolorow, Orange, & Atwood, 2001a). What good psychoanalytic clinicians do is not to dive beneath the surface of the patient's experience to tell him ("interpret") what he is *really* feeling, but to discover what is being excluded from consciousness by attending in meticulous detail to the patient's *experienced* subjectivity. This is a mode of listening that in some ways parallels what is characteristic of *any* good listener, but it is distinguished from more everyday forms of listening by a central concern with attending to what *does not* appear in consciousness, as well as to what is muted, experienced without the expected affect, or given a particular spin that seems not to be consonant with how the person is behaving or with other aspects of what he is experiencing.

Such a view of psychoanalytic work constitutes, in essence, a bringing into more explicit focus what has long been at the heart of clinical practice but has been obscured by the influence of the archaeological model, with its images of the really crucial material as deeply buried, as well as by the abstractions and reifications that were the legacy of Freud's metapsychology. Those images and abstractions implied that the aim of the work was to bypass the "superficial" conscious experience of the patient in order to discover and interpret what lies below. But with the possible exception of traditional Kleinian practice, most clinical work from a psychoanalytic perspective has really *not* been about interpreting material that until the analyst's intervention had been thoroughly and permanently barred from conscious experience (recall the quote from Freud earlier in this chapter regarding the infrequency with which patients recall thoughts or experiences that had been thoroughly forgotten or inaccessible previously). Rather, it has entailed tracking, in sensitive and finely detailed fashion, the patient's actual experience and using that very effort as the foundation for achieving greater knowledge of what is *not* conscious.

The aim of the psychoanalytic clinician is to enter into the patient's world, but it is not an entering in the sense of going "inside" a realm that has been hidden behind a wall and is thoroughly inaccessible to conscious experience. It is an empathic *immersion in* the patient's experience, an immersion that leaves the patient feeling *understood*, not "interpreted" (see Bromberg, 1993, and Stolorow et al., 1987, for a similar view of the psychoanalytic process).

It is consciousness itself that is the royal road to the unconscious. It is through attending to the variable qualities and contents of consciousness, noticing what comes into focus sharply, what is experienced in only a dim or blurry fashion, when the focus and quality of conscious experience shifts, either abruptly or subtly, when the patient's subjective experience seems wholehearted and when it is hedged, muted, or affectless, and so forth that the clinician comes to understand the nature of what is being defended against. The unconscious is not so much a *hidden* realm, fully formed and lying unseen below, but rather an *unarticulated* set of potentials for fuller experience, a set of proclivities and inclinations that guide and shape experience without the patient's fully elaborating, acknowledging, or endorsing them (cf. Stern, 1997). Understanding of the unconscious is always an inference based on close study of the vagaries of consciousness.

The move toward a greater and more comfortable embrace of phenomenology, as Stolorow (1997b) has pointed out, is not a move away from concern with the unconscious, but, much as I have already discussed, a *reconceptualization* of the unconscious, a reconceptualization closely related to the shift in emphasis from repression to dissociation that has been one of the concerns of this chapter. The new focus on multiple, complex, and shifting degrees of access to and articulation of experience derives from closer attention to the actual experiences of patients rather than a vision of the dynamic unconscious as a "subterranean locale" (Stolorow et al., 2001b, p. 44) and the therapeutic process as "an archaeological excavation of ever deeper layers of an isolated and substantialized unconscious mind" (Stolorow et al., 2001b, p. 47). The reader can readily see the close parallels between this emerging point of view and the critique of the archaeological model presented in the previous chapter.

Increasingly, psychoanalytic clinicians, instead of *diving under* the person's experience, guided by a normative and standardized theory, are *diving into* that experience. Instead of attempting to demonstrate to the patient how he is *deceiving* himself, they aim to invite him to see how he is *restricting* himself, how some aspects of his experience are not being given the same respect, attention, or articulation as others. In that sense, rather than *dismissing* conscious experience as but a cover for what is "really" underneath, they attempt more fully to *explore* conscious experience, and in the process to expand and deepen it (cf. Shapiro, 1981, 1989, 2000).

Conscious experience, the "surface" of the psyche, is, for many clinicians, no longer viewed as just the husk to be discarded in order to go "deeper." The surface may provide its own deep insight into the person's psychology, an insight that is at least as important and profound as that associated with exploration of the underlying meaning. Consider, for example, the following two dreams, similar in that in both the "latent content" may be seen to include a symbolic representation of the penis, but significantly different in their implications and in the larger psychological meaning they convey. In one dream, the male patient is waving a sword triumphantly and then the scene shifts and a jet plane is taking off and "piercing the sky." In the second dream, a different male patient *also* dreams of a jet plane taking off, but then continues the dream with the plane losing attitude and crashing into a swamp. To "interpret" that the plane (or the sword) is a penis, and the swamp a vagina loses much of the meaning of the dream. The more profound meaning, we might say, lies not in the "latent content," but in the *surface* qualities of the descriptions. There is a big difference between a penis that pierces the sky and one that "loses altitude" and lands in a swamp. Similarly, there is a huge difference between a "vagina" that is represented by a swamp and one that is symbolically represented by "a cozy nest, warm and snuggly" (an element from still another male patient's dream). We might well anticipate that the patient's sense of self, sex life, and relations with women will be considerably different in the different cases. (See also in this connection Erikson's [1954] illuminating discussion of one of Freud's most intensely examined dreams.)

The rhetoric that for many years was closely associated with the defense of traditional psychoanalytic approaches to theory and practice depicts such emphasis on the details of conscious experience as a retreat from the "hard-won" insights Freud achieved against great resistance. But a strong case can be made that it is the archaeological mode of thought and the associated rush to *dig under* conscious experience that is the retreat—a retreat from what is perhaps the chief virtue of the psychoanalytic method, its intense attention to and immersion in the subjective world of the other. The rush to interpret the "underlying" fantasy is perhaps most evident in traditional Kleinian practice, but it is a temptation that at one time or another probably ensnares almost every psychoanalytically informed clinician, a gravitational pull exerted by theory on practice that requires both awareness and sophistication to resist.

What, in actual practice, good psychoanalytic clinicians do most of all is explore the subtle nuances of subjective experience, and it is that very attention to what *is* experienced that enables them better to understand what is being omitted. From such a vantage point, at once phenomenological and psychoanalytic, Stolorow (1997b, p. 341) has pointed out that "the very boundary between conscious and unconscious is . . . a fluid and evershifting one, a product of the changing responsiveness of the surround to different regions of the child's emotional experience."[12] In strikingly similar fashion, from the vantage point of multiple self-states, Davies (1996) emphasizes that "what is conscious and what is unconscious at any particular point in time will emerge fluidly out of the particular constellation of self- and object-related experience that crystallizes in the foreground of interpersonal experience at any given moment" (p. 562). This idea of a fluid boundary between what is conscious and what is unconscious, Stolorow and Atwood (1989) point out, "contrasts sharply with the traditional notion of the repression barrier as a fixed intrapsychic structure, 'a sharp and final division' (Freud, 1915a) separating conscious and unconscious contents" (p. 369).

Putting these various observations together, we may say that close attention to the actual experiences of people in psychoanalytic sessions reveals the traditional conception of the unconscious as a separate, cordoned-off region of the mind to be a rather crude conceptual tool. It is an idea that was of great value in the early years of psychoanalytic inquiry as an initial way to grasp a newly appreciated phenomenon, but it is insufficiently supple to provide an adequate account either of the aims of the dynamic psychotherapist or of the richly variegated nature of human experience and behavior in all its many contexts.

VARIETIES OF INTERSUBJECTIVITY

The phenomenological emphasis of Stolorow, Atwood, and Orange has been closely linked with another concept that has been central to the entire evolution of the relational movement—intersubjectivity. As

---

[12] I would add that this depiction holds for the adult as well as for the child.

Stolorow et al. (2001a) note, however, the term "intersubjectivity" has been used in distinctively different ways that at times imply and derive from quite different theoretical positions. Benjamin's (1990) "object relations" version of intersubjectivity, Ogden's (1994) neo-Kleinian version, and Orange et al.'s (1997) contextual version have much in common, but they also differ in sometimes important ways.

A key feature of Benjamin's version of intersubjectivity is her emphasis on the developmental thrust toward—and simultaneous resistance to—recognizing the other as a fully human *subject,* a center of agency, hope, and feeling. For her, intersubjectivity "refers to that zone of experience or theory in which the other is not merely the object of the ego's need/drive or cognition/perception, but has a separate and equivalent center of self" (Benjamin, 1990, p. 35). In contrast to many other theorists who identify strongly with the object relations tradition, Benjamin, while attentive to the dimensions of human experience in which we do experience and treat other people as objects, addresses the limitations of a theoretical vision in which all human relations are conceptualized as "object" relations. She argues that "the unfortunate tendency to collapse other subjects into objects ... is a symptom of the very problems in psychoanalysis that a relational theory should aim to cure" (p. 34). In a felicitous linguistic play with a famous passage from Freud, she contends that "the inquiry into the intersubjective dimensions of the analytic encounter would aim to change our theory and practice so that *'where objects were, subjects must be'*" (p. 34, italics added).

Benjamin also maintains, as an essential feature of her approach to intersubjectivity, that recognizing the other as a subject, as an experiencing being and a center of agency, is essential for the first person to fully experience *his or her own* subjectivity (see also Benjamin, 1988, 1996, 1997). But, much as in the important work of Fonagy and his colleagues on the very similar concepts of mentalization and reflective function (e.g., Fonagy, 2000, 2002; Fonagy & Target, 1997, 1998; Fonagy et al., 2002, 2003), she emphasizes that this capacity is a developmental achievement and one that is often "only unevenly realized" (p. 35).

In presenting her object relations version of intersubjectivity, Benjamin suggests that the defining task of relational theorizing is "to account both for the pervasive effects of human relationships on psychic development and for the equally ubiquitous effects of internal psychic mechanisms and fantasies in shaping psychological life and interaction" (Benjamin, 1990, p. 35). This conception of the theoretical agenda of the relational paradigm converges significantly with the core aim of the cyclical psychodynamic point of view discussed in the last chapter and the analysis in terms of schemas, assimilation, and accommodation discussed in this one. But there are important differences as well between the cyclical psychodynamic viewpoint and Benjamin's version of intersubjectivity, which she describes as "an object relations perspective based on the complementarity of intrapsychic and intersubjective aspects of self-development" (p. 33).

In contrast, I would argue that the concept of complementarity is only a way station between the views Benjamin rightly criticizes (those that view as *dichotomous and opposing* perspectives such notions as drive and object relations, ego and id, or intrapsychic and interpersonal) and a more thoroughly integrated view in which the impact of the actual others in our lives and the role of our ongoing and/or preexisting psychological structures and tendencies are understood not just as "complementary," but as *mutually constitutive.* Unlike, say, the wave or particle views of matter, which, at least at our present stage of knowledge, do require a conception of complementarity to incorporate all the observations, the roles of so-called "inner" and "outer" determinants *appear* to be competing or contradictory only because of certain characteristics of the original conceptual foundation of psychoanalytic thought. Stolorow et al. (2001a) have described one of those characteristics as a residual Cartesianism that places limits on the degree to which some relational viewpoints are able to transcend the subject–object dichotomy.

Relational theories converge in their pursuit of the general agenda that Benjamin describes—accounting for "the pervasive effects of human relationships on psychic development and for the equally ubiquitous effects of internal psychic mechanisms and fantasies"—but they *differ* in the details of how they approach the task. In part, these differences follow from not very well appreciated ambiguities in the terms and concepts that embody Benjamin's seemingly consensual statement. One such ambiguity lies in the word *development.* Does this refer only to *early* development, before the experiences with others become "internalized"? In this direction lie relational theories that retain significant elements of the archaeological model of buried psychological strata inaccessible to the influences of more contemporary experiences (which through their lens appear to be "superficial").[13] The theoretical

---

[13] Benjamin's (1990) concern that without "sustaining contradiction" between the intrapsychic and the intersubjective what results is "a triumph of the external" perhaps reflects a variant of this view.

perspectives I described in Chapter 4 as "excluded middle" theories fit in this category. In contrast are those theories that conceive of development as a process of continuous construction (Zeanah et al., 1989), in which the structures of psychological life are constantly evolving in relation to their transactions with new experiences, even as they powerfully shape and influence those new experiences (see, e.g., the discussion above of schemas, assimilation, and accommodation).

Similarly, what precisely is meant by "internal" psychic mechanisms? This is one of those tropes that has become so utterly familiar in psychoanalytic discourse that it is no longer really noticed or interrogated theoretically. Is the term understood merely as a way of indicating that the structures belong to or are a characteristic or property of a particular individual, brought with him from situation to situation, rather than his experience being solely and *reactively* a product of the intersubjective field? Such an understanding of "internal," as discussed in previous chapters, is perfectly consonant with the version of relational thinking that informs this book. As Mitchell (1993a) and Schafer (1976) have pointed out, however, spatial metaphors are both pervasive in psychoanalytic thought and potentially problematic. "Internal" is one such spatial metaphor, and if not examined closely, it can readily lead to an unwitting equation of "inside" with "buffered from the influence of 'external' events." If "internal" is understood in *this* fashion, it contrasts sharply with the understanding of *contextual* structures at the heart of the cyclical psychodynamic point of view,[14] with the contextual form of intersubjectivity emphasized by Stolorow, Atwood, and Orange (1999; Orange et al., 1997; Stolorow et al., 2001b), and with the intersubjective and contextual emphasis of much theorizing on multiple self-states.

One unusual feature of the particular version of intersubjectivity elaborated by Stolorow and his colleagues, distinguishing them from most other leading psychoanalytic writers, is their highlighting of the ways in which the unconscious influences on our experience and behavior include not just motives or thoughts that are repressed or otherwise defended against (the traditional dynamic unconscious), but the structures of meaning and interpretation through which we apprehend the world, which *also* are often unable to be articulated and consciously experienced—and which have equally momentous consequences. As they put it:

---

[14] See also the discussions of the contextual unconscious in Wachtel and Wachtel (1986) and of the contextual self in Wachtel (1995).

In the absence of reflection, a person is unaware of his role as a constitutive subject in elaborating his personal reality. The world in which he lives and moves presents itself as though it were something independently and objectively real. The patterning and thematizing of events that uniquely characterize his personal reality are thus seen *as if they were properties of those events rather than products of his own subjective interpretations and constructions.* Psychoanalytic therapy can be viewed as a procedure through which a patient acquires reflective knowledge of this unconscious structuring activity. (Stolorow & Atwood, 1984, p. 101, italics added)

This expansion of the meaning of clinically relevant unconscious processes—including as a central feature of the work not just the traditional repressed or dynamic unconscious but the *unconscious organizing principles* (which *may not* be repressed, but still require extensive exploration to enable the person to modify the problematic patterns of his life)—converges with the emphasis of the Boston Process of Change Study Group (e.g., Lyons-Ruth, 1998, 1999; Stern et al., 1998; Stern, 2004) on "implicit relational knowing" (see Chapter 10). It offers as well an important point of convergence between the psychoanalytic point of view and the discoveries of contemporary cognitive science, which highlights the critical and pervasive role of mental processes that are unconscious but not repressed (cf. Bucci, 2000; Eagle, 1987; Hassin, Ulemann, & Bargh, 2006; Kihlstrom, 1984, 1987; Shevrin, 1992).

Stolorow and Atwood differ from the vantage point of most cognitive science research, however, in several important respects. Where much of the Zeitgeist of contemporary cognitive science is explicitly or implicitly antipsychoanalytic and distinguishes sharply between its conception of unconscious or implicit processes and that of psychoanalysis (e.g., O'Brien & Jureidini, 2002), Stolorow and Atwood conceptualize these fundamental organizing processes not as an *alternative* to the psychoanalytic unconscious but as a complementary and *additional* factor in our mental life. Additionally, rather than viewing these implicit processes as neural substrates that are virtually impossible to notice or reflect upon, Stolorow and Atwood take as one important goal of the therapeutic process to help the person achieve at least some degree of awareness of these organizing structures and the way they shape our experience of the world and our perceptions of the options available to us. Finally, in a view that particularly unites them with other thinkers in the broad relational spectrum, their understanding of these organizing structures is not as residing inside an isolated mind or brain but as inherently and continuously intersubjective.

INTERSUBJECTIVITY AND ACTION

In attempting to further illuminate the relation between the cyclical psychodynamic version of relational theory depicted in the last chapter and the related theories discussed in this one, it is clarifying to consider the particularly central role of *action* in cyclical psychodynamic theory. From a cyclical psychodynamic vantage point, intersubjectivity is evident not only in the realm of perception, representation, or subjective experience but, equally importantly, in the realm of action. No theorist, of course, would deny that our actions make a difference in our lives or that the ways that others react to us are very strongly influenced by the ways we act toward them. But the legacies of both the phenomenological tradition and the long-standing intrapsychic emphasis of psychoanalytic thought have given a primary focus to the ways that people *perceive* and *experience.* In the cyclical psychodynamic approach to relational theory and practice, there is an explicit emphasis on complementing this focus with an equal focus on the crucial role of people's mutual *actions* in the intersubjective field.

Attention to the dynamic systems that constitute the nature of our living-in-the-world (see, e.g., Ghent, 2002; Stolorow, 1997a, 1997b, 1997c; Thelen & Smith, 1994; Wachtel & Wachtel, 1986; Wachtel, 1997) highlights the role of people's mutual actions and interactions in creating and maintaining the patterns in their lives. The role of actions, moreover, is critical not only in maintaining overt *behavioral* patterns but also in the patterns of representation and subjective experience that have more typically been at the center of psychoanalytic discourse. Just as our behavior is determined by the ways we unconsciously construct the world, the ways we construct the world are constantly being modified or maintained by the events we encounter from moment to moment, events that in significant measure we also *bring about* through our behavior (and, to complete the circle, through the subjective interpretations that *lead us* to act in the way we do). It is not a matter of one or the other, of one being more important or fundamental, but of their being part and parcel of a single process of *living in the world.*[15]

---

[15] It should be clear that when I refer to a "single process" I am not negating the idea I emphasized earlier—the very considerable variability in behavior and experience from context to context. Rather, in referring to a "single process" I am pointing to the unity—the intertwinedness, if you will—of the *causal* factors, the way in which perception, affect, motivation, existing representations, *and* action are all part of one continuous loop that can simultaneously be described as stable and predictable and as constantly evolving.

This is not to place actions at the center and treat representations and subjective experience as peripheral or to posit a one-directional view of cause and effect with actions as cause and self and object representations as effects. Such an account would be as simplistic, incomplete, and inaccurate as a focus that is exclusively on the causal role of "internal" experience and that *leaves out* the crucial role of actions (a much more common state of affairs in psychoanalytic discourse, even if rarely avowed explicitly). What is crucial, from a cyclical psychodynamic vantage point, is the mutual, *bidirectional* interplay between subjective experience and mental structures on the one hand and actions in the real world on the other.

We do not persist in our old ways of perceiving and experiencing simply because they have been "internalized" (and thenceforth are there because they are there). That persistence requires a repeated set of *transactions* with others, transactions in which one's own behavior—and its role in eliciting particular behaviors from the other—is crucial. To reprise the terminology I introduced earlier, understanding the persistence of the key patterns in people's lives requires an understanding of the ways in which we induce others (usually without awareness or understanding of the process) to play the role of "accomplices" in those patterns. A purely "internal" accounting does not address this dynamic. Rather, a full and adequate account of the individual as a person *living-in-the-world* is an account in which everyday actions and what might be called deep subjectivity are equally present but in which it is acknowledged that we do not really understand either without understanding the other. The case of Richard described in the last chapter and the further case material in the chapters that follow are illustrations of how this way of thinking proceeds in understanding individual human beings and the lives they lead.

8

■ ■ ■ ■ ■

Exploration, Support,
Self-Acceptance, and the
"School of Suspicion"

In the last chapter, I emphasized the importance of *acceptance* in effective clinical work and related the emergence of a more accepting approach toward the patient to a number of key concepts in the evolving relational point of view. In this chapter, I want to further articulate the nature of a clinical approach that is rooted in promoting the patient's self-acceptance and reappropriation of cast-off or rejected aspects of the self. In so doing, I will discuss some of the confusions that have existed in the field for many years regarding the nature of "support" in psychotherapy and will examine how an emphasis on a more accepting and less adversarial clinical stance intersects with a number of prominent trends in relational thought.

In a provocative depiction of the experience of the psychotherapy patient, Leston Havens has commented, "In the current interpretive climate of much psychotherapeutic work, patients sit waiting for the next insight with their fists clenched. Small wonder, for it is rarely good news" (1986, p. 78). Havens's description may have a touch of humorous exaggeration, but it also was a serious attempt to address a problematic feature of the way that the therapeutic process was conceived and undertaken by many therapists. For many years, psychotherapy was approached as a largely adversarial process. The patient's resistances were assumed to be strong and pervasive, however cooperative his manifest attitude might appear. As a consequence, efforts on the therapist's part to act in ways that might be viewed as kindly or helpful in any other context were seen as aiding the resistance and thus impeding the progress of the therapy. Certainly not all therapists operating from traditional assumptions were cold and distant, but ideas of neutrality and anonymity, images of the therapist as like a mirror or a surgeon (Freud, 1912a), and prohibitions against "gratifying" the patient's regressive longings all contributed to significant limitations on the therapist's simple human responsiveness.

A key contribution of the relational movement in psychotherapy, from its earliest roots in the work of writers such as Ferenczi, Fairbairn, and Winnicott, to its most recent formulations in the hands of contemporary relational theorists, has been an alternative, less adversarial and more nurturant and affirmative vision for the conduct of psychotherapy. Of course, not all relationally oriented therapists practice in the same fashion. The emphasis by Fairbairn on the therapist as providing "an actual relationship with a reliable and beneficent parental figure" (1958, p. 377), for example, or the emphasis by Winnicott (1960) on "holding" and the provision of needed relational experiences, comport much more closely with the approach described here than do, say, Kleinian attempts to tell the patient about his supposedly primitive and destructive inclinations toward his objects.[1]

Regarding the latter, Orbach (2004), a prominent British proponent of the relational point of view, provides a particularly scathing description:

> Returning to live and work in the United Kingdom (in 1984 in the heyday of Kleinian practice) I discovered that the patient—for much of British analysis—had become not so much an individual to be engaged with, as someone whose defense structure needed to be excavated to show the patient how much of his or her internal world was beset by envy and destructiveness. . . . The countertransference material was evaluated for what the patient "did," and "put into"; for how he or she "showed contempt" or "attacked" the analyst or the analysis. I got the feeling that there was a maddening kind of "got-

---

[1] So too do more recent relational contributions such as those of Mitchell (1988a, 1993a), Frank (1999), Fosshage (2003a, 2004), Aron (1996), Stern (1997), Maroda (1999, 2002, 2004), Hoffman (1998), and many others.

cha" operating. The patient, who invariably didn't know the rules of therapy, would somehow transgress them. He or she would comment on the books on the therapist's shelves (envy of the analyst's knowledge or distrust of the analyst's capacity to think without props), say hello on bumping into the therapist in the street (invading and inappropriate), talk too much (controlling the space), talk too little (not allowing anything to penetrate), feel too much (being unable to think), or not have sufficient affect (defending against desperation, devastation, depression), compliment the therapist for how the therapy was helping (seductive and avoiding), arrive early (overanxious) or late (controlling), or induce in the therapist the desire to care for him or her (manipulating the therapist)—all of which were inevitably interpreted as evidence of [patients'] defenses against being in therapy in the way the analyst wanted them to be. (p. 398)

One reads this rather shocking account with the fervent hope that it is an exaggeration; Orbach clearly does not believe it to be so. She offers it as the background for her own embrace, as a welcome and urgently needed alternative, of the emerging relational point of view as it was being developed by Mitchell and others in the United States. It serves as well as a vivid representation of the kind of clinical approach—*whatever* theoretical label is applied to it—that this chapter (and this entire book) is devoted to challenging and moving beyond. But it is important to be clear that it is not only Kleinian analysts who can manifest perhaps unwitting cruelty in the service of confronting the patient with the truth they believe he has disowned. The unacknowledged tone of reprimand in clinical interpretations is widespread in our field (see Wachtel, 1993; Wile, 1984), and is by no means absent in the work of theorists and therapists who are part of the overall relational synthesis. And, of course, the Kleinian point of view is itself widely regarded as a part of that synthesis, and has influenced in significant (and not always sufficiently examined) ways the language and assumptions of the entire spectrum of object relations theorists and practitioners.

Another caveat to bear in mind in addressing the differences between traditional and relational ways of approaching clinical work is that, at the other end of the spectrum, classical or Freudian accounts of the therapeutic process also exhibit quite considerable diversity of thought and practice. The aim of this book is to provide an alternative to the adversarial and withholding mindset that has falsely been equated with being deeply exploratory. That mindset does seem to me to be more prevalent in classical than in relational practice. But there are many noteworthy contributions from Freudian analysts that reflect the humane edge of the classical approach and its continuing efforts to extend clinical practice well beyond the easily caricaturable formulations that were once so prevalent. These include Loewald's (1960) depiction of the analyst as a new, good object, Stone's (1961) emphasis on "physicianly concern," Schafer's (1983) discussions of the "conditions of safety" required for good psychoanalytic work, and Wallerstein's thoughtful examinations of the ways that the findings of the Menninger research project require modifications of traditional psychoanalytic assumptions about clinical technique (e.g., Wallerstein, 1988, 1989). Without appreciation of these and many other advances within the Freudian paradigm, the critical dialogue between classical and relational points of view is reduced to a falsely dichotomous polemic.

Nonetheless, it is necessary to point out that the mainstream Freudian paradigm has manifested considerable ambivalence toward carrying through on its most humane and forward-looking insights. In a statement that Frank (2005) notes is "one of the most widely quoted passages in all of psychoanalysis," Anna Freud (1954) comments that

> we should leave room somewhere for the realization that analyst and patient are also two real people, of equal adult status, in a real personal relationship to each other. I wonder whether our—at times complete—neglect of this side of the matter is not responsible for some of the hostile reactions which we get from our patients and which we are apt to ascribe to "true transference" only. But these are technically subversive thoughts and ought to be "handled with care." (pp. 618–619)

That such acknowledgment of the reality of the analyst's presence and impact as a person and of a personal relationship between two equals should feel so "subversive" and need to be "handled with care" speaks volumes about the difficulties psychoanalysis has had in fully incorporating its own most advanced understandings of what is really transpiring in the room and of what is required for a genuinely therapeutic result to be achieved. It will be apparent as I proceed that, reflecting my immersion in the alternative paradigm that is the topic of this book, I do not share this ambivalence regarding acknowledging the reality of my participation. Nor do I see any difficulties in principle, whether clinical or theoretical, in acknowledging the relationship between myself and the patient or in offering support, encouragement, or any of the other elements that, in almost every other form of human relationship, contribute to the well-being of both parties. There are, however, ways in which the particular nature of a *therapeutic* relationship transforms in certain ways the meaning and nature of the support and encouragement that are given. In particular, it is important that my emphasis on creating a more humane, "present," and supportive environment in the therapy not be misread as glossing over or avoiding the more difficult aspects of the patient's life, his character, or the dilemmas he faces. Ultimately, the only way to be truly supportive and affirmative in the therapeutic context is to provide the patient with the experience of being fully understood, of having what at least *he* experiences as the dark side or the weak side acknowledged and known. Without this acknowledgment and recognition, what the therapist takes to be support or affirmation is likely to feel hollow to the patient. It may even leave the patient feeling less accepted than before, as the therapist's seeming avoidance of the "hard parts" is experienced (whether consciously or not) as proof that who the patient really is, what he *really* is like, is unacceptable.

The aim of the work I am describing is *to make room for the very thoughts and feelings that the patient finds most frightening and shameful.* This cannot be done if one attempts to "cover over" those thoughts and feelings. Rather, what is required is that patient and therapist together *immerse themselves* in these experiences, understand them, help them move from the often incipient and inchoate state in which they are presently represented (cf. Stern, 1997) toward a means of expression and articulation that enables the patient to confront the actual dilemmas he faces in his life. (See also in this latter regard Stolorow & Atwood, 1984.)

What I am advocating is thus not an avoidance of the "hard stuff," but rather, an understanding of how *better to get at* the hard stuff, or how better *to work with* the hard stuff; how, that is, to call the patient's attention to the hard stuff in ways that *make a difference* in his life. And that, I hope to show, requires promoting not merely insight (though insight is indeed important), but self-*acceptance*. It is not enough to *know* that one is feeling or wanting something, not enough, even, to know it "emotionally" rather than just "intellectually." For real therapeutic change to occur, the patient must become not just more conscious but less self-rejecting.

WHAT DOES IT MEAN TO BE SUPPORTIVE
IN PSYCHOTHERAPY?

Much of what I wish to convey in this chapter (and indeed, in this book) can be understood as about how to be more supportive of the patient while being deeply exploratory at the same time—or, conversely, how to be thoroughly and keenly exploratory while being warmly supportive and helpful at the same time. In the literature of psychotherapy, the terms "support" and "supportive" have usually been taken to imply an approach to therapeutic practice that is sharply contrasted with exploratory or "depth-oriented" therapeutic work. Support is usually conceived of as a trade-off, a *compromise.* It may be necessary, may even be the best clinical course for a particular patient, but it is usually understood as best because of some *limitation* that restricts the possibilities for more thoroughgoing clinical change. That limitation may lie in the patient's diagnosis (e.g., he may be viewed as too severely disturbed to bear the stresses of fully exploratory clinical work). It may lie in other dimensions of the patient's ego functioning, in his motivation for treatment, even in the cultural assumptions with which he enters the therapy. It may lie in restrictions due to time or economic resources or the patient's stated goals for the treatment. But in one way or another, the decision to undertake the therapy "supportively" is usually taken to mean that the breadth and depth of therapeutic change will be limited as a consequence. To borrow a phrase from the economists, support is usually viewed as a "regrettable necessity."

This attitude is widely evident in the literature. Werman (1984), in his book on the practice of supportive therapy, for example, states that "insight-oriented psychotherapy is based on the assumption that the patient possesses psychological equipment of adequate quality. . . . *In contrast, supportive psychotherapy assumes that the patient's psychological equipment is fundamentally inadequate* (p. 13, italics in original). Rockland (1989) states that "exploratory psychotherapy seeks to uncover unconscious mental contents, whereas supportive therapy covers them over" (p. 16). And in discussing a major Menninger Foundation research project—which found, to the surprise of most of the senior psychoanalysts and researchers who participated, that the expected superiority of "exploratory" therapy over "supportive" therapy did not materialize and that the expected sharp distinction between them in practice was absent as well—Wallerstein (1989) states as the rule which had typically guided clinical work undertaken from a psychoanalytic perspective (and which was assumed by the Menninger staff prior to the project) the following: "Be as expressive as you can be and as supportive as you *have to* be" (p. 203, italics added). Based on the findings of the Menninger project, Wallerstein raises serious questions about this widely held assumption.

An instance of the stance that support entails a compromise of therapeutic depth that is especially pertinent to the present discussion appears in Nancy McWilliams's influential textbook, *Psychoanalytic Diagnosis* (McWilliams, 1994). McWilliams's discussion of this issue is particularly interesting to consider here because her description of her work with more disturbed patients—which she explicitly contrasts with her approach to "neurotic-level" patients—is notably skillful and sensitive and because with *these* patients, she works in a way that is very consonant with the approach described in this book, whereas with "neurotic-level" patients she explicitly denies them—on theoretical grounds that are precisely those I wish to reexamine here—the kind of support she freely (and skillfully) offers her more disturbed patients.[2]

Discussing self-disclosure, for example, a topic I will take up in more detail in Chapter 11, McWilliams presents self-disclosure as a quintessential feature of therapy that is "supportive," and argues, in this context, that "the technique of supportive therapy is *diametrically opposite* that of uncovering therapy" (1994, p. 73, italics added), which she regards as the treatment of choice for patients who are less disturbed. With healthier patients, she argues, "one avoids emotional revelations so that the patient can notice and explore what his or her fantasies are about the therapist's affective state. With more troubled clients, one must be willing to be known" (p. 73).

In elaborating on this point—a very traditional one in the literature of psychoanalytically oriented therapies—McWilliams offers an interesting illustration that can help to clarify how the relational approach described in this book differs from more traditional ideas of how best to approach the therapeutic process. It is natural, she says,

> for the therapist to feel irritated with any patient at various points during treatment, especially when the person seems to be behaving self-destructively. A perception that one's therapist looks annoyed would be upsetting to any client, but it is mortally terrifying to more deeply

---

[2] As I will discuss below, the spirit of her more recent book, *Psychoanalytic Psychotherapy* (McWilliams, 2004), is significantly different, and reflects, I believe, a substantial shift in the central tendency in psychoanalytic thought in the ensuing decade.

troubled ones. If a neurotic-level person asks, "Are you mad at me?" one helpful response would be something along the lines of, "What are your thoughts and feelings about what it would mean if I were mad at you?" If the same query is made by a potentially psychotic patient, the therapeutic reply is something like, "You're very perceptive. I guess I *am* feeling a little irritation—as much with myself as with you. I'm a bit frustrated that I can't seem to help you as fast as I would like. What was your reason for asking?" (pp. 73–74)

What strikes me about this comparison is that her suggested response to the more disturbed patient seems a fine illustration of how a sensitively responsive therapist works, whereas the version suggested for the healthier patient seems cliched and deadened and much less likely to help or engage the patient. The comment she frames for the more disturbed patient acknowledges the *reality* of the patient's perception. It *validates* the patient's experience, and also, in its acknowledgment of the therapist's feelings, conveys the message that feelings of irritation or frustration (implicitly, on *either* party's part) need not destroy a relationship. It thus contributes to making such feelings less frightening, more able eventually to be assimilated and accepted by the patient as well.

The comment suggested for the healthier patient, in contrast, is much less forthcoming, displays much less of the "unwavering emotional honesty" that McWilliams notes is required for work with severely disturbed patients but seems to imply is not so essential with healthier patients. Besides not specifying what her irritation is in response to, the comment is also evasive, "cagey"—"What are your thoughts and feelings about what it would mean *if* I were mad at you?"

Why would a therapist view this last comment as superior to the more "supportive" version? In part the answer has to do with what I referred to in a previous chapter as the "default position," the implicit rules that long governed psychotherapeutic practice.[3] Because this way

---

[3] I refer through much of my discussion to the default position because I believe that it captures better than do terms like "classical" or "Freudian" the traditional clinical stance in comparison to which many therapists feel they must justify their innovations. The default position is *not* in fact exclusively a "Freudian" conception. One of the key issues I want to explore and make manifest is that much work that is undertaken from a relational perspective *also* faces the gravitational pull of the default position, and thus the "apolitical" name "default position" seems to me more suitable for the effort to clarify potential therapeutic options than does any term that is closely associated with a particular theoretical label.

of working has become, sometimes without being acknowledged as such, a kind of standard against which proper technique is measured, therapists feel they must justify deviating from it. Importantly, they often do not experience a similar burden of proof for maintaining it. It is true that the healthier patient can "take it" better, and thus that the *urgency* of providing support is greater for the more disturbed patient. But *everyone* is vulnerable in certain realms, and those realms happen to be the very ones patients come to therapy to work on. The feelings, perceptions, or inclinations we attempt to bring to the patient's awareness in exploratory psychotherapy are feelings that the patient feels acutely vulnerable about experiencing. If such feelings are *not* our focus, then we are looking in the wrong direction. Consequently, even though "neurotic-level" patients have greater ego strength or emotional resources in general, if we are *really* to work in depth, our work must go to where the patient has *not* felt able to tolerate the feeling, to where he has shrunk from the feeling for most of his life and feels acutely threatened by it.

To be sure, the less forthcoming (less "supportive") version of the therapist's response is not necessarily harmful to the therapeutic process. At times, it is all that is needed to facilitate the patient's explorations, and I certainly make comments of this sort not infrequently in the course of my own work. To cast *every* comment in the "supportive" forms I will champion in this book would feel very wordy and artificial. It would also start to sound monotonous to the patient. *Variety* in our language is essential if we want the patient to keep hearing what we are saying. Even the makers of car alarms have (to the great annoyance of city dwellers) learned that they must make the sounds *change* fairly frequently if we are not to tune them out; and even so, we all have had the experience of only "noticing that we had stopped noticing" when the alarm stops and the *silence* becomes a new, fresh stimulus. (Less often recognized is that this same caveat regarding variety in our therapeutic language holds for the persistent use of the "default" style of communicating as well. If we constantly "sound like a therapist" in our comments to our patients, what we say begins to lose its information value and to be attended to less acutely.)

But if "default"-type comments can be useful and acceptable as part of our overall repertoire, they are nonetheless often insufficiently robust in their capacity to aid the patient in accepting and assimilating conflicted inclinations and experiences. In much clinical writing and discourse, the implicit assumption seems to be that the more "strin-

gent" or restrained the therapist's approach is, the better, and the purpose of diagnostic assessment is very largely to find out how much the
patient *can take*.[4] And the assumption lying behind *that* assumption is
that greater stringency promotes greater insight and self-exploration
and is therefore ultimately in the patient's best interest. (Recall here
Wallerstein's rubric noted above: Be as expressive as you can be and as
supportive as you *have to* be.) From this vantage point, although more
disturbed patients *may not be able to tolerate* the rigors of this version
of exploratory therapy, and so must be offered a different approach,
the watered-down brew that must suffice with them should not be
offered as the "full strength" therapy to those whose constitution permits the stronger stuff.

In contrast, my own view is that the highly skillful, empathic way
McWilliams approached her psychotic patient in the example discussed
above—a way of working that is paralleled in different ways in other
examples in her discussion of "supportive" work—is what is most useful, with some variations, for almost all patients. McWilliams notes, for
example, in introducing her clinical vignette that "to prove that one is a
safe object is not so easy." But she argues that for a "neurotic-level"
patient, "it is usually enough to interpret the transference, that is to
comment on how the patient is mixing one up with some negative person from the past or some projected negative part of the self." With
severely disturbed patients, in contrast, "one must repeatedly *act* different from the patient's most frightening expectations." Here again, it
seems to me, McWilliams reserves for the most disturbed patients what
is of great value for *all* patients. As I will discuss in more detail in
Chapter 10, a wide range of theorists have pointed to the therapeutic
value—if not the therapeutic *necessity*—of providing patients with new
real experiences that differ from their problematic expectations (e.g.,
Fairbairn, 1958; Fosshage, 2005; Frank, 1999; Kohut, 1984; Loewald,
1960; Mitchell, 1993a; Stern, 1997; Weiss & Sampson, 1986; and, more
controversially, Alexander & French, 1946). These writers do not
restrict this aspect of the work to psychotic patients alone.

Based on her excellent recent book on psychoanalytic psychotherapy (McWilliams, 2004), I am confident that McWilliams herself also
provides—with *almost all* of her patients—a fuller emotional responsiveness than is embodied in the default position, and that providing a

---

[4] Stein (1979), for example, refers proudly to the "austere and demanding discipline" that
characterizes psychoanalytic work.

new kind of relational experience for her patients—that is, *acting differently*—is an important part of what she offers them. As she notes in that book, "That we are inherently social creatures who mature in a relational matrix and require relationship in order to change is suggested by the well-established empirical finding that the alliance between patient and therapist has more effect on the outcome of therapy than any other aspect of treatment that has been investigated so far" (McWilliams, 2004, p. 41; see also in this regard Frank, 1999, 2005, and Norcross, 2002).

This contrasts quite sharply with the view, expressed in her 1994 book, that if "supportive" interventions are applied with less disturbed patients, they place limits on the depth that the therapy can achieve, and that, indeed,

> both self-disclosure and advice giving are aspects of supportive therapy that make it *"irreversible."* If one has misdiagnosed the patient in the direction of underestimating his or her health, one cannot become more invisible again. Therapy can shift from an uncovering style to a more expressive one, or from expressive to more supportive treatment (when an initial diagnosis was too optimistic), but one cannot restore a potential to analyze transference when one has become more "real." (McWilliams, 1994, p. 76, italics added)

This idea of "irreversibly" ruining the treatment or "spoiling" the transference by being too real or too self-revealing harks back to the arguments of Gill (1954) discussed in Chapter 2. Much of this book (including the discussion in Chapter 2 of Gill's own very perceptive critiques of his previous position) is addressed to the limitations of such a point of view.

Thankfully, the process of therapy is considerably more "forgiving" than is implied by writers who portray an inviolable "frame" to the therapeutic process that is breached only at great peril to the work. Far from irreversibly restricting the progress of the therapy, the therapist's departures from grace, so to speak, are regarded by many contemporary theorists as at the very heart of what is therapeutic about what transpires. Influential discussions of the importance of addressing breaks in empathy (Kohut, 1984), resolving ruptures in the therapeutic relationship (Safran & Muran, 2000), or analyzing transference and countertransference enactments (Frank, 1999; Renik, 1993a, 1993b) all speak not only to the nonirreversibility of most therapist "errors" but to the *centrality* in the process of the therapy of addressing those very experiences. Put differently, such "errors" are not only inevitable but part of the "basic stuff" from which therapeutic change is fashioned. Indeed, in her more recent book on psychoanalytic psychotherapy, McWilliams (2004) makes this point herself, noting that "mistakes (or what clients experience as mistakes) are inevitable, no matter how experienced one is, and they can be addressed in a conversation that has considerably more therapeutic power than the (strictly hypothetical) 'ideal' response would have had" (p. 48). She further adds at a later point, "If one tries to be virtually invisible, the result will be either to behave so stiffly that the patient's comfort will suffer, or to lie to ourselves about what is possible, or both. . . . It may help to remind oneself that what we know empirically about therapeutic effectiveness is that outcome is much more highly correlated with an attachment to a vivid individual person than with the application of any specific techniques" (p. 182). (The word *vivid* here is especially noteworthy.)

The approach described in the present book is much closer to McWilliams's later conceptualization of the therapeutic process than to the position taken in her earlier discussion of the problematic implications of "support." The present approach derives from a different vision and a different set of assumptions than those that posit a sharp distinction between supportive and exploratory approaches. Central to the clinical approach described in this book is the assumption that being supportive and being exploratory or depth-oriented are not alternatives but complementarities, two sides of a single process. To the degree that either is lacking, the other suffers as well. With insufficient support, exploration is stymied, or it becomes an antitherapeutic and even potentially covertly sadistic activity. With insufficient exploration, support becomes a superficial exercise in reassurance that fails genuinely to reassure.

This is a quite different conception of support than is embodied in the typical discussion of "supportive" therapy in the literature, and it is essential that the reader be clear about this difference if she is to grasp what I am advocating. Far from implying "covering over" or "bolstering of defenses" conceived of as an activity that is in sharp contrast to the "*un*covering" that is the aim of more exploratory approaches, the support envisaged here entails the provision of *the necessary relational nutriment to make genuine insight possible*. The aim is to expand the patient's awareness and, at least as important, to expand his sense of who he is, what he feels, what he is capable of, what it is permissible for him to experience. My argument with more traditional approaches to attaining therapeutic insight is not with the value of insight per se, but with how it is approached.[5] My contention is that some of the features of traditional therapeutic practice that were designed to promote insight actually have the opposite effect, making it more *difficult* for the patient to experience the self-acceptance that is the very ground of insight and that is as well a crucial value in its own right.

In this respect, my position parallels in important ways Fairbairn's (1958) contention that "the actual relationship existing between the patient and the analyst as persons must be regarded as in itself constituting a therapeutic factor of prime importance. . . . [providing] the patient with an opportunity . . . to undergo a process of emotional development in the setting of an actual relationship with a reliable and beneficent parental figure" (p. 377). "Beneficent," it should be noted, is a term that clearly implies something more than merely "neutral."

TRANSCENDING THE HIDDEN ELEMENT OF REPRIMAND

In reconsidering the meaning of support in psychotherapy and challenging the frequently assumed antithesis between support and exploration, we begin to lay the foundations for a fundamental shift in therapeutic stance and aim. One way to describe this shift, which is at the very center of this book's concerns, is that the basic aim of the therapy is not so much to *discover* what experiences and inclinations have been cast out of consciousness as to help the patient *feel more comfortable and accepting toward them.*

As I have discussed in detail elsewhere (Wachtel, 1993), there is a strong, if unrecognized, undercurrent in the practice of psychotherapy that gives many comments that therapists make a chiding or undermining tone. That pejorative tone is well captured in the quotations by Havens and by Orbach earlier in this chapter. It is evident, I believe, in much clinical work deriving from the default position, and it is another of the reasons why I preferred McWilliams's "supportive" approach to dealing with patients' mistrust (acting in a way that demonstrates one

---

[5] As will be apparent below, I do also wish to question what I believe to be a frequent *overemphasis* on insight, a single-minded focus on promoting insight that can impede the mobilization of *other* therapeutic processes that are at least as important (see also in this regard Fonagy, 1999; Fosshage, 2005; Frank, 1999; Mitchell, 1993a; Wachtel, 1997).

is trustworthy while proceeding with exploring the experience of mistrust) to her more "exploratory" approach with "neurotic-level" patients ("It is usually enough to interpret the transference, that is, to comment on how the patient is mixing one up with some negative person from the past or some projected negative part of the self"). The problem with commenting on how the patient is "mixing up" the present reality of the therapist's benign presence and the negative reality of the past is that it implies that the patient's perceptions are *wrong*.[6]

The ways in which therapists' comments can be unwittingly pejorative was illustrated for me in a different, but very interesting, way a number of years ago, in a nonclinical setting but one very closely related to the assumptive world that guides therapeutic work. The setting was a program meeting of a psychoanalytically oriented clinical training program. At the previous meeting, several students had, with considerable difficulty and not a small dose of courage, spoken up and expressed anger about a number of ways that they felt the faculty had been insufficiently supportive and attentive. At the next meeting, after some time had passed without any overt reference to the fairly dramatic events of the previous meeting, one faculty member, who was clearly trying to be helpful and to bring everyone back to paying attention to what had transpired the time before, said, "There was a lot of aggression expressed at the last meeting. I wonder why no one is talking about it."

What struck me about the comment was that referring to "aggression" rather than "anger" had a dimension of delegitimatizing the students' complaints. "Anger" has a much clearer connotation of being angry *at* something; "aggression" has more of an implication of something from within, something that "comes out" rather than something that is *brought* out by events. The faculty member's intent was to open up the topic for further discussion, but her mode of framing it had the potential for a chilling effect on the flow of dialogue, a subtle element of reprimand and invalidation. The example seems especially instructive because the tone of the faculty member's comment *did not* seem to me to stem from any malign intention on her part but rather from habits of thought and language that are so thoroughly woven into the fabric of our clinical theories and clinical discourse that they simply feel "natural" to many people who have

---

[6] I will discuss below how to encourage the patient to explore potential *alternative* ways of seeing things without dismissing the way he does see things as wrong or as a "distortion."

been clinically trained in the psychoanalytic tradition. But there is a very significant difference between referring to people's anger and referring to their "aggression." The first is likely to be associated with interest in what they might be angry *about,* and hence treats their feeling as at least potentially justified and related to actual events that need to be addressed. The second *interiorizes* the understanding, making it something about the persons who harbor these feelings rather than about their grievances.

BEYOND ABSTINENCE AND RENUNCIATION: TOWARD A LESS JAUNDICED VIEW OF HUMAN NATURE

An important additional source of the insufficiently supportive and potentially undermining approach I am critically examining in this chapter is a jaundiced view of human nature that has lain, sometimes unnoticed, at the foundations of psychoanalytic thought and influenced much of the structure of its assumptions both about people's motives and about how to proceed clinically. At the heart of psychological disorder, I have been suggesting, is self-mistrust, the fearful sense that our innermost thoughts, feelings, and desires are dangerous and bad. From this vantage point, therapy is in large measure a process by which that fear and self-mistrust can be overcome and greater self-acceptance achieved. Such a view of psychological disorder, of course, is premised on the idea that the patient's fears of his feelings, thoughts, or wishes are *unrealistic* fears, that they are indeed fears to be "overcome." There is, however, a strong thread in psychoanalytic thought that starts from a significantly different premise, namely that our innermost thoughts and feelings, the most direct expressions of what we most deeply desire, *are* dangerous and would indeed create havoc in our lives and in society as a whole were they to be expressed in unmodified form; that is, in a form that is truest to what they really are. In *Civilization and Its Discontents,* for example, Freud (1930) depicted our most fundamental desires and inclinations as incompatible with the requirements of civilized life unless they are quite significantly modified and "tamed." As Philip Rieff (1979) put it in his characteristically wry way in his classic work, *Freud: The Mind of the Moralist,* "Psychoanalysis prudently refrains from urging men to become what they really are; the new ethic fears the honest criminal lurking behind the pious neurotic" (p. 322).

One of the key contributions of writers such as Fairbairn, Winnicott, and Kohut—all important contributors to what was eventually to become a broad relational synthesis—was to shift our understanding of the young child's fears, avoidances, and self-alienation away from a vision of the child's innately recoiling from what might be called the "objective" danger of uncontrollable impulses. Instead, their focus was on the vulnerable child's sensitive, and to some degree accurate, registration of actual parental intolerance of or unresponsiveness to the child's affective life. This was an important corrective to the theoretical perspectives of both Freud and Klein, who located the source of the child's anxieties in characteristics that were biologically innate and, in their most fundamental nature, subjectively unacceptable and innately destructive to social harmony.

One consequence of the adverse view of human nature that for so long lay at the heart of psychoanalytic thought was the assumption that the desires and feelings that emerge when one probes deeply into the unconscious are desires that must in large measure be *given up* if one is to lead a healthy and productive adult life with other people. To be sure, a crucial aim of psychoanalytic work was to liberate the individual from the excessive restrictions that arose from the *wholesale* rejection of the impulses resulting from their repression, and to substitute a more limited and discriminating approach that allowed at least for partial gratification. But nonetheless, once the forbidden desire was brought to light, it was in significant measure its *renunciation* that was seen as essential to promoting cure and to enabling the patient to move on in his life. This element of renunciation, the need to give up the infantile desire or fantasy and "grow up," has been noted by a wide variety of influential psychoanalytic writers. Some of them endorse it, some criticize it, but all are in agreement as to its prominence in the traditional psychoanalytic understanding.

Dewald (1972), for example, in an important statement of the classical psychoanalytic approach, states that it is the patient's "persistent wish for this gratification of childhood fantasies that sustains and maintains the neurosis today. When this awareness is ultimately fully appreciated and recognized by the patient, it will represent an important step towards final resolution of the neurosis, inasmuch as it then indicates to the patient that she carries within herself the potential for *renunciation* of the childhood demands and thus for resolution and cure of the neurotic suffering" (p. 375, italics added). Friedman (2002), in a related vein, describes the essence of the process of working through and the key to the mutative power of the psychoanalytic method as "revivifying old attachments (in the relationship to the analyst) and then *killing them off*" (p. 541, italics added).

Mitchell (1986), with a somewhat different theoretical intent, similarly points out that "Freud saw the analytic process in terms of *renunciation*; by bringing to light and renouncing infantile wishes, healthier and more mature forms of libidinal organization become possible" (p. 115, italics added), and Lachmann and Beebe (1992), discussing the traditional drive model of therapeutic action, state that it assumes that "by analyzing rather than gratifying [the patient's] wishes, the analyst promoted their *renunciation* and replacement by ego autonomy and frustration tolerance." They go on to say that although there have been attempts to update this model, "its basic assumptions and its concrete linkage to treatment and structure formation have continued to influence psychoanalytic theory and practice" (p. 134, italics added).

Aron (1991a) elaborates still more fully on this tendency and its implications for the clinical process, pointing out that "Freud often wrote that once the unconscious conflicts between impulses and defense were made conscious, then, in the light of secondary process thought, the patient would have to *renounce* or *condemn* the infantile wishes" and adding that "Waelder (1960) wrote that once the drive was recognized as part of oneself, it would be condemned, 'consciously denied gratification,' so that after a while it would gradually be 'given up' " (p. 88). Still more pointedly, he further adds that,

> The traditional view of the analytic process emphasizes an ethic of renunciation and sacrifice in the service of health and maturity. . . . The focus is on pleasures which needs to be *relinquished* and *abandoned*. [This] focus . . . lends itself to the abuses of a "maturity morality." Patients can easily come to feel that the analyst wants them to "grow up." Patients are likely to feel that the analyst is judgmental and is awaiting the day when they stop acting childishly and begin to act maturely. This is not a projected transference fantasy which needs to be analyzed as a distortion. It is often an accurate perception of the analyst's attitudes rationalized by theoretical beliefs. (pp. 90–91)

Approaching the matter from the vantage point of Kohut's self psychology, Basch (1995) makes a similar point with a particularly vivid example; indeed one that—although representing the view of an actual candidate in training in a prestigious institute—seems to take the traditional stance to the point of absurdity:

> A candidate I was supervising presented the following excerpt from his patient's material: Once on the couch, the patient said, "Well, I did it. Did you see the papers?" The patient was referring to a major achievement that had come to fruition after much planning, hard work, and anxiety and was now being publicly acknowledged and celebrated. "Of course, I said nothing," the candidate assured me. After a minute or so of silence, the patient associated, in an angry tone, to his ungiving, emotionally distant father.
>
> I asked the candidate, "What were you thinking during the patient's silence?" "I wondered what he was trying to get away with," my student replied. "What do you mean, 'trying to get away with'?" "You can't give in to the patient," was the reply. (p. 367)

Basch refers to this stance by the analyst as part of the "ritual of abstinence" that characterizes much psychoanalytic work: "whatever the patient wants or seems to want in the way of a response must, on principle, be thwarted" (p. 368). He traces this stance on the part of many analysts to the assumption that patients are constantly striving for "surreptitious" gratification of their instinctual desires and that permitting this gratification to occur will prevent the buildup of tension necessary for the patient to acknowledge, rather than satisfy, his infantile longings.

The conception of the therapeutic process at the heart of this book, in common with the ideas of Lachmann, Beebe, Mitchell, Aron, Basch, and Kohut described in the last few pages, represents an alternative to this vision of frustration, abstinence, and renunciation as the path to meaningful therapeutic change. The aim is not self-repudiation or renunciation, even in the service of a more workable compromise that allows at least for the gratification of "derivatives" of what we most fundamentally desire. Rather, it is greater self-acceptance *at the core*. It aims at a *reappropriation* of feelings and desires that have *already been* repudiated and need, so to speak, to be repatriated.

It is certainly necessary for the therapist to work with her eyes fully open. The history of our species—to this very day—makes it clear how readily cruel aggression or callous disregard for the interests and welfare of others may be displayed by human beings, both on the massive scale of war and nations (and, I should add, of the free-market economy) and on the more intimate scale that is likely to be the main focus of the events discussed in psychotherapy. Nothing in the emphasis on affirmation and self-acceptance emphasized in these pages implies denial of these painful realities of human life. But it does point to a different vision of how to help people move beyond the darker side of our human potential than the vision of renunciation that (often without full articulation and awareness) has so often underlain the rules of clinical work. Obviously empathy, caring, and acceptance are not the exclusive province of the way of working described in these pages. But as I proceed, I believe it will be apparent that I am describing a significant departure from the traditional attitude of the psychoanalytic psychotherapist, a departure that is part of a growing shift in the profession whose potential has still not been fully realized.

PSYCHOANALYSIS AND THE "SCHOOL OF SUSPICION"

The jaundiced view of human nature that I have here been discussing is embedded in a larger philosophical context that has both shaped and been given its most recent form by the psychoanalytic point of view. This larger context includes assumptions not just about the content or key dispositions of human nature but about what it means *to inquire profoundly into* that nature. Characterizing the essential quality of that larger vision, Paul Ricoeur (1970), in one of the most influential philosophical inquiries into psychoanalysis yet to appear, views Freud (along with Nietzsche and Marx) as one of the three great pillars of what he calls the "school of suspicion." Their shared approach, he argues, is a "hermeneutics of suspicion," in which the central concern is "the *unmasking, demystification, or reduction of illusions*" (p. 9, italics added). If we seek the intention that these three thinkers had in common, he says, "we find it in the decision to look upon the whole of consciousness primarily as 'false' consciousness" (pp. 32–33).

It is important to be clear that Ricoeur does not introduce these ideas as a *criticism* of psychoanalysis, nor of Marxian or Nietzschean thought. Rather, Ricoeur views the seemingly destructive or invalidating attitudes embodied in these thinkers' ideas as a necessary prelude to deeper or more radical change:

> These three masters of suspicion ... are, assuredly, three great "destroyers." But that of itself should not mislead us; destruction, Heidegger says in *Sein und Zeit,* is a moment of every new founda-

tion. . . . All three begin with suspicion concerning the illusions of consciousness, and then proceed to employ the stratagem of deciphering; all three, however, far from being detractors of "consciousness," aim at extending it. (1970, pp. 33–34)

Ricoeur's analysis brilliantly illuminates the liberating intent and dialectical complexities in these three thinkers' mode of analysis. But his apt characterization of psychoanalysis as part of a larger "school of suspicion" nonetheless calls to our attention a dimension of Freudian thought that is often overlooked and that can have problematic implications when applied clinically. Stripping away the patient's false consciousness was, after all, essentially the aim of Basch's supervisee discussed above, and it is an aim that can mask or rationalize harsh, insensitive, or depriving behavior on the therapist's part, as it did in the example Basch offered. In that case, the patient's associations to his distant, emotionally ungiving father were doubtless overdetermined and, in part, probably did reflect and even clarify the conditions of his childhood. But, as Basch clearly implies, they also were an implicit comment (in an atmosphere in which only an indirect reference was likely to feel safe) on *the therapist's* distant and ungiving stance; and they pointed, in *both* their referents (that is, to the distant past and to the occurrences in the therapist's office right at the moment), to an atmosphere in which it is difficult to grow and thrive.

The attitude of suspicion that is often prominent in psychoanalytic thought has been remarked upon not only in philosophical reflections such as Ricoeur's, but by writers more directly associated with the psychoanalytic tradition or with therapeutic practice. Messer (2000), for example, discussing the practice of brief psychodynamic therapists, states that "like psychoanalysts, they adopt an *attitude of suspicion* toward the patient's statements, taking nothing for granted. They challenge the patient's illusions, although not in as thoroughgoing a way as in psychoanalysis" (p. 67, italics added). Similarly, Peter Wolff (2001), in a paper presented to the Rapaport–Klein Study Group, a prestigious group of research-oriented psychoanalysts, states that "psychoanalysis is grounded in an 'epistemology of suspicion.' It accepts no thing at face value. Instead, it assumes that behind every apparently rational statement, behind every reasonable action, behind every innocuous mistake, behind every irrational action, and behind most cultural conventions, there lurks a hidden wish or unacceptable motivation," and he adds, echoing the key assumption of the school of suspicion, that "in order to emancipate us from our illusions, the method therefore exposes the hidden meanings . . . of our personal secrets." In a similar spirit, Roy Schafer (1997), one of the most respected contemporary psychoanalytic thinkers, in commenting on the contemporary Kleinian approach to clinical practice, commends as one of its important and valuable features its "policy of suspicion" toward the patient's account of his experiences (p. 3).

To be sure, none of the writers I have just quoted intend the term *suspicion* to mean something malign. The "suspicion" that the psycho-analytic way of looking or listening implies could be seen as simply another way of referring to the unconscious, to the idea that what we *say* we are feeling or *think* we are doing is far from the whole story and must be carefully probed if both patient and therapist are not to collude in an illusion that is ultimately the source of the patient's suffering. The problem arises in the implicitly adversarial cast that this "suspicion" may give to the therapeutic work, in the potential for invalidating of the patient's conscious experience as a "false" or "distorted" consciousness, in the readiness to see "resistance" when the patient views things differently from the therapist, and in the temptation to view the patient as benighted and needing the therapist to disabuse him of the distortions that constitute his conscious experience.

In my own work, I do *a lot* of probing, and I do assume, quite regularly, that what the patient is saying is unlikely to tell the whole story. But my aim in this is to *expand* the story, to help the patient to see that *there is more to him* than he has assumed, that there are further potentials not yet realized, further feelings not yet given their fair due. It is not to show him that his perceptions of himself are "illusory" or that what he shows the world is a "false self." The assumption that the patient's perceptions are illusory, that he is *hiding* something, that his consciousness is a *false* consciousness—rather than an *incomplete* or *partial* consciousness—can create a mindset for the therapist and an experience for the patient that is *invalidating*, that *dismisses* the patient's experience rather than expanding upon it. It implies that he wants something else *instead* of (rather than *in addition to*) what he thinks he wants, and thus that his understanding of himself is *wrong* rather than incomplete.

In workshops and in supervision, I have attempted to highlight the differences between these two ways of addressing the patient's experience (and of attending to the unconscious dimensions that are not yet represented in awareness) by calling attention to the difference between speaking of what the patient "really" wants and what he "also" wants. It has been my experience that clinicians quite frequently refer to what the patient "really" wants—both in the way that they talk *about* the patient and even in the way they talk *to* the patient: "I think what you're really feeling is. . . . ," "I think the feelings you're describing toward your friend are really feelings you have toward me," "I think what you're really saying is. . . . ," and so forth. In contrast, one can explore unconscious inclinations just as fully by making comments such as "It sounds like you're feeling worried about her but you're also feeling angry," or "I wonder if that feeling that your friend is not leveling with you is something that you're feeling with me too," or "I wonder if another part of what you're trying to say is. . . . " Such comments look just as much at what is left out, but they do not dismiss the person's conscious experience. Rather, they *expand* it.[7]

THE ADVERSARIAL POTENTIAL OF THE INTERPRETIVE STANCE

Interpretation has always been at the very center of the psychoanalytic approach to clinical work. But although many attempts have been made to define precisely just what interpretation is and to clarify how interpretations may be distinguished from other ways that the analyst or therapist participates in the process (see, e.g., Bibring, 1954; Laplanche & Pontalis, 1973; Moore & Fine, 1990; Nichols & Paolino, 1986), the term has had such prestigious connotations in psychoanalytic discourse[8] that in contemporary usage it is not uncommon for therapists to refer to virtually everything they say to the patient as an "interpretation." This tendency may be particularly evident among students, who are insecure about whether they are practicing in a properly "professional" way, but it is evident among experienced practitioners as well. In a recent contribution, for example, Friedman (2002) noted that "if you asked an analyst what he did, he would say, 'I interpret' " (p. 544).

---

[7] I have suggested, only partly facetiously, that one can predict the likelihood that a therapist will be helpful to her patients by calculating her "also to really" ratio.

[8] Bibring (1954), for example, portrayed interpretation as "the supreme agent in the hierarchy of therapeutic principles characteristic of analysis" (p. 763), and Laplanche and Pontalis (1973) maintained that "interpretation is at the heart of the Freudian doctrine and technique" and that "psycho-analysis itself might be defined in terms of it" (p. 227).

In principle, there is nothing inherently problematic in the expanding usage of the term. Meanings of terms inevitably evolve and change over time, and the linguistic community evolves along with those changes. Indeed, in many ways this informal loosening of the term's usage has been a vehicle for the loosening more generally of some of the restrictive rules that had impeded therapists' responsiveness to their patient's needs. Because interpretation has been such a highly valued activity in the psychoanalytic world, the protective coloration offered by calling whatever one says an "interpretation" can make psychoanalytically oriented therapists more willing to go outside the bounds of what had previously been standard practice.

But implicit in the very process of designating a larger and larger range of the therapist's comments as "interpretations" is an affirmation of the idea that *interpreting* is what the therapist ought to be doing. Few therapists continue to pursue the old ideal of resolving the patient's difficulties through "interpretation alone" (e.g., Gill, 1954; Eissler, 1953), but aspects of this older ideal often persist in unexamined fashion. Attempting as much as possible to make their comments "interpretation-like," for example, therapists may be less forthcoming in manner than is optimal, more emotionally restrained and close to the vest, more mysterious, anonymous, and "neutral." Since the aspects of his experience about which the patient needs greater clarity are particularly the ones that are associated with anxiety, shame, or guilt, merely pointing them out in neutral fashion may be insufficient.

Let me illustrate with a brief clinical example. A therapist consulting me described a difficult session in which the patient was clearly upset about something that had happened with her boyfriend, but seemed hesitant to say what it was. She alluded a number of times to what had occurred, but each time, instead of further elaborating, she said things like, "I'm just being a big baby. It's no big deal." In response, the therapist said to the patient, "I think you are avoiding telling me what happened because you're viewing me the same way you viewed your parents. You're expecting me to tell you to calm down or that you're overreacting, just the way they did, and so you're doing what you've always done when you anticipate that—just shutting yourself up." Following this comment, which he thought would be helpful, the session had seemed to unravel. There was little coherence to the rest of the session, and what little there was seemed to center on the patient's periodically talking about herself in a painfully self-disparaging fashion. The comment that was intended to help seemed to make her feel worse.

What I believe was central in the unraveling of this session was that this comment about the patient's anticipating a critical response from him could itself be experienced as critical. The therapist was looking only at the *content* of the interpretation, what might be called its purely "informational" dimension (the dimension, we might say, which *made it* an interpretation in his eyes). He was attempting, in essence, to *enlighten* her about what she was doing, to inform her as a benignly neutral observer. What he did not notice was the way in which his comment could convey that she was doing something wrong *right now,* both by mistrusting him and by confusing him with her parents, failing to be "realistic" or to transcend her previous patterns. And there were many signs that, although she dared not say so, and probably could not articulate it even to herself, to this vulnerable woman the therapist's comment was a message that once again she had done something wrong.

Had the therapist in this case been less concerned with framing his comment to the patient in a manner that sounded like an "interpretation"—"neutral" in tone, framed as if it were simply reporting an observation, and pointing to how the patient was repeating the past (the latter being a common, though not necessarily essential, feature of those remarks thought of as "interpretations")—he might have instead said something like, "It seems like it's hard to really believe that I could hear what you're telling me and feel differently about it than your parents did." This comment aims to illuminate roughly the same pattern, but it does so in a somewhat different way that can have quite a significant difference in its impact on the patient. Instead of saying you're doing *the same* thing with me as you did with your parents (that is, nothing has changed; you're doing the same thing you always have), it implicitly points to something that is potentially *different,* to the possibility of the other person's *interest* in her experience and capacity to hear and take seriously what was upsetting her. It goes beyond the neutral, "just the facts, Ma'am" style commonly associated with "interpretations," and implicitly *empathizes* both with the pain she is experiencing and with the *difficulty* in moving beyond it ("it's hard" to believe the therapist feels differently). Moreover, it implicitly conveys considerably more than the neutral version does that the therapist *does* feel differently. This, of course, also makes it a "two-person" comment rather than just an "observation" of the patient from a point outside the relational field. It brings the therapist into the picture, says something about the therapist as well as the patient.

Sometimes these dimensions need to be highlighted even further. Depending on the particular patient or the particular point in the treatment, it may be necessary to further transcend the hedged, neutral, "interpretive" stance of the default position. There are a wide range of options for ensuring that the patient gets the message that the therapist *does* experience her upset (and her wish to communicate it) differently from her parents. One might, for example, say very explicitly to the patient something like, "You know, in fact I want very much to hear what had upset you, and I *haven't* felt that you're someone who makes too big a fuss, but I guess you got the message so often when you were growing up that you were just too much for your parents, that your feelings were a burden to them, that it will take a while for you to be fully convinced about how I feel." (This example, of course, raises the venerable question of so-called self-disclosure, a topic I will take up in Chapter 11.)[9]

It may be noted about this last version that the phrase "it will take a while" also serves to convey acceptance of the patient not yet being there and to express an expectation that she *will* get there. It conveys a *trajectory* rather than a static state of affairs. It enables the patient to experience her not being there yet not as meaning she is incapable of getting there or is taking too long, but as part of a process that the therapist is conveying quite clearly takes time.

From the vantage point of the default position, these various dimensions of reassurance and encouragement place limits on the depth and breadth of change that can be achieved. They are seen as truncating the therapeutic work by preventing the patient from encountering the full extent of her despair, anger, or stubborn refusal to take a risk. In this view, for example, by the therapist's being so explicitly receptive and encouraging of the patient's expression of feelings that she fears are unacceptable, the patient's *anger* at being treated dismissively is inhibited or circumvented, and thus her understanding and exploration of the depths of that anger is foreclosed. In contrast, if

---

[9] Of course, there is no foolproof way to ensure that the patient will experience the therapist's comment in the fashion the therapist intends. It is reasonable to assume that the *probability* of a helpful experience will vary with the way the comment is put to the patient, but the subjective element can never be eliminated, and ultimately the comment means *what it means to the patient.*. As I further describe below, the process of therapy includes very considerably the therapist's tracking of how the patient actually does experience what she said and then attempting to clarify and elaborate in the same spirit I have been describing (that is, through inquiring, for example, *how else* the therapist's comment might be experienced rather than attempting to demonstrate that the patient *mis*perceived the comment or its intent).

the therapist remains more ambiguous, the anger has room to mobilize and come out. But such a view assumes the anger is simply "inside," something already there that must "come out" if the patient is to achieve deep and lasting change. From a two-person view, in contrast, matters are more dynamic than that. The patient's anger is not just something "inside," but a response to what is transpiring between her and the other person. It is not a fixed inner attribute, always there but sometimes hidden, but rather is stirred in certain interactions (whether consciously or unconsciously) and not in others.

Such a view does not ignore or brush over the patient's anger, nor does it treat it as an artifact that has little to do with her and is only related to what the therapist is doing or to the external situation. There is plenty of room in this way of thinking (depending on what actually emerges from clinical exploration) to conclude that the patient is someone who has the *personal characteristic* of being prone to get angry in certain situations, or that she is prone (consciously or unconsciously) to experience a wider range of situations as infuriating than most people. But that proneness is not an acontextual file cabinet that "stores" static internal representations of object relational scenarios or affect states. It is a dynamic and *interactive* tendency, which is both fully hers *and* a function of the particular context in which she finds herself.

This way of viewing whatever anger (or any other feeling) emerges in the course of the work points us to be alert not only to the patient's dynamics, but also to the therapist's role in the pattern that is observed. In the case being described, for example, it is very possible that the therapist, on some level, experienced the patient's alluding several times to an important experience with her boyfriend but not elaborating on it as teasing or as frustrating, and that the nature and tone of his interpretation was not just a function of the default position but was also in part a reflection of these feelings. As a consequence, he may, indeed, *not* have been as receptive as he otherwise might have been, and the patient may well have picked this up, and further inhibited her elaboration of the story as a result. This would be one more instance of the self-fulfilling nature of intersubjective patterns that I have been describing in the last few chapters. As in my earlier discussion of the "race against time" that characterizes many interpersonal transactions, one of the potentially unfortunate consequences of the way that each person evokes a particular skewed sample of the other person's possible ways of acting or feeling is that feelings or actions on the part of one or both parties that were *not* inevitable, come to *seem* inevitable to either one or both persons. They come to feel as though this is just "the way she is," "the way the world is," "what my life is like," "the kind of person I am," and so forth. Including the therapist's participation in this dynamic pattern, we might speculate that the patient did repeat an old pattern of hers but did so in part because the therapist got drawn into it as an "accomplice." That is, the patient may have evoked in him (again not necessarily with awareness on either of their parts) the same kind of response she *frequently* evokes in others by her ambivalent efforts to reach out and, simultaneously, to *protect herself from* reaching out. The teasing or frustrating quality of such behavior, and the response in the other that it evokes, then "confirms" her mistrust and sets the stage for the next round of the pattern, and the therapist's "interpretation" becomes a part of the process of that perpetuation.[10]

UNFORMULATED EXPERIENCE AND TRANSCENDENCE OF THE ADVERSARIAL STANCE

For many years, the patient's underlying aims and fantasies were viewed as like a text written in a foreign language, needing to be *interpreted* to him in order for him to understand them, but already written, already "there." In recent years, however, this view has increasingly given way to the view that there is *not* a single latent meaning, just waiting to be dug up and deciphered. Rather, what is there to be interpreted, to have its meaning brought out, is a set of still evolving *potentials* for experience and further articulation, what Gendlin (1996) has referred to as a felt meaning and Stern (1997, 2002, 2004) as an unformulated experience. The target to which the interpretive effort is directed, one might say, is less like a completed text (even a not yet read or discovered text) than at most *a scribbled outline of preliminary notes* for a text. Viewed from this vantage point, the interpretive process is not one of finding a singular meaning that has simply been "hidden." It is a process of helping an experience to emerge and articulate itself in a way that it never fully has before.

---

[10] Of course, the evocative pull of the patient's behavior is not inexorable. It will be more likely to evoke a problematic response from some people (including therapists) than from others. This is another dimension of the two-person perspective.

This point of view has been a particular concern of constructivist, intersubjective, and other relational thinkers. It has perhaps been developed most fully in its clinical and theoretical implications in Hoffman's (1992, 1998, 2006) elaborations of the constructivist point of view and Stern's (1997, 2004) discussions of unformulated experience. From this vantage point, interpretation is not a "seeing into" what is really there or "seeing through" to find what is underneath and hidden. Rather, it is a "seeing with" the patient to discern together how his experience might be further articulated and where he might be inclined to go. Though useful interpretation is constrained by the facts of the actual history and actual neural processes ongoing in the patient (cf. Westen & Gabbard, 2002a, 2002b), there are *many* potential interpretations that fit the material, and the criterion for choosing among them is not so much whether it is "correct" or "exact" (Glover, 1931) as whether it is *useful, helpful,* facilitative of the patient's growth and increasing comfort with himself. It will *not* be helpful if it does not in some way reflect and make contact with the patient's experience. But there is more than one interpretation that can do so, and some are more likely to promote growth and change than others (cf. Wachtel, 1993).

An interesting illustration of the interpretive possibilities of this way of thinking is offered by Stern (1997). The patient is a man in his thirties who is in the midst of a divorce and is "feeling so sad and bereft that he can scarcely imagine a different kind of future." Stern tells us:

> In his dream he is driving very carefully on an icy mountain road. Around him thick snow is falling. It is silent and cloudy, and the landscape is dull and colorless—black, white, and shades of gray, evoking (in his associations) his depression over his divorce. As he rounds a turn in the road, which hugs the shoulder of the mountain, the sun appears very suddenly, shining brilliantly in a cloudless and intensely blue sky, and he is faced with a breathtaking mountainside of glittering snowfields and intensely green trees. It seems to him at that moment, inside the dream, that this vista is the most beautiful thing he has ever seen, and he is filled with a feeling of great happiness and fulfillment. (p. 33)

What does this dream "mean"? I would imagine that every reader could come up with at least several possible interpretations for the dream, based in part on your theoretical predilections, on which features of the dream you take to be figure or ground, on how "symbolic" you intend to be, and, in actual practice (as opposed to reading the dream in a book), on your understanding of the patient and of where he is at the moment. A good case could be made for many of these interpretations as "right" from the point of view of making sense of the material in a meaningful, coherent, and perceptive way. But only some of them will be "right" from the vantage point of helping the patient to grow beyond the state of despair with which he had been struggling.

Stern chose to make the interpretation that "the dream is a way of depicting previously unimagined inner resources that the patient will be able to use to make a new life" (p. 34). One of the first things to notice about this comment is that it is *not* an exposing of a forbidden wish or an unmasking of the patient's false consciousness. It has more the quality of what I have called an "attributional interpretation" (Wachtel, 1993; see also Chapter 12 of this book). That is, it attributes to the patient a capacity, an understanding, or an inclination to move in a positive direction that the patient has not yet realized (in both senses of the word "realize"), and in so doing it *enables* the patient to move forward in a way that he had not before. At the same time, it is important to be clear that the offering Stern describes is not just a gratuitous comment that is "made up" to make the patient feel better. It is based on close attention to the details of what the patient actually described. Stern reports that the patient was deeply moved by his comment and that he experienced the interpretation as true to his experience.

We may also note that, although Stern's comment has a different tone and content from most interpretations described in the literature, it does fit within Laplanche and Pontalis's (1973) definition of interpretation as "bringing out the latent meaning" of the patient's material. But the nature both of the assumed latent meaning and of the process of bringing it out differs considerably from what characterizes work rooted in the default position. As I have already noted, Stern's comment—his interpretation, if you will—centers not on something primitive that the patient is hiding but on an unrealized potential in the patient that is in the process of emerging. At the same time, although Stern pays attention to a different aspect of what the patient is saying than is common in psychoanalytic interpretations, it is no less latent— indeed, even no less *submerged*—than the themes that are more commonly found in analyst's interpretations. We have the sense that the patient is *surprised* by what Stern has said. Although it instantly resonates for him, it was not something that he had consciously articulated for himself previously, although he had expressed it vividly in an alternative form in the dream.

There is nothing in the conceptual shift from presuming fully formed fantasies or desires that are simply "hidden" to articulating as-yet *unformulated* experiences that implies a lack of interest in or capacity to address the more usual foci of psychoanalytic inquiry. In this instance, Stern chose to look elsewhere than in the ritualistic direction of finding the "primitive" or negative, but we may safely assume that in the course of his work Stern's attention is also regularly drawn to the implicit contents that are more common in psychoanalytic discourse—to an angry feeling, a sexual wish, an unacknowledged feeling of jealousy or envy, and so forth. Nothing in choosing to address the dimension he did implies excluding the other dimensions or settling for a prettied up or euphemistic avoidance of the hard truths. But what *is* implicit in his position is that if one chooses to focus on the darker side, one is no more grounded in the "real" bedrock, no "deeper" (see also Wachtel, 2003a) than if one chooses, as he did in this instance, to bring forth the as yet unappreciated and unacknowledged feelings of hope and new direction.

BEYOND UNEARTHING AND UNMASKING

If the formulations that for so long were at the center of psychoanalytic theory and practice are just "the way things are," if dangerous and ultimately unacceptable oedipal feelings or Kleinian destructive rage at the breast are what "really" lie beneath our apparently civilized facade, then we have little choice but either to confront that painful truth or bury it. This is, of course, the traditional distinction between expressive and supportive treatment, treatments that tear down defenses or those that shore them up.

The basic structure of inquiry, of both Freudian and Kleinian thought, is adversarial. Short of "superficial" supportive treatment, which brings a measure of comfort at the price of "covering over" the person's deepest and most genuine subjectivity, there is nothing to do but to find a way to force the person to confront and acknowledge what he *doesn't want* to acknowledge; indeed, to own up to a truth that in some way not only *feels* shameful but *is* shameful. (See, in this regard, Weiss & Sampson, 1986; Weiss, 1998; Silberschatz, 2005.) If, on the other hand, human nature is less singularly determinate, less readily defined in terms of a few fundamental and virtually inevitable fantasies or desires, then our understanding of the therapist's task and the available options may be quite different. If what "lies beneath" is not a fixed set (or seething cauldron) of inherently destructive and antisocial tendencies, but rather what Stern has depicted as unformulated experiences—inclinations that are continually emerging and taking shape in response to the ongoing and itself evolving context—then instead of wresting these experiences from the unwilling clutches of the person who is secretly harboring them, we may *invite* them out and help them to take a shape that the patient is comfortable with and that works in his life.

The revised theory of anxiety, which I discuss in more detail in the next chapter, provided a potential alternative to this adversarial view. It offered a means of articulating much more clearly an understanding that was in certain ways implicit in Freud's conception of resistance from the very beginning—that the resistance was not a perverse expression of the patient's stubbornness or uncooperativeness but rather an expression of the anxiety that was the primary force in the patient's difficulties in the first place. The patient retreated from certain thoughts, feelings, and memories and kept them hidden not because he was "resisting" the analyst's efforts but because they felt *dangerous*. This is an important corrective, and to the degree that it leads the therapist to *help the patient feel less afraid of his deepest impulses and feelings* (rather than confining herself to pointing out to the patient that he is hiding something or what it is he is hiding), it represents, in my view, the progressive thrust of clinical theory and practice. But there are many indications that the older, more adversarial vision of resistance persists. A simple clinical example will illustrate what I have in mind. It illustrates as well how (notwithstanding the limits discussed in earlier chapters) the two-person perspective associated with the relational point of view is an important element in transcending the critical view of the patient that I am addressing in this chapter.

A student therapist was struck by the degree to which her patient kept an emotional distance from her, preventing her from having meaning or impact for him. The patient came faithfully to sessions, was never late, even spoke quite fluidly and seemingly openly about his daily experiences. But he seemed to have no emotional response— indeed, he seemed not to care when the therapist, first because of the flu and then because of jury duty, had to cancel several sessions over a period of a few weeks ("It's okay, I understand. Things come up in your life and you just have to attend to them."). He also failed to show the feelings that the therapist anticipated either before or after the summer break when the therapy had to stop ("That's just the way the clinic works. I understand. Why should I have any feelings about that?"), and he generally exhibited a manner in the sessions that was diligent, dutiful, but left the therapist feeling that she was not really a meaningful person in his life, just someone who provided a service.

Concerned that this attitude on the patient's part was in the service of resistance and was preventing him from being able to really benefit from the therapy, she said to him, "Have you noticed that nothing I say seems to have any real meaning or impact for you? I think you're trying to keep me at a distance, that you don't want to get too close to me or let me have too much emotional meaning for you."

Let us assume for the sake of the discussion that the therapist's description of the patient's distancing from her did accurately capture at least one aspect of what the patient was up to or what the meaning of the pattern was. What the foregoing discussion has emphasized is that accuracy alone is an insufficient criterion for evaluating whether a particular comment or interpretation is clinically useful. There is a range of equally "accurate" ways of depicting what is conflictedly being expressed in the patient's behavior, a range of ways of contributing to the greater articulation of what is as yet still somewhat unformulated. None of them simply identifies "what is there." Each contributes to *shaping* what is there, each gives a slightly different push to the patient's experience and to the articulation of his desires. We are in a much better position to craft comments that are effective and therapeutic when we are clear about that impact, rather than hiding behind the illusion that we are simply "telling it like it is."

In thinking about the particular interpretation that the therapist made in this instance, we may note to begin with that it was, in essence, a "one-person" interpretation. That is, although it includes the therapist in one sense (*she* is the one being kept away; the interpretation is about an interaction between two people), in another sense it is structured as an observation that the therapist makes of *the patient*, an observation of what *the patient* is doing, with no consideration of the part that the therapist's own behavior or own characteristics might play in it. This becomes clearer if one considers an alternative framing that addresses the same observation on the therapist's part in a significantly different way: "I have the sense that I don't feel trustworthy to you, that it's necessary to keep me away in order to feel safe." Here the patient's keeping the therapist away is still the focus of the comment, but the onus is removed from the patient. The question of whether the patient is "distorting," is being "irrational," is inappropriately imposing images and expectations from his past upon the present, is here not a matter of presumption but of exploration. This framing allows for the possibility that the patient's mistrust *makes sense* in light of something the therapist is actually doing and of the meaning to the patient of that behavior on the therapist's part. (At the same time, the comment does not presume that the therapist simply "is" untrustworthy. It is not a masochistic "it must be my fault" comment by the therapist, but a comment that leaves open for exploration how the interaction between them has left the patient feeling as he does.)

There are at least two important advantages to this way of approaching the task of calling attention to and clarifying what is going on. First of all, it transcends the attitude of suspicion discussed earlier in this chapter while retaining what is valuable about it. A question is *still* introduced about the patient's experience; he is still invited to explore what this is about. But the automatic presumption of error, irrationality, or the beclouding of consciousness by archaic fantasies and perceptions is not there. Second (since the *possibility* of error and misperception based on the patient's past and his defenses—as opposed to the *presumption* of such occurrences—is indeed important to explore), the alternative I am suggesting to what the therapist actually said is likely to be *more* effective in exploring this possibility. When the patient's perception is not totally dismissed, as it is when only *his* contribution to the experience of mistrust is the focus, he is more likely to be able first of all to acknowledge that he *is* feeling mistrustful and second to *consider and examine* his take on what is transpiring between them.

Gill (1979) has made a similar point in discussing the importance of beginning the exploration of transference experiences with what it was about the therapist or what she did that was the basis for the patient's perception. Thus, for example, Gill states that if the patient experiences the analyst as harsh, "this is, at least to begin with, likely best dealt with not by interpreting that this is a displacement from the patient's feeling that his father was harsh but by an elucidation of some other aspect of this here-and-now attitude, such as what has gone on in the analytic situation that seems to the patient to justify his feeling" (p. 265). Gill's point is not that we should back off from exploring the full range of possibilities that dynamic therapists have always examined. Rather, it is that, first, it is more *respectful* of the patient to begin with his experience of what actually has been going on and second, that the patient is much more likely to *hear* what one is saying, to give it serious consideration rather than defensively dismiss it, if his perception is, to begin with, taken seriously.

INTERPRETATION AND AMPLIFICATION: TWO MEANINGS OF UNDERSTANDING

There is an old joke about our field that almost all readers will have encountered. Two psychoanalysts pass in the hall. They both say hello, and as they walk on, each thinks, "I wonder what he meant by that?"

What is this joke about? Why do people think it is funny? The joke, I think it is clear, is about precisely the attitude of suspicion that has been a central topic of this chapter. It would not be funny if what the audience implicitly assumed both analysts thought "the meaning" was was that the other was trying to be friendly, that the other liked him, even that "hello" really meant, "I'd like us to get together for lunch next time." The humor depends on the audience knowing that each analyst assumed that the hello *really* meant something aggressive, or shameful, or sexual, or was a defense against such a meaning.

This view of psychoanalysis is reflected as well in the comments that practically every psychotherapist has probably encountered at some time or other at a wedding or cocktail party when, in the course of meeting someone, she mentions that she is a therapist—"You're not going to analyze me, are you?" We know, when we hear that, that the person saying it (in slightly apprehensive, if nominally jocular tone) does not mean, "You're not going to understand my point of view with exquisite empathy, are you?" The comment clearly means, "You're not going to see through me and know all my shameful secrets, are you?" If the person making the comment is a little more sophisticated (or a little more skeptical) about the psychoanalytic enterprise, it may also mean, "You're not going to take perfectly innocent remarks and turn them into something shameful, are you?"

The apprehension implicit in the joke and the cocktail party banter reflects, in essence, the legacy of what I have called the default position. At various points in this book, I have discussed ways in which the default position impedes the process of self-acceptance and reappropriation of cast-off aspects of the self that is central to the healing process of psychotherapy. Assumptions about the "primitive" and often destructive nature of the underlying motives and fantasies that direct our behavior; the assumption that the "archaic" psychological structures and inclinations of our earliest years persist in essentially unmodified form as the "real" sources of our behavior and experience throughout life; a stance of skepticism and mistrust toward the patient's account of his experience; a depiction of the patient as fixated or arrested at an early "developmental level"; a suspicion that the patient is attempting to wrest inappropriate gratifications from the therapist and that he is thereby attempting to evade his responsibilities in the work; a hesitancy to provide "support" to the patient; an implicit view that he must "grow up" if he is to get better—these and similar attitudes are deeply woven into the fabric of psychoanalytic thought, beginning with Freud, and they extend into many corners of the contemporary psychotherapeutic scene. All of them, I suggest, are unnecessary for a full and accurate account of the patient's psychological reality and are counterproductive to the pursuit of therapeutic growth and relief from suffering.

It has been a guiding assumption of psychoanalytically inspired therapeutic work that the key to the patient's getting better is understanding himself. It is worth our noting here that the word *understanding* has more than one meaning. The meaning most often emphasized in the literature of psychotherapy has been that associated with the idea of insight, having an *accurate* grasp of what one is wanting and feeling and what is really going on in one's life. But there is another meaning of the word, the meaning implied when we describe someone as an "understanding" person. This second meaning of understanding is both a requirement for the effective psychotherapist—who must manifest understanding in *both* senses—and a quality that the therapy must help the *patient* to achieve toward his own inclinations and experiences.

This second sense of understanding—the sympathetic, on-the-patient's-side way of viewing his experiences—has been impeded by the attitudes I have been examining in this chapter. All too often, the pursuit of insight in therapy has been more than just a matter of helping the patient get in touch with the truth about himself. It has been an effort to get in touch with the *cold, hard* truth. The assumption has been that beneath the patient's conscious experience of himself lurk motives and fantasies that are primitive and often destructive.

The alternative described in this book, largely rooted in the evolving relational paradigm, but critical of certain versions of relational thinking that retain unnoticed elements of the default position, aims just as fully as the traditional approach at illuminating the patient's experience, going beyond the limits of the patient's conscious view of himself. But it does not aim to unmask, to reveal illusions, to "interpret" the patient's underlying aims and assumptions as more primitive or infantile than he realizes. Rather, as I have emphasized, it aims to *expand* his conscious experience of himself, to show there is *more* to him than he has thought. For that reason, I suggest that it is preferable to refer to the comments we make to patients in this pursuit as *amplifications* rather than interpretations. Especially given the history of our field, "interpretation" too readily lends itself to a conception of the therapist as a Delphic knower who *translates* for the person what he is too unenlightened to see himself. *Amplification* still implies attention to unconscious processes, still retains the view that the person does not know "the whole truth" about himself. But it implies a process of building on what the patient already does know. In that sense, it *takes seriously*, rather than dismisses, the patient's conscious experience.[11]

At the same time, this alternative way of thinking and speaking about the process takes seriously as well the idea of the unconscious, an unconscious that must be plumbed to know *even more* about the person and to enable him to know *even more* about himself. In the process, what is discovered will almost certainly include aspects of the self that, at least initially, are regarded with anxiety or shame. The therapist must not retreat from the exploration of these more conflict laden aspects of the self. Overcoming the defenses that have kept these aspects of the self persona non grata is a central dimension of the therapist's task.

Indeed, not only must the therapist address the feelings that the patient is *subjectively* ashamed of, she must also take seriously that some of the feelings and inclinations that have developed under the conditions of self-restriction that the therapist is seeking to ameliorate do have potentially harmful implications either for the patient or for others. The appropriate alternative to the default position and the attitude of suspicion is not a Pollyanna-ish or euphemistic denial of the dark side of human nature. It is an understanding that that dark side is

---

[11] Lewis Aron (personal communication) has pointed out to me that Jung has used the term "amplification" in a somewhat similar way. See also Samuels (2000).

no more "real" or "fundamental" than the aspects of experience and behavior that we admire or readily accept. It is, as well, an attempt to understand how the latter can be crushed by the weight of shame and self-rejection, how a life lived in a self-rejecting way can *become* a life lived aggressively and hostilely, can *seem* to be (and in certain ways can actually be) a life that is lived self-indulgently or impulsively. The skill of the good psychotherapist does not lie in helping the patient to "grow up" and renounce the infantile impulses that are revealed through the harsh light of the clinician's lens, but in helping the patient "grow beyond" the tendencies that have arisen as a result of the anxieties and restrictions that accrued in the course of development. For that to happen, the second meaning of understanding must be a central feature of the therapeutic relationship.

9

Insight, Direct Experience, and the Implications of a New Understanding of Anxiety

One of the most significant contributions of the relational point of view has been the construction of a theoretical viewpoint and the creation of a theoretical climate in which the attitude of suspicion discussed in the previous chapter could begin to be overcome. From this newer vantage point, the problems patients bring to psychotherapy derive not from the primitive and destructive nature of our fundamental biological drives, but from the ways in which people learn, in the course of growing up, to view with horror and revulsion some of the feelings and vital desires that are part of the basic core of the self. Given how dependent we are (not only early in life but throughout the life cycle) on our attachment to the central figures in our lives, any sign that we are displeasing these attachment figures, or that certain features of our emerging selves are threatening to them and difficult for them to relate to or accept, can trigger a retreat from our own experiences and inclinations and an attempt to be who these crucial figures need us to be. From this vantage point, therapy is less a matter of the "unmasking, demystification, or reduction of illusions" depicted by

Ricoeur (1970) than a process by which the patient's fear and self-mistrust can be overcome and greater self-acceptance achieved. Insight and self-awareness are by no means irrelevant to this process; to enable the assimilation and acceptance of these experiences, they must be brought into the open and directly experienced. But the larger purpose is transformed in this alternative vision, and the overcoming of guilt, shame, and constricting anxiety moves to the center.

In this chapter, I want to explore the question of how we can most effectively help our patients to overcome that anxiety, guilt, and shame. In doing so, I will elaborate on some potentials in the relational paradigm that have thus far not been widely appreciated or implemented. These potentials include not only considerations that help us to move beyond what I have been calling the default position, but also possibilities for psychoanalytic understanding to be fruitfully combined with the methods and insights of other therapeutic approaches. I have written about these integrative possibilities previously (e.g., Wachtel, 1977, 1987a, 1997; Wachtel & Wachtel, 1986). Here I wish to elaborate on them further and to clarify how the reformulations deriving from the relational paradigm contribute to and extend them. In particular, I want to examine closely a major revision in the psychoanalytic understanding of anxiety that occurred many years ago but whose implications for clinical practice have still not been well assimilated into psychoanalytic thought, even by many relationalists.

THE UNNOTICED REVOLUTION

With the publication of *Inhibitions, Symptoms and Anxiety*, Freud (1926) launched a major revolution in psychoanalytic thought. Unfortunately, very few analysts noticed. To be sure, the revisions in the theory of anxiety that were introduced in that work were almost immediately incorporated into the general theoretical structure of psychoanalysis and into the psychoanalytic literature. But when it came to the *therapeutic* applications of these theoretical revisions, their radical implications were much slower to be recognized. Indeed, they remain largely unappreciated and unacknowledged to this day. The mainstream of psychoanalytic thought continues to ground its approach to the therapeutic impact of psychoanalysis in an older set of assumptions, centering on the uncovering of repressed material, enabling the patient to gain insight about aspects of himself that he had previously hid from his awareness.

The new understanding introduced in *Inhibitions, Symptoms and Anxiety* did not explicitly downgrade the role of insight into our repressed impulses. But the logic of the new theory did suggest, when closely examined, that even more central to achieving therapeutic change is the *overcoming of anxiety* associated with those impulses. Much of the revised understanding of therapeutic process and technique discussed in the last chapter implicitly builds upon this new conceptualization of the role of anxiety. The move away from an adversarial and withholding approach to the patient, the deemphasis on discovering what the patient is hiding and the corresponding attention to aiding the patient in reappropriating cast-off and rejected parts of his own experience, represents a significant change from the original tenor and theoretical foundations of psychoanalytic work.

Prior to 1926, Freud had viewed anxiety primarily as a discharge phenomenon. It was a consequence of repression and of the damming up of libidinal tension that repression brought about. In this regard, anxiety was understood not dissimilarly from neurotic symptoms such as hysterical conversion reactions, with the exception that the discharge occurring by way of anxiety was an essentially automatic, almost physical result rather than, as with symptoms, a meaningful and symbolic psychological event. Anxiety, one might say, could not be similarly "translated"; it was more to be endured. In *Inhibitions, Symptoms and Anxiety*, however, Freud reversed his understanding of the relation between anxiety and repression. Explicitly revising his earlier view, he stated that anxiety was not the *result* of repression as he had previously believed but rather the *cause*; it was to avoid the anxiety that would otherwise ensue that the individual repressed the forbidden impulse.

This was a highly significant modification. As he put it in that work:

> It is no use denying the fact, though it is not pleasant to recall it, that I have on many occasions asserted that in repression the instinctual representative is distorted, displaced, and so on, while the libido belonging to the instinctual impulse is transformed into anxiety. But now an examination of phobias, which should be best able to provide confirmatory evidence, fails to bear out my assertion; it seems, rather, to contradict it directly. (Freud, 1926, p. 109)

In reviewing this change a few years later in his *New Introductory Lectures*, Freud (1933) stated further that "the surprising result [of our further studies] was the opposite of what we expected. It was not the repression that created the anxiety; *the anxiety was there earlier; it was the anxiety that made the repression*" (p. 86, italics added).[1]

Perhaps the most important implication of this revised conceptualization was that (without this being clearly noticed in the psychoanalytic community, or even by Freud himself) it significantly modified the role of repression itself. In this new formulation, repression moved from being the absolutely central fulcrum of the psychoanalytic understanding of neurosis and of personality development to becoming a *consequent* phenomenon that depended on something else more fundamental—namely, anxiety.

Freud (1914b) had earlier described repression as the very cornerstone of psychoanalysis. And, from that vantage point, it was clear that *undoing* repression, enabling the patient to become *conscious* of what had been repressed, was the cornerstone of the therapeutic method that derived from it. But if anxiety lies *behind* or *underneath* repression; if, as Freud (1933) put it, anxiety *makes* repression, then repression no longer lies at the very foundation. The cornerstone has been shifted. Repression remains important, to be sure, but *anxiety* becomes the new cornerstone.

This shift in the very cornerstone of psychoanalysis could—and should—have led to a fundamental revision in the understanding of what is necessary and sufficient for therapeutic change. If undoing repression, making the unconscious conscious, is the most fundamental aim and necessity of the therapeutic process, then all other ways of helping people to feel better must be subordinated to promoting insight. If, on the other hand, undoing *anxiety* is most fundamental, then quite different strategies emerge as possibilities. Even more important than bringing the repressed impulses to awareness is making them feel safer, enabling the person to *be less afraid* of his feelings, thoughts, and wishes.

In part, the revisions proposed in *Inhibitions, Symptoms and Anxiety* built upon earlier revisions presented in *The Ego and the Id* (Freud,

---

[1] Freud had, of course, recognized from the beginning that repression was *motivated* and that repression was an act designed to prevent or diminish psychological distress. In this respect, his conceptualization remained consistent. But the relation between anxiety, which he viewed for many years as a *product* of repression, and the pain and "unpleasure" that he viewed as lying behind repression remained unclear for many years.

1923), in which Freud introduced the "structural theory" (Arlow & Brenner, 1964) of ego, id, and superego. To many psychoanalytic scholars, it was *The Ego and the Id* that was the more fundamentally important work, and indeed it was a major watershed in a number of respects. Of particular significance for clinical practice, *The Ego and the Id* shifted the focus of psychoanalytic thought from the specific concept of repression to the broader and more variegated concept of defense— a term Freud had introduced very early in his work, but which took on new and major significance in *The Ego and the Id* and, even more, in Anna Freud's (1936) *The Ego and the Mechanisms of Defense*, which built very significantly on its foundation. Both of these landmark works emphasized the *wide range* of ways that people keep threatening or unacceptable material from becoming a full part of their experienced sense of self; repression is but one of the ways we can accomplish this. Sometimes, it is possible to obliterate the offending thought or feeling from consciousness altogether, and repression both suffices and dominates. But in many instances we *do not* completely block the unwanted thought or feeling from awareness. Rather, we marginalize it, rationalize it, become aware of it as an "idea" without actually feeling it very much, and so forth. "Making the unconscious conscious," it became clear, was often not enough, because a wish or fantasy could be conscious and yet still defended against quite significantly and powerfully.

But although the introduction of the structural perspective brought important modifications in technique, centering especially on the analysis of defenses as a necessary complement to the analysis of the repressed material itself, it also needs to be said that, in contrast to its significance for metapsychological theory, *The Ego and the Id* left the conceptual foundations of the *therapeutic* enterprise largely untouched. The basic aims of "uncovering," of "discovering," of promoting "insight" through interpretation remained largely as before.

The theoretical reworkings of *Inhibitions, Symptoms and Anxiety*, on the other hand, implicitly pointed to a rather fundamental revision, one in which the very aims of insight and interpretation were removed from their position at the absolute core of the therapeutic process. Insight remained of great value and importance, but the logic of *Inhibitions, Symptoms and Anxiety* suggested that it could no longer be viewed as the single most important element in the work. That becomes the overcoming of anxiety, the mastery of the fear that made the person engage in self-deception, defensive misrepresentation, or dulling of affective experience in the first place.

Consider, for example, the idea that one must interpret and work through the defenses before interpreting the repressed material itself (e.g., Fenichel, 1941; Greenson, 1967). The typical premise for this idea, rooted in the assumptions of ego psychology and the structural theory, was that without doing so, the still-intact defenses would once again render the material inaccessible and little would be permanently altered. What had been uncovered would once again be buried. The mode of addressing those defenses, however, remained that of "interpreting" them. In that sense, the role of insight in the psychoanalytic understanding of the therapeutic process, far from being downgraded, could be seen as having been extended even further. Now what was needed was not only insight into the repressed material but insight into the repressive or defensive effort itself.

The revised theory of anxiety introduced in *Inhibitions, Symptoms and Anxiety,* however, provides a conceptual tool for a different— and deeper—understanding of why interpreting unconscious material without addressing the defenses that have kept it unconscious is unsatisfactory. It is not so much that the aim of interpreting defenses is completely wrong; it is certainly the case that simply interpreting or "bringing to light" what has been repressed, without addressing the ways in which the person has maintained the recovered thought or desire in a state of repression, is unlikely to be of much enduring therapeutic value. But the call to interpret defenses before interpreting what is being defended against is only a *partial* advance based on only a *partial* understanding. As a consequence it is also misleading and potentially an impediment to more effective practice. The more fundamental reason that material that has been "unearthed" and talked about in one session can readily be resubmerged not long after is the patient's continuing *anxiety* about the defended-against material and the failure to overcome or diminish that anxiety. When *that* is accomplished, when the person is helped to become *less afraid* of the thought or feeling or desire that is being defended against, *then* it can be accepted and integrated and there will be no need to re-repress it.

SHOULD WE DISTINGUISH BETWEEN ANXIETY AND FEAR?

In the discussion thus far, I have used the terms fear and anxiety more or less interchangeably. In contrast, much of the psychoanalytic literature draws a rather sharp distinction between the two concepts. There have been many bases offered for this distinction: for example, apprehension regarding something external versus something that is part of oneself; fearful affect that is specific versus vague and undifferentiated; wariness and unease whose object can be named versus whose object is unclear and perhaps unconscious. Sometimes, the distinction is also rooted in the difference between fear as a consciously *experienced* affect and anxiety as a psychological impetus that may often operate silently and invisibly, leading us to avoid thinking certain thoughts or feeling certain feelings without even being aware that we are doing so, much less that we are afraid of them. This latter conception builds on Freud's concept of signal anxiety, and it is rooted in the observation that so long as we do successfully avoid thinking the forbidden thought or feeling the forbidden feeling, we are aware neither of the avoidance nor of the threatened discomfort that lies behind the avoidance. (Of course, to anticipate the discussion immediately below, it is also the case that fear too leads us to avoid many situations quite automatically without any awareness that we are doing so.)

These distinctions between different varieties of apprehension and experienced threat are important to keep in mind in refining our clinical formulations. They aid us both in making those formulations more nuanced and differentiated and in generating communications and interventions that the patient will experience as responsive to his specific subjective experience. But I nonetheless find forced and unconvincing the argument that fear and anxiety are fundamentally different phenomena. This way of thinking is both overly dichotomous and question begging. If one *chooses to call* the experience of dread before an external object or situation "fear" and the experience of dread induced by one's own thoughts or feelings "anxiety," one cannot argue with the definition per se. The reason it is so tempting to resort to "argument by definition" is that it is invulnerable to empirical adjudication.

But drawing such a sharp distinction is clinically counterproductive. It deprives us, when thinking about how to deal with "anxiety," of any of the knowledge that has been gained by studies of how people overcome fear. Moreover, because some authors distinguish sharply between anxiety and fear and others do not, and because the criteria for the distinction can vary from author to author, it becomes difficult to evaluate or compare differing clinical observations or research findings. Thus reports in the research literature that document the powerful clinical utility of methods such as exposure to what one is afraid of (see below) have very largely been ignored by psychoanalytic clinicians as irrelevant to the ways that anxiety is conceptualized in their work. As I shall discuss shortly, however, there is much in the rapidly accumulating findings regarding the efficacy of exposure in treating overtly fearful states that is pertinent in clinically important ways to addressing the less conscious anxieties that are the more common focus of therapists operating from psychoanalytic or humanistic/experiential orientations.

It is certainly true that the anxieties likely to be the primary concern for these therapists differ in a number of important ways from the anxiety that is manifested in phobias or in panic attacks. Often the anxiety that lies at the heart of the patient's difficulties is not itself the complaint that the patient brings, and its powerful role in shaping his behavior and his life options may be largely out of awareness. The patient's complaints may range from depression to numbness to a lack of real connection with people to a vague, general sense that something is wrong but without the instantly identifiable element of anxiety that calls out so acutely in a phobia or panic attack. In these cases, the triggers for the anxiety (whether consciously experienced or not) are usually not specific phobic objects or specific external situations but perceived threats to the person's ties to beloved or needed objects, threats that are often evoked by the stirring of certain thoughts, feelings, or perceptions of self or other. There need not be an "objective" danger of abandonment to evoke the dread. All that is required is that the person *perceive* the stirring of the feeling or desire as a threat to a key relationship or to the ongoing sense of self. Operating unconsciously, the anxiety may only become evident or experiential when the thoughts or feelings that are its triggers threaten to emerge into awareness. Nonetheless, as we will see, much can be learned about the dynamics of overcoming and mastering these more relationally rooted anxieties by attending to the discoveries that have been made in the treatment of more manifest forms of anxiety.

In what follows, I will attempt to build bridges between clinical approaches that have evolved from different directions and are rooted in different sets of observations. It will be evident, however, that quite different challenges are posed for the clinician depending on whether the primary focus is on such disorders as phobias or panic disorder or is on the broader set of complaints—about unsatisfying relationships, crises of meaning, absence of zest and vitality in living, painful feelings of self-doubt or worthlessness, and so forth—that are a central part of the caseload of many therapists. It will also be evident as I proceed that clearer understanding of the dynamics of fear and anxiety provides the clinician with valuable conceptual tools for approaching related distressing affects such as guilt and shame, which similarly operate not just in consciously experienced fashion but as the often invisible driving force behind defenses and the constriction and misrepresentation of experience.

HOW IS ANXIETY OVERCOME?

Shifting the primary emphasis of the therapeutic work from achieving insight to overcoming anxiety brings to focal awareness a crucial question: precisely how *do* we overcome anxiety? In considering this question, it may be useful to start, as Freud did in 1926, by taking a closer look at phobias and other disorders in which anxiety is most obviously a part of the picture. If we consider phobias and other anxiety disorders from a contemporary vantage point, attending to the clinical and theoretical advances that have been achieved in the eight decades since the publication of *Inhibitions, Symptoms and Anxiety*, it is evident that a key element in overcoming anxiety—perhaps *the* key element—is *exposure* (see, e.g., Zinbarg, Barlow, Brown, & Hertz, 1992; Foa & Kozak, 1986; Foa & Meadows, 1997; Deacon & Abromowitz, 2004; Richard & Lauterbach, 2006). When the individual suffering from a phobia is repeatedly exposed to the source of his fear without the anticipated negative consequences, this *experiential* demonstration of the safety of encountering what was previously fearfully avoided is likely to be more powerful than any merely verbal or cognitive effort to persuade the person that there is no danger or than any effort to "interpret" the meaning of the fear.

Much the same conclusion emerges from research on other disorders in which the conscious experience of anxiety is a central feature. In panic disorder or in posttraumatic stress disorder, for example, there is similarly an enormous body of evidence for the effectiveness of exposure as a therapeutic agent (e.g., Zinbarg et al., 1992; Keane, 1995, 1998; Nemeroff et al., 2006; Foa, Huppert, & Cahill, 2006). Although there remains considerable controversy over the exact mechanisms that account for the reduction of anxiety in exposure, with different proponents arguing for the importance of extinction, habituation, counterconditioning, self-efficacy, and so on, there is widespread agreement and very substantial evidence that repeated exposure to what one fears is a powerful—if not essential—path to anxiety reduction.

In certain respects, the value and importance of this approach to overcoming anxiety has long been recognized by psychoanalytic thinkers as well. Discussing the treatment of severe obsessional disorders, for example, Freud (1919) advocates using the influence of the analyst to "forcibly suppress the compulsion of the disease" (p. 166), an approach that is barely distinguishable from the contemporary behavioral exposure technique of response prevention. Similarly, he states that "one can hardly master a phobia if one waits till the patient lets the analysis influence him to give it up" (p. 165). Referring in particular to those with agoraphobia who have altogether abandoned going out alone, he states, "one succeeds only when one can induce them by the influence of the analysis to . . . go into the street and to struggle with their anxiety while they make the attempt. One starts, therefore, by moderating the phobia so far; and it is only when that has been achieved at the physician's demand that the associations and memories come into the patient's mind which enable the phobia to be resolved" (p. 166).

Even more directly pointing to the role of exposure, Fenichel (1941), in his influential early volume on psychoanalytic technique, states that "when a person is afraid but experiences a situation in which what was feared occurs without any harm resulting, he will not immediately trust the outcome of his new experience; however, the second time he will have a little less fear, the third time still less" (p. 83).

But the exposure strategy becomes more complicated to pursue when we move from the realm of phobias to the kinds of "problems in living" that take up most of the time of practicing therapists. The body of evidence pointing to the powerful impact of exposure on anxiety reduction is enormous; but precisely how to bring about the exposure, or even *what* the person needs to be exposed *to,* is a question that poses considerable challenges. Most of the formal research on the clinical effectiveness of exposure has concentrated on *external* fears rather than the patient's fears of his own thoughts and feelings, the fears that lie at the heart of more complex disorders and complaints. When the object of one's fear is a clearly identifiable external object or situation, such as dogs or flying on airplanes, arranging for exposure to what one fears is relatively easy. Straightforward cognitive-behavioral exposure techniques usually suffice and are usually the treatment of choice in such cases. Complexities arise, however, as we move from the phobias to such complaints as troubling relationships, dissatisfaction with one's job or career, feelings of meaninglessness, or low self-esteem.[2]

To begin with, in such cases, it is harder for the therapist to know what experiences the patient needs to be exposed to. The occurrence of defenses that obscure what it is that is being avoided makes it difficult to identify just what the target of the exposure should be, as does the inherent ambiguity of most emotional and interpersonal experiences. How to *read* such experiences is not usually "given" in the experience itself, which is one of the reasons why some form of interpretation (though not of the sort examined critically in the last chapter) remains an important part of the therapeutic effort. Moreover, even where the therapist does have a pretty good idea what it is that the patient needs to be exposed to, it is not so easy to bring that exposure about. If the person is defending against a particular feeling or experience, then he can (without even being aware of doing so) prevent himself from *having* that experience.

One of the most problematic features of anxiety is that because we tend to avoid what we are afraid of, we never get to see if it might no longer be dangerous. This is, of course, a central way in which defenses, though they protect us from immediate discomfort, perpetuate our difficulties. The thought or feeling that we defend against is prevented from occurring, and as a consequence we cannot reevaluate whether the ominous consequences we anticipate will really follow.

Sometimes, of course, the inclination being defended against *does* occur, notwithstanding the defensive effort. That is the import of the expanded understanding of defenses discussed earlier in this chapter in relation to the introduction of the structural theory. Much defensive effort does not render the material being defended against thoroughly invisible or accomplish a complete avoidance of awareness or expression. But these various mental maneuvers are categorized as defenses because they do serve in one way or another to blunt the experience or render it, to use Sullivan's (1953) apt term, "not me." Defenses such as intellectualization or isolation enable the person who is verbally aware of a wish or attitude or aware of the *cognitive* representation of an affect nonetheless not to *feel* the feeling or the inclination and thus not

---

[2] Even when the presenting problem is a phobia, it should also be noted, it is not infrequently the case that in the very process of working on the phobia—especially if this is done sensitively with an acute ear for the nuances of communication, rather than in a mechanical manner—the patient comes to see other issues in his life that he would like to work on which require a more complex approach.

to fully experience it as his own. Projection enables perception of anger, or dependency, or lasciviousness, or what have you to be represented in consciousness, but, again, not as one's own. Rationalization may enable conscious representation of both the wish or feeling *and* the affect, but redescribes what is being experienced in such a way that both psychological ownership and genuine awareness and understanding are impeded. And so it is with any other psychological process that merits being described as defensive; the feeling, thought, or inclination does not occur as a *fully experienced* event or as something that *belongs to me.* And in thus succeeding in avoiding the full experience of what one fears experiencing, one at the same time loses an opportunity to test out whether the fear is still merited.

The import of these repeated avoidances is difficult to overestimate. They prevent us not only from learning to overcome the anxiety (that is, from testing out whether it really is, or continues to be, dangerous to experience the forbidden feeling or desire), but also from accumulating experiences in *expressing* those feelings or wishes. With experiences and inclinations that are *not* being avoided or distorted because of guilt or shame or anxiety, we learn, through a long series of trial and error exchanges with others, to gratify our desires in the world, to express and regulate our affective experiences, and to test out our perceptions of others' feelings, motives, and reactions to our own behavior and expressions of affect. But for the segment of our experience that is avoided or cast aside, we do not have that opportunity, and the cast-out parts of our experience and psychological life cannot be similarly refined and integrated into our transactions with others. As a consequence, they remain a kind of terra incognita—inhibited, avoided, unacknowledged—as well as a continuing source of unease, both subjectively and interpersonally.

In helping the patient to overcome these persisting fears and to liberate and bring to light the inner tendencies that have been suppressed and fearfully avoided, a crucial component of the therapist's skills entails doing what is necessary to evoke and bring to full experiential contact the avoided thought, wish, affect, or experience of self or other. When the therapist successfully "interprets" what the patient is avoiding or is experiencing in an unacknowledged way, she is, in essence, bringing the patient into closer contact with (*exposing* him to) the previously avoided experience. Most dynamic therapists, however, are unlikely to think in terms of exposure per se and hence are not specifically directed toward bringing exposure about. If the therapist is thinking too much in terms of insight or bringing repressed material to consciousness, then she may end up being too verbal or cognitive and insufficiently experiential (a matter that I take up further in the next chapter). The general and long-standing idea that insights must be emotional and not just intellectual helps here, because it overlaps in important ways with the idea of exposure, though from a different angle. But framing the task *explicitly* as one in which promoting exposure is a key element can add significantly greater clarity and focus to the therapist's efforts and enable the therapy to be conducted in ways that are both more experiential and more effective in helping the patient finally overcome the anxiety that has been at the root of his self-alienation.

Phrases such as *"try to picture* the experience of telling your mother you aren't coming over for dinner," or *"what is it like to experience* that shaky feeling of telling Rick you'd like to spend more time with him?" or *"put yourself back* in the situation where you were trying to tell Joan that she had hurt you" are closer to the exposure paradigm and can help to immerse the person in a more alive and emotionally vivid fashion in the conflictual experience that needs to be encountered. New insights may certainly arise from this effort; the emphasis on exposure does not imply lack of interest in promoting insight. Indeed, much as with exploration and support, as discussed in Chapter 8, the two emphases enhance each other. The immersion—and the reduction in anxiety that follows from the immersion—is likely to promote new insights and the emergence of affective experiences that were previously warded off and kept out of awareness. But there is nonetheless something important added when the emphasis is not so much on "discovering" as on *experiencing,* and on the *repeated* experience, the testing over and over of whether in fact the previously avoided experience is safe.[3]

---

[3] The reader may note here a parallel to the concept of working through, which also points to the need for *repeated* efforts to address the particular conflict or issue. But although the concept of working through reflected an understanding that the one-time "aha" experience of attaining an insight was rarely sufficient for enduring therapeutic change, most discussions of working through continued to be rooted in the belief that it is insight that is most essentially responsible for cure. The present account, in contrast, highlights repeated *exposure* to the previously avoided experience, leading to reduced *anxiety* about that experience and hence greater acceptance and assimilation of the experience, as a key element when working through is successfully achieved. It thus leads to subtly different ways of promoting the working through process. See Wachtel (1993, 1997) for further discussion of the different ways of conceiving of working through and how understanding the central role of overcoming anxiety changes our understanding of the process of working through.

In applying this perspective, however, to the anxiety and dread arising from the (usually unconscious) sense that the perceptions, affects. thoughts, and desires that form the very core of the self are in conflict with the need to maintain a tie to the world of needed and vitalizing objects, the concept of exposure must be reconceived as a two-person process. That is, instead of the patient needing to accumulate exposure to something *outside* of the therapeutic relationship (high bridges, small spaces, pigeons, dogs, etc.), he must accumulate exposures to the kinds of *relational experiences* he has fearfully avoided. Central to those experiences are the patient's own warded-off thoughts, feelings, and longings as they arise in interactions with key others. Those psychological events must be mobilized and experienced in the transaction for the patient to be exposed to the real sources of his anxiety, with the consequent possibility of overcoming that anxiety. But the total configuration includes as well, as an important and intrinsic component, the emotional participation of the other (and, in the process of therapy, particularly of the therapist)—her experience of and attitude toward the patient; her capacity to perceive, understand, and relate to the full range of the patient's experience; and the subtle (and often unconscious) emotional cues that derive from her experience and are communicated in the transaction between them. For the patient to be persuaded experientially that having the forbidden thought or feeling will not be disastrous to the foundational relationships in his life, he must have an experience *in the relationship* that he can let those thoughts, feelings, and desires emerge *and that the other will continue to be there.* That "being there," it is important to understand, is more than just being there physically or even than being there in a nonpunitive way (though obviously that is important). It requires that the other be *engaged*; that she *really see* the feared wish or feeling and that she *relate* to it; that comfort in the interaction between patient and therapist not be achieved by smoothing over the rough spots, by making invisible (and, in that sense, "unspeakable") what is difficult for either party.

This does not mean that the therapist must approve of or like everything about the patient. That is generally an impossible goal in an intense relationship that truly engages all aspects of the person, and holding such a goal would only serve to motivate hypocrisy and denial on the therapist's part. Rather, it means that the therapist must *see* and *understand* the conflicted and dreaded aspects of the patient's experience, and that her *overall* acceptance of the patient not be achieved on the basis of excluding or "not noticing" what is uncomfortable (for either party) to notice. This is close to what I understand Rogers's (1957) concept of unconditional positive regard to be—not an approval of everything the person does, however insensitive, immoral, or aggressive it might be, but an acceptance of the person as he is, a readiness to view him clearly and wholly and, to the degree possible, to see things through his eyes.

Such a view of the therapeutic process brings together the qualities of empathy and insightful understanding that are highlighted in the training of psychoanalytic and experiential therapists and the skill in promoting exposure that I have been discussing in this chapter. The therapist can promote exposure to what the patient *needs* exposure to—that is, to the truly *relevant* experiences—only if she *sees* or senses or intuits what vital parts of the patient's inner life are being avoided and repeatedly cast aside as a result of the anxiety they arouse. These are the experiences that the patient needs to be able to confront and assimilate, but they are rendered difficult to see by the very avoidance that the anxiety repeatedly brings about. The therapist's skill consists in good part in both her own identifying and drawing out these hidden and avoided experiences and in helping *the patient* to see and understand them more clearly. But it also consists in helping create the conditions in which the patient is able to repeatedly *expose* himself to those experiences so that the attendant anxiety can be mastered and overcome. The exposure, as noted earlier, must be very largely within a two-person framework of experience, but it must be an experience of exposure nonetheless.

Over the years, this dimension of exposure and direct experience was ignored or greatly underestimated in the psychoanalytic literature, which tended to overemphasize insight in a way that served as a faith-based explanation for therapeutic change. In more recent years, however, there has been increasing appreciation and acknowledgment that "something more than interpretation" (Stern et al., 1998) is needed to maximize the potential for growth-promoting change. That something else or something more has begun to be addressed in important and useful ways, particularly with regard to the central role of new relational experience (e.g., Aron, 1996; Fosshage, 2005; Frank, 1999; Mitchell, 1993a) and of implicit relational knowing (Lyons-Ruth, 1998). I shall be discussing these concepts in some detail in the chapters that follow. But I wish here to complement these perspectives with an emphasis on the utility of an expanded, two-person or intersubjective version of the exposure paradigm. The importance of direct exposure has been powerfully supported by evidence from the treatment of phobias and other disorders in which the patient's anxiety is on the surface and is readily seen as a crucial target of the therapeutic effort. In what follows, I want to show how exposure plays a central role in more subtle or characterological sources of distress as well.

INTERPRETATION AND EXPOSURE:
A CLINICAL ILLUSTRATION

The differences between a dynamic therapy that centers on interpretations and one that centers on exposure to and *experiencing* the avoided and forbidden are illustrated in the following example, which also clarifies how promoting exposure can at the same time enhance the traditional aims of exploration and self-understanding. It illustrates as well the convergence between the paradigm of exposure and the concern with *self-acceptance* that is so central to the approach I am describing. In addition, the case material illustrates a number of other ways in which the therapeutic interaction is subtly altered by the point of view I discuss in this book. Although these other dimensions are not as focally relevant to the issue of exposure per se, they are nonetheless of considerable importance in the overall clinical approach of concern here. I will therefore comment as well on these additional dimensions as they arise in the material to be discussed.

The patient, Nancy, a woman of 38, had been having difficulty getting fair credit for what amounted to coauthorship with a collaborator, Linda, who wanted merely to acknowledge Nancy as someone who had provided helpful input. Complicating the situation for Nancy was that she also thought of Linda as a friend and so felt especially awkward about the potential conflict between them. More generally, Nancy was someone who was prone to feel selfish and petty *whenever* she asked for her fair share, and as a consequence she was frequently taken advantage of and, despite considerable talents, was somewhat thwarted in her career. She began the session saying, "I don't know how I feel today." I responded by saying, "Tell me more about the experience of 'I don't know.' What does that feel like?"

In approaching this opening to the session, I took the "I don't know" as not simply a statement of ignorance but as a likely statement of conflict.[4] That is, what I heard in her communication, what I took to be its meaning, was not so much that she literally *did not know* what she was feeling, but that she was in conflict about it, wary about whether it was safe to focus on it and to discuss it. I was thinking as well that, very likely, part of that wariness was a concern about what beginning to talk about what she was feeling *would lead to,* a hypothesis that was very shortly confirmed when her response to my inquiry led not only to her beginning to express and talk about feelings that were distressing to her, but right to thoughts about a situation in which she was acutely uncomfortable.

Within a few seconds of my expressing interest in the actual experience of "not knowing" what she was feeling today, Nancy said that she was feeling rather anxious and irritated and began to talk about the situation with Linda, her coauthor. In elaborating on her views of the nature of the collaboration between them, she said, with some heat, that she deserved at least 40% of the credit, maybe more. "Linda did have certain connections that I didn't have, but it was my idea to begin with, and I've done *a lot* of the work on it as well, maybe more than she has."

Why was Nancy so readily able to say what she was feeling just a few seconds after saying she "didn't know" what she was feeling? Put differently, why was my expression of interest in the experience of "I don't know" so rapidly followed by her "knowing" what she was feeling? We may note to begin with that my asking her to "tell me more about" the experience of "I don't know" conveyed an *interest* in her experience. Most simply and directly, it conveyed that I was prepared to hear more, that I was not put off by what we both were implicitly sensing lay in wait (that is, the anger and irritation that she referred to almost immediately after my comment).

My comment conveyed an interest in Nancy's experience in a second way as well, a way that probably added to her sense of security in the situation and thus further contributed to tilting the balance of forces and producing a rapid movement from "I don't know what I'm feeling" to a discussion of what she *was* feeling. By asking her to *tell me more about the experience* that led her to say "I don't know," I was both acknowledging that there *was* an experience and communicating an impression that it was interesting in its own right. In other words, I

---

[4] One could also, of course, view her "I don't know" as an indication of resistance. I discuss below why I did not approach it from this vantage point.

was not responding so much to an absence (as would be the case if I were thinking mainly in terms of "resistance") as to a presence. I did not *challenge* her "I don't know," I *went into it.*

This was especially important in the work with Nancy, because as I shall elaborate below, Nancy was very prone to feel, about many different aspects of her experience, that "I don't do things very well" or "I'm not doing this very well." Had I focused on the way she was *avoiding* telling me what she was feeling, this would have been one more instance of this. It would likely have been countertherapeutic not only in the sense of making her feel worse about herself, playing into her difficulties in a way that compounded them, but also in the sense that it would likely have closed off rather than opened up the channels of expression and communication.

To be sure, if one chose, one could certainly understand her "I don't know" from the point of view of resistance. It was a way of (at least temporarily) blocking access to an important, if conflicted, experience, and it was indeed an aim of the work to enable her more readily to discuss such experiences. In my approach to her "I don't know," however, I was not trying to get her to notice or acknowledge her resistances. I did not "interpret defenses." Instead, I tried to promote an experience of approaching, staying with, experiencing the state of mind that she *was* in, and to do so in a mode that valued that experience as itself communicating something, rather than implicitly disparaging it as resistance.

The experience (the presence rather than absence) that I attended to initially was not the one that she may have thought was required or expected in therapy—telling me "what she was feeling"—but it was a presence nonetheless. That is, the experience of uncertainty, of befuddlement, of blockage, of "I don't know," was itself an experience, and in inquiring the way I did, part of what I conveyed was that it was as legitimate an experience as any other. Telling me she didn't know what she was feeling was in fact telling me what she was feeling. The feeling of "I don't know" *was* the feeling at that point, and although it was a product of conflict—and was simultaneously the gateway to and the locked door in front of still other feelings that we would indeed eventually have to get to—it was a "real" feeling nonetheless.

One might certainly argue that in some sense Nancy "did" know what she was feeling, since she could readily identify it as soon as I made my comment. It is not my view, however, that in a directly experiential sense she "really" knew but was just not saying. I believe that her immediate experience *really was* "I don't know what I'm feeling," and that it reflected the sense of blockage that resulted from her anxiety and apprehension. Put differently, or from a slightly different perspective, just beneath the inhibitory operations that blocked her awareness of what she was feeling, the statement expressed a not yet articulated sense of "I don't know . . . *where this might go*" or "I don't know . . . *if what I'm feeling is acceptable*" or "I don't know . . . *what I'd feel if I took the lid off.*"

Turning to a slightly different dimension of my response to Nancy's opening comment, we may note that although my asking her to tell me more about the *experience* of "I don't know" could be seen as the functional equivalent of asking her for her "associations," there is a subtle difference that I think is important at a moment of vulnerability such as that we are addressing here. Asking about her *experience* in a certain sense *validates* her experience, and aims to go *further into* her experience. Asking for associations, in contrast, or saying something such as, "*What comes to mind* about that experience?" can seem to imply that what she is saying now is not good enough, that we must go *somewhere else* to find the "real" meaning. While it is certainly the case that very commonly in the course of my work, probably almost every day, I ask patients, "What comes to mind?" it is nonetheless important to be aware of the small nuances in meaning that can, at moments when the patient is feeling very vulnerable, leave the patient feeling marginally more or less supported in the effort she is making. I am reminded here of a case reported by Greenson (1967). Although he had never expressed a political opinion in the analysis, the patient knew he was a liberal Democrat because, unwittingly, whenever the patient said anything positive about a Republican, Greenson asked him for his associations, whereas he did not if the patient said something positive about a Democrat. Asking for associations, the patient recognized, was a way of expressing disapproval, of indicating that this particular attitude needed looking into.

Sometimes, instead of asking for associations, therapists ask for the patient's *fantasies* ("What's your fantasy about what I'm feeling?" "What's your fantasy about where I'm going on vacation?") Words like *fantasy* are so familiar, so much part of the discourse of most dynamic therapists, that it can be easy to overlook the ways in which such language can subtly undermine and disparage. Although one can argue that the technical meaning of the psychoanalytic concept of fantasy simply refers to an unconscious structure of thought or feeling, and does not necessarily imply that the patient is wrong or foolish, the everyday meaning of the term often implies that a fantasy is illusory or delusional, "just a fantasy." Indeed, even the way it is used by psychoanalysts carries this implication much of the time. From a constructivist viewpoint, in which the nature of what is "realistic" and what is error or fantasy is largely a matter for discussion and negotiation, the idea that the contents of the patient's mind are "fantasies" is an anachronism, a holdover from the objectivist vision in which the analyst views rationally and realistically the *irrationalities* of the patient. One can continue to pursue understanding of the patient's unconscious or not fully formulated assumptions and structures of thought without prejudging them as "fantasies." Indeed, we do best clinically when we examine how, even if idiosyncratically and often in symbolized and indirect form, the patient's "fantasies" reflect acutely the life circumstances and relational events that the patient encounters (cf. Gill, 1982; Wachtel, 1993).

Returning specifically to the issue of exposure, it is interesting to note that as the session unfolded, it became apparent that Nancy's description of her contribution to the writing of the book and what she viewed as appropriate credit for that contribution was quite different telling it to me in the session from how she had discussed it in her conversations with Linda herself. As Nancy elaborated on her actual conversations with Linda, it was clear that she did not make her case nearly as strongly or clearly with Linda as she had with me. So I said to Nancy, "See if you can put yourself back in the situation with Linda. See what it feels like to say to her what you have just told me: 'Linda, this was my idea to begin with. You never would have thought to do this at all if I hadn't come up with it, and I've done at least as much work on it as you have. I deserve to be listed as a coauthor.'"

When Nancy did begin to imagine such a conversation, she became increasingly aware of her anger at Linda, and increasingly *uncomfortable* about the anger. I then said to her, "Okay, let's go back into that situation and see what it's like when you're angry, just let it go in whatever way your feelings take you. You can decide later how you want to actually present it to Linda, or for that matter, whether you want to at all. For now, our aim is just for you to experience what it's like for you to feel angry and, frankly, for you to *feel less afraid* of being angry, so you have more room to make choices that work for you."

Note that this was not an *interpretation*. I did not point out to her the anger that she had been hiding from herself, nor did I point out that she had been *avoiding* anger or *avoiding noticing* her anger. To be sure, I had been thinking for a while about her struggle with angry feelings, and I did have as an aim to help her to be more comfortable and accepting toward such feelings, and hence more able to acknowledge them consciously. Moreover, explicitly pointing to feelings that the patient has not yet allowed himself to consciously experience is by no means an activity outside the range of my everyday clinical work (though, as discussed in the previous chapter, I am very concerned that such comments not be made in a tone that implies laying bare the patient's illusions or self-deceptions, but rather in a way that *invites* or *makes room for* or *makes more acceptable* the experience that has been cast out of consciousness). But in this particular instance I did *not* comment on Nancy's anger until she herself had discovered the experience. Rather, what I did was first create conditions (beginning with my acceptance of and interest in her "I don't know") in which she would feel safer and more self-affirming, and hence would be more likely to let herself discover and acknowledge the anger. Then, once the anger was out in the open some, I encouraged her to *expose* herself to the experience of anger, to engage in an *experiential* exercise of making the anger feel safer rather than a primarily *verbal* exercise of "interpreting" it. I asked her to *put herself into* the situation of being angry in much the way one asks a phobic patient to approach the situation that *he* fears.

In thinking about approaching the material Nancy had defended against in a way designed to help her reduce the anxiety and shame that kept her unable to accept these experiences, it is important to note that one of the key painful experiences for this patient was the experience of "I'm not doing this very well" or "I don't do things very well." Treating her "I don't know what I'm feeling" as a resistance, as something problematic that needed to be overcome, would have played into and aggravated this already painful inclination to feel she had not done things right. In contrast, viewing her statement as a legitimate communication in its own right helped to enable her to feel just a fraction stronger or more capable, and thus was a further contribution to tipping the balance toward exploration of still other feelings.

I have discussed elsewhere (Wachtel, 1993) a similar kind of process that has been particularly helpful in working with patients with schizoid or obsessional tendencies. With these individuals, one sometimes encounters the situation in which the patient says he is not feeling anything at all. Often, this is stated in a way that conveys a painful sense of emptiness or of "not being all right," and although there may also be overtones of resistance in the message, the main sense the therapist has is of the patient's vulnerability. This can make it difficult to address the experience with the patient because any attempt to focus on it heightens the patient's sense of inadequacy and of not being normal, at times even of not being quite human.

However, following an approach similar to how I addressed Nancy's experience of "I don't know what I'm feeling," one can at times be strikingly helpful by accepting and starting with the experience that the patient does have. For example, if it seems appropriate to what is presently transpiring, one might say something like, "What I'm sensing from what you've been saying is that it's very painful to view yourself as someone who has no feelings, that it makes you feel like an incomplete human being. But I'm also struck that that painful sense of lacking feelings is itself a feeling. In fact, it seems to me at this moment like a *very strong* feeling; you're feeling *a lot* that you're inadequate, that you're not like other people, and it feels very *bad*. What's coming across to me is not that you don't have any feelings but that it feels to you that you have the *wrong* feelings, that you're *supposed to* have a *different* feeling."

This kind of commentary, I have found, is often quite striking to these patients. Even in patients whose defenses include an excess of sophistication and cynicism, it often evokes a sense almost of wonderment: "You mean my awful feeling right now is a *feeling*? It *counts*?" And when I respond, say, with "Well, what do you think?" there may be almost giddy laughter preceding a comment such as, "Yeah, I guess it is." Once this step is achieved (obviously, as in almost everything in the process of therapy, not as a once-and-for-all single transformative event but as part of a series of such transactions), then it is often possible to explore how the patient learned to dismiss some of his feelings as "not counting" or as the "wrong one." Starting with validating the less welcome feelings (feelings of coldness or indifference, of wanting to get away from people, of pretending to feel what is expected), one can often over time help the patient to regain access to a wider range of feelings. Indeed, once feelings of love or caring, for example, are removed from the realm of "what I'm supposed to feel"—which is not infrequently what has quashed them—they often begin to emerge in a version that feels more like the patient's own.

I had the opportunity to observe a particularly interesting instance of this process a number of years ago:

A patient reported that his father died, and said he had no feelings. He felt we should talk about his father's death, but didn't know how to because he didn't feel anything about him. From clues in the session and from what I already knew about him, I suggested that it wasn't true that he didn't have feelings about the death. He just wasn't feeling *grief* at the moment. Instead, he was feeling a sense of relief at his father's being gone and a defiant feeling of "I don't care." The patient broke into a nervous laugh and said, "Yes, that's right! But is that a feeling?" He began to reflect that maybe he wasn't "good," but he was a "real person" after all. A variety of meaningful and affect-laden associations began to occur to him and, interestingly, later in the session he did directly experience feelings of grief and loss. It seems likely to me that had I focused on his defensive way of warding off feelings (however "accurate" my interpretations), he would have had considerably more difficulty getting in touch with the range of feelings that the death stirred in him. (Wachtel, 1993, pp. 123–124)

THE PERPETUATION OF EARLY FEARS

One might wonder why fears and anxieties that are rooted in the helplessness of early childhood do not disappear over time as the dependent infant grows into an increasingly capable child and then an adult. In part, of course, the answer is that they do. It makes little sense to describe every adult, even those who seem to live full and rich lives, as an emotional cripple, living within a cage created by the fears of early childhood. And we know that many common fears and symptoms— including fears of monsters lurking under the bed or frenzied emotional "meltdowns" that would be a sign of severe pathology in an adult—are absolutely normal parts of early childhood and are clearly "outgrown" by most individuals over time (at least in their overt or original form).

Moreover, there exist countervailing forces in the course of development that push toward growth and change rather than the perpetuation of childhood limitations. Some authors have conceptualized these countervailing forces as reflecting a biologically innate tendency toward personal growth and self-actualization that will be expressed naturally by the personality if it is not actively blocked and impeded. Others have discussed how the parents' efforts to provide consistent and loving attention or empathic resonance help the child to structure his emerging desires and fantasies and, over time, to experience them as relatively safe and consonant with the self. It is true that parents can place demands on children or seem to make their love contingent in ways that lead the child to be wary of his emerging thoughts, desires, and feelings. But they can also be "good enough," in Winnicott's (1975) felicitous phrase.

There are many ways, however, in which the consequences of our early fears can persist, and virtually none of us escape completely unscathed from the prolonged dependence that is the state of child-hood for our species. Understanding the complexly interacting psychological processes and events that maintain these persistences, including very centrally the vicious circles that are at the heart of the process, is of central concern for the practice of psychotherapy. I have already discussed the way in which the defensive avoidances brought into play by these early peremptory fears prevent us from testing the waters to see if the danger no longer exists in such a dire way and how they interfere with our learning to modify and modulate conflicted desires, preventing us from finding safer and more acceptable—as well as more gratifying—ways of expressing them. But there are still further problematic consequences to our learning to escape from the emo-tional states we come early in life to experience as dangerous. For one, by excluding in this way some of the fundamental emotional building blocks of human experience, we impair both our vitality and our ability even to really know what will bring us satisfaction. This is one of the reasons why attaining a measure of insight remains an important goal of the therapeutic effort, notwithstanding the importance of going beyond the *almost exclusive* focus on insight that for so long impeded therapeutic practice. Moreover, avoidant retreat from certain features of our emotional life also prevents access to some of the cues and sub-tle experiences that are the foundation of successful "intuition"; we are thus rendered less adept socially, less able to negotiate the daily interac-tions with others in a way that brings real satisfaction and security. And ironically, these efforts to protect our ties to others and our sense of self by restricting affective expression and awareness end up leaving us *more* vulnerable, as we find ourselves less able to deal effectively with situations that ordinarily evoke the "missing" emotional state and therefore more anxious when those situations arise. Indeed, what may happen is that fears that may initially have been "unrealistic" can increasingly become realistic as a consequence of the very ways that the person deals with them. Our defenses protect us from anxiety in the immediate moment, but increasingly they become a way of perpetuating the very state of vulnerability they were designed to quell.

In a certain sense, then, we may say that Freud's original formulation, that anxiety is a result of repression or defense, was not as completely wrong as he said it was in 1926. Although it is true that anxiety comes before repression and is its primary cause, it is also the case that once repression and other defenses and self-restrictions are in place, they in turn generate or perpetuate anxiety in their own right by the way that they render the person more vulnerable and less capable. Once again, what we encounter here is a vicious circle, in which anxiety generates defenses that in turn generate still more anxiety and hence still further defensive efforts. Or, as family therapists sometimes put it, the solution becomes the problem.

10

■　■　■　■　■

Enactments, New Relational Experience, and Implicit Relational Knowing

In the last few chapters I argued that both depth of exploration and effectiveness in promoting desired change are enhanced by a clinical approach that is considerably more engaged, encouraging, and accepting than the default position that for so long dominated the thinking of psychotherapists. In place of the rather standoffish, cautious, "objectivist" stance that aims to confront the patient with the truth he has denied and buried; that is suspicious of his motives and wary lest the patient "manipulate" the therapist into providing "infantile" gratifications; that seeks, ultimately, to persuade the patient to renounce his childish longings and face reality, the approach described here aims to help the patient reappropriate the aspects of his self-experience and affective life that have been cast aside under the pressure of anxiety, guilt, and shame. It regards support not as antithetical to effective self-exploration but as the very ground of such exploration, providing the safety and encouragement necessary for exploration to proceed in a manner that truly expands the self.

As I have noted in earlier chapters, in discussing writers such as

Stone (1961), Loewald (1960), and Schafer (1983), this evolution in clinical thinking is not the exclusive contribution of the relational movement. Clearly, though, that movement has helped to accelerate and enhance this evolution and to increase its acceptance in the psychoanalytic community. Even among relational thinkers, however, departures from the default position have at times been conflicted and hedging. As Crastnopol (2001) has put it:

> Most of us relationalists received some training in a more classical model and have internalized important elements of that approach, both theoretical and technical. These unarticulated, unconscious assumptions and beliefs act sotto voce to modulate our clinical choices in ways we may grasp only imperfectly, or not at all. As a result, the continuing influence of these earlier analytic values and guidelines on our work is not sufficiently formulated and transmitted in relational teaching or writing. (p. 390)

In this chapter, I will further examine both how relational thinking has contributed to the transcendence of the default position and how, nonetheless, some of the holdover assumptions that Crastnopol alludes to have frequently constrained relational thinkers from fully pursuing the clinical implications of their conceptual innovations. I will elaborate in particular on how an understanding of the pervasive role of vicious circles in the maintenance of problematic psychological patterns and experiences fits together with an emphasis on deep understanding and empathic immersion in the experience of the other. I will discuss as well how this synthesis points to a therapeutic approach that is less centered on the therapist's role as interpreter and more attuned to her role as a participant in new relational experiences that promote change via *implicit* reworking of internal working models and other relational schemas. Such an approach is more focused on the immediate affective and experiential interchange that has variously been called, among other conceptualizations, corrective emotional experience (Alexander & French, 1946), new relational experience (Frank, 1999), moments of meeting (Stern et al., 1998), passing the patient's tests (Weiss & Sampson, 1986), new object experience (Loewald, 1960), repairing ruptures in the therapeutic relationship (Safran & Muran, 2000), and "an actual relationship with a reliable and beneficent parental figure" (Fairbairn, 1958, p. 377).

THE THERAPEUTIC RELATIONSHIP
AND NEW RELATIONAL EXPERIENCE

For most of its history, psychoanalysis has been essentially an *interpretive* discipline. Interpretation was valued above all other interventions, and, indeed, a range of influential writers advocated approaching the therapeutic task, whenever possible, via interpretation alone. In discussing interpretation in his influential textbook of psychoanalytic technique, Greenson (1967) called interpretation "the single most important instrument of psychoanalytic technique. Every other analytic procedure prepares for an interpretation, amplifies an interpretation, or makes an interpretation effective" (p. 97). When other influences and interventions were introduced—Eissler (1953) called them parameters—they were generally viewed as needing to be "resolved" by *themselves* being interpreted.[1]

At the same time, there has, from the very beginning, been an appreciation that the interpretive effort is embedded *in a relationship,* and that that relationship is itself a crucial part of the process. Indeed, in a noteworthy quotation, Freud stated, "What turns the scale in [the patient's] struggle is not his intellectual insight —which is neither strong enough nor free enough for such an achievement—but *simply and solely* his relation to the doctor" (1917, p. 445, italics added). Notwithstanding the seeming implications of this apparently rather definitive statement, however, Freud also repeatedly insisted that this source of influence was only temporary and could be resolved through interpretation, and that is the view that has dominated psychoanalytic thinking over the years. In essence, the primary function of the relationship was not to be a direct source of change in itself but to bind the patient to the analyst, to prevent him from running away when the going got tough and to make him more accessible to the *interpretations* that the analyst offered. As Freud put it in elaborating on the role of the relationship in his understanding of the analytic process, "In so far as his transference bears a 'plus' sign, it clothes the doctor with authority and is transformed into belief in his communications and explanations" (1917, p. 445).

---

[1] Even the increasingly prominent concern with making a case for there being "something more than" interpretation (e.g., Stern et al., 1998) speaks, by that very language, to interpretation as the standard or benchmark against which other kinds of interventions are measured or in relation to which other interventions are "additional."

The terms "intellectual insight" and "explanations" in the quotations from Freud in the last paragraph are noteworthy. Although Freud recognized—and indeed emphasized—that intellectual insight alone could not do the job, that what is now generally referred to as *emotional* insight is needed, it is not difficult to discern an air of *regret* in Freud's statement that intellectual insight is not sufficient to do the job. Belief in the analyst's *explanations,* as Freud here put it quite explicitly, remains at the heart of Freud's view of cure, and one of the problems with relying on interpretation as the primary engine of the therapeutic process is that so often what interpretations amount to are explanations. They may be explanations of the *origins* of a pattern (essentially, "You are feeling or doing this now because such and such happened in your past") or of the *reasons* for it in the present ("You are feeling or doing such and such because unconsciously you feel or want *x*").

I have, of course, somewhat exaggerated the explanatory or intellectual dimension in these last two illustrations. Comments of this type were not that rare in the earlier years of psychoanalytic practice, but today, one hopes, therapists are a bit more subtle. At the same time, writing as recently as 1996, Aron could state that "the international consensus among psychoanalysts" is that "the analyst's task is to interpret, that is *to explain* the patient's behavior and associations" (p. 95, italics added). My aim in what follows is to highlight the *experiential,* in contrast with the *explanatory* dimension of the therapist's participation, the way in which change is promoted most of all by *what actually happens between people.* This experiential dimension certainly does not exclude reflective awareness and the struggle to understand both oneself and the other. These are essential features of human psychological functioning, especially in the realm of relations between people and the experience of self. All experiences are experiences *as registered and interpreted by the individual.* But, as I shall elaborate below, much of the processing of experiences that goes on in the mind or the brain is procedural rather than declarative. It is the latter that is essentially emphasized in the traditional conception of interpretation as "[making] conscious the unconscious meaning source, history, mode, or cause of a given psychic event" (Greenson, 1967, p. 39) and in the common emphasis on explicit recall of early experiences and fantasies (Fonagy, 1999). But increasingly it is being understood that the process of therapeutic change is very largely a matter of *procedural* learning (e.g., Fonagy, 1999; Stern et al., 1998). I shall have more to say about this distinction later in this chapter.

Mitchell (1997) has argued that although interpretations are traditionally viewed as the central source of therapeutic change, interpretations *cannot* achieve this on their own because they can only be heard through the very categories the analyst is trying to change via the interpretation and because the analyst is inevitably drawn into the very pattern she is trying to interpret. Consequently, Mitchell concludes, "There must be something else on which the analyst can rest his weight while he is tugging on his interpretive bootstraps. . . . But whatever else is out there, in the analytic situation, has been generally invisible to our available conceptual repertoire, and *the preservation of Freud's now anachronistic model of therapeutic action, of interpretation leading to insight as the basic mechanism of change, lulls us into not really looking*" (1997, pp. 47–48, italics added).

That tendency not to look was very strongly reinforced by the reaction of the psychoanalytic community to the introduction by Franz Alexander (e.g., 1950, 1953, 1954, 1956, 1961; Alexander & French, 1946) of the concept of the corrective emotional experience as an alternative explanation for the source of therapeutic change. For Alexander, the key lever of change lay in *direct experience* that contradicted long-held expectations rather than in interpretations that *explained* them as rooted in the past. In Alexander's view, the insights that patients achieved in psychoanalytic therapy were at least as much a *product* of the changes in the patient's presenting difficulties as their cause.[2]

In one of his clearest statements of the basic principle, Alexander (1961) stated, "The cognitive act, namely the intellectual *recognition* of the difference between past and present is secondary to the actual *experiencing* of this difference in interacting with the therapist. In this view the emphasis shifts from insight to experience, although the role of insight as a secondary but often powerful consolidating factor is by no means denied" (p. 307).

At the time Alexander introduced his innovations, he was profoundly anathematized and virtually excommunicated from the psy-

---

[2] A very similar view has been expressed by Fonagy (1999), this time based on an additional 50 years of accumulated clinical experience and on the findings of cognitive science: "Analysts and patients frequently assume that remembering past events has caused change. I believe that the return of such memories is an epiphenomenon, an inevitable *consequence* of the exploration of mental models of relationships. . . . It provides an explanation but is therapeutically inert" (p. 218, italics added; see also Ghent, 1995, p. 486).

choanalytic community.[3] Alexander's approach to patients was depicted as artificial, ungenuine, and manipulative, and to this day, even writers who are strong advocates of acknowledging the long neglected role of new relational experiences in the therapeutic process continue to deride Alexander's contribution. Thus Mitchell (1997) calls Alexander's approach "a custom-designed posturing opposite to the emotional style of the parents" and depicts it as "contrived and manipulative" (p. 16). Greenberg (1996) refers to "Alexander's simplistic and overdrawn theory of 'corrective emotional experience' " (p. 195), and Frank (2005) states, "Mainstream psychoanalysts attacked [Alexander's] 'flexible' approach as nonanalytic—correctly, in my view, in so far as the analyst's stance was inauthentic and manipulative" (p. 22).

For decades, this scornful (Gill, 1994) attitude toward Alexander's "heresy" (Friedman, 1986, p. 333) impeded the evolution of psychoanalytic thinking about the therapeutic process. When the "dreaded" (Friedman, 1997, p. 1227) specter of the corrective emotional experience was raised, most analysts retreated. Writing more than 40 years after Alexander introduced his innovations, Friedman (1988) noted that "the 'bad' example of Franz Alexander, with his 'corrective emotional experience,' is held up as a warning to theorists who talk about nonconceptual, discursive, noninterpretational elements in therapy" (p. 521), and Frank (1999), writing still a decade later, noted that the "suppressive influence . . . survives to this day [and] has prevented the full emergence of many participatory and helpful forms of psychoanalytic activity" (p. 192). In the same vein, Mitchell (1997) notes that "by using Alexander as a foil, 'classical' psychoanalytic technique was reshaped and reaffirmed as the unique standard methodology [what I have called in this book the default position] for several decades to come. Psychoanalysis and proper analytic technique were preserved as noninteractional and nonsuggestive, as offering a unique situation within which the inner dynamics of the patient simply emerge in their pure form, uncontaminated by external influence" (pp. 15–16; cf. Wachtel, 1982a).

At the same time, it must be noted that Alexander's new under-

---

[3] The reaction to Alexander's innovations in the late 1940s and for decades afterward paralleled the response to earlier innovations by Ferenczi (e.g., 1955; Ferenczi & Rank, 1925). That response, and the relatively recent resurgence of interest in Ferenczi's work, has been well described in Aron and Harris (1993). See also Aron (1996), Bonomi (1998), and Dupont (1988).

standing of the therapeutic process never really disappeared. It became, rather, the insight that dared not speak its name. Influential psychoanalytic writers repeatedly put forth formulations that closely resembled Alexander's forbidden idea, but usually with a terminology that obscured the similarity. Thus Alexander's formulation is paralleled in important respects by Fairbairn's view that what is therapeutic in analysis derives from the analyst providing "an actual relationship with a reliable and beneficent parental figure" (1958, p. 377), as well as by Loewald's (1960) emphasis on the importance of the analyst being a new good object, Kohut's (1977) account of the analyst as offering himself as a new and more empathically responsive self-object, and Weiss and Sampson's (1986) depiction of therapeutic progress being promoted by the therapist's passing tests set by the patient (see Eagle, 1993; Wachtel & DeMichele, 1998). Parallels are evident as well, in a variety of different forms, in the emphasis on new relational experience across virtually the entire spectrum of approaches that constitute the contemporary relational point of view.

But the continuing taboo associated with the concept of the corrective emotional experience, *even if it has* been rediscovered and reconfigured in other terms, means, as the quotations from Friedman and from Frank on the previous page illustrate, that a "do not enter" sign is still posted at a crucial juncture of psychoanalytic thought and discourse, restricting creative thought in unnoticed and unpredictable ways. We know, from our clinical work most of all, that when any line of thought or association is forbidden, it leads to further restrictions— restrictions that are impossible to predict but that follow from the way that danger signals are also aroused by otherwise acceptable ideas that are *associated with* the forbidden thought, and then ideas associated with *those* ideas. In this way, even when thought looks free and unrestricted, there are invisible magnetic fields that pull people's thinking away from potentially dangerous directions *without the thinker experiencing overt distress or knowing he is avoiding.* This idea is embodied both in Freud's (1926) concept of signal anxiety and in Sullivan's (1953) of the anxiety gradient, and it is something we should take as seriously in evaluating the nature of theory development (especially in a field in which transferential and personal identity bonds are so powerful) as we should in evaluating the impact of covert avoidances on the lives and the thinking of individual patients. When there are black holes, forbidden thoughts, ideas that cannot be named, there is inevitable constriction. We may "work around" the restriction by finding new names (new relational experience instead of corrective emotional experience, for example), but when there is still something "forbidden" in the air, there is, inevitably, a price to pay. To be sure, there are certainly grounds on which to take issue with particular aspects of the way that Alexander framed his version of the corrective emotional experience, and ways in which the contentions of manipulativeness and lack of genuineness that were the focus of his critics to the exclusion of everything else did have some basis in things Alexander actually said and did. He wrote, for example, that "not every analyst is a *good enough actor* to create, convincingly, an atmosphere he wants" (Alexander, 1961, p. 331, italics added), and there were ways in which his clinical stance could seem to be characterized as a kind of preplanned role-playing rather than the responsive, continually evolving engagement that is more characteristic of contemporary therapists who advocate new relational experience as a key therapeutic factor.

Alexander's ideas, however, are rarely given the kind of benefit of the doubt that Erikson (1963) was referring to when he said of Freud's libido theory, "True insight survives its first formulation" (p. 64). There are certainly ways in which Alexander's "first formulation" was a bit cruder than those that were offered by other innovators some years or decades later, building on his contribution, whether acknowledging so or not. Today we are accustomed to taking many of Freud's formulations, as well as those of other early psychoanalytic pioneers, as brilliant first steps that required further refinement. The meanings of Freud's recommendations that the analyst should be like a mirror or like a surgeon, or of venerable concepts like the blank screen, or neutrality, or even transference and countertransference are continually being reworked and redefined as psychoanalytic thought evolves, and today's usage of these terms often bears at most only a family resemblance to the way they were first formulated and stated in the literature. Were these concepts subjected to the same prosecutorial mindset that has persistently been applied to the concept of the corrective emotional experience, the psychoanalytic literature would look strikingly different today.

Alexander's understanding of the difficulties in achieving the appropriately "corrective" stance with the patient was limited by the development of the field at the time. Although in certain respects he was one of the pioneers of two-person thinking—both in his emphasis on the relational experience as an important therapeutic factor and in his appreciation (Alexander, 1961) that the patient's transference reactions were in part a response to the actual behavior and characteristics of the therapist—he also largely manifested the same objectivism that characterized virtually every psychoanalytic thinker of his era. As a consequence, his innovative and progressive aims—for example, to replace the one-size-fits-all approach, in which "neutrality" and "interpreting" were advocated for all patients, with a more specific and differentiated approach in which the particular needs, vulnerabilities, and history of the patient determined how the therapist constructed the relationship—were combined with an underestimation of the difficulties and complexities in achieving these aims.

The therapist does not stand outside the patient's relational field, assessing the patient's needs from a vantage point of dispassionate expertise. She is inevitably drawn in, sometimes caught in the emotional force field sufficiently that, for a period of time, she becomes a participant in the problematic pattern, an "accomplice," as I have called it. The process whereby we can, over time, gain sufficient reflective distance on the pattern in which we and the patient are mutually caught is a difficult one to conceptualize (Stern, 2003). But it does seem that, at least to some degree, good therapists do precisely this, and in thereby managing to respond differently to the patient than others in his life have tended to, they contribute to changing the pattern.

Because of the strong presumptions in the psychoanalytic community of his day regarding the superiority of interpretation, neutrality, and the promotion of insight over all other forms of therapeutic intervention, Alexander emphasized *non*interpretive approaches to providing a corrective emotional experience. In a theoretical climate of rather pervasive and stultifying orthodoxy, it was natural that recognition of the powerful therapeutic role of new relational experiences in their own right would be formulated as an *alternative* to the prevailing approach. But from a contemporary vantage point, we may note that interpreting too is a form of interacting (e.g., Stolorow & Atwood, 1997; Gill, 1991; Aron, 1996; Mitchell, 1997; Hoffman, 1998) and is itself a new way of responding to the patient that is likely to differ quite substantially from how his parents interacted with him or how other current figures in his life respond. In this sense, an interpretation too can be a new relational experience. This is in part the idea embodied in Ogden's (1994, 2004), Benjamin's (2004), and Aron's (2006) conception of the therapeutic or analytic "third." It is also closely related to Stolorow, Brandchaft, and Atwood's (1987) depiction of the therapeutically effective new relational experience as being an experience of being deeply and accurately understood by the other, a formulation that can be seen as uniting the interpretive tradition and the tradition of the corrective emotional experience. But offering "something different" by offering an interpretation is only one of the many possible alternative responses; it is not always the most effective and at times is not benign. To the degree that an "interpretive" response reflects (as it not infrequently does) a stubborn persistence of the default position, a refusal to interact (or at least to acknowledge interacting), it can be experienced, depending on the patient's particular developmental history and the representations of relationships that evolved as a result, not as a *corrective* emotional experience, but as a *repetitive* emotional experience; that is, as an enactment of earlier, pathogenic interactions with the parent.

In a contemporary relational variant on Alexander's essential idea, Mitchell (1997) describes a process in which the therapist's response needs to be different for different patients but in which that response evolves out of the moment by moment engagement between the two participants. The shifting emotional state of each, as well as between them, means that no one way of interacting and engaging is likely to be appropriate for the entire course of the work, and Mitchell's understanding of the process is clearly one in which the therapist's genuineness is crucial, as is her attention to the nuances of the relational state between them. At the same time, it will be apparent that Mitchell's description here overlaps considerably with Alexander's original conception. He describes the therapeutic process as one in which patient and therapist

> struggle together to find a different kind of emotional connection. There is no general solution or technique, because each resolution, by its very nature, must be custom designed. If the patient feels that the analyst is applying a technique or displaying a generic attitude or stance, the analysis cannot possibly work. Sometimes *making interpretations* works analytically, not simply because of the content of the interpretation, but because the patient experiences the interpreting analyst as alive, as caring, as providing fresh ways of thinking about things, as grappling deeply with what is bothering him. Sometimes *refraining* from interpreting works analytically, because the patient experiences the quiet analyst as alive, as caring, as providing fresh ways to be together that don't demand what may have come to feel like the inescapable corruptions of language. Sometimes *patience* seems called for: a sustained involvement over time that is evidence

of a kind of relationship different from past abandonments. Sometimes *impatience* is required: an exasperation that conveys a sense that the analyst can envision something better than the patient's perseverative patterns and cares enough not to take the easy way out and passively go along. (Mitchell, 1997, p. 58, italics added)

Here we see what might be regarded as the mature expression of Alexander's original formulation, a version of the idea of the corrective emotional experience that is integrated with an understanding of the therapist's participation and immersion in the patient's experience and, implicitly, of the need to keep groping toward a better state even if one is groping to some degree in rather dim light. Contemporary understanding suggests that we are engaged in continual adjustments and refinements in relation to the patient, and that what we thought was the properly corrective stance at one point in the evolution of our understanding may, upon reflection, turn out to have been counterproductive and that, moreover, the very experience generated by *one* "corrective" response on the therapist's part brings forth a different personal and relational configuration that may now need a *different* kind of response. We rarely get it right "once and for all," but the work proceeds by making midcourse corrections—indeed, can be seen as *very largely consisting of* the midcourse corrections. As both Kohut (1984) and Safran and Muran (2000) have suggested, progress comes not so much from avoiding mistakes as from making therapeutic capital out of those mistakes, from repairing the breaks in empathy and ruptures in the therapeutic alliance that are an inevitable (and ultimately very important) part of the process.

A CLINICAL ILLUSTRATION

I would like at this point to illustrate and elaborate on some of the considerations put forth thus far in the chapter by offering a clinical example. In doing so, I will also be able to point to ways in which the particular version of relational thinking that guides this book—the cyclical psychodynamic theory, with its emphasis on the central role of vicious circles in maintaining the problems people bring to psychotherapy—gives a particular cast to the clinical interaction and to the way that the therapist attempts to help the patient extricate himself from the tangle in which he is caught. The patient, Michael, was a graduate student who had an unusually prickly, sometimes even paranoid-seeming manner. His father had been exceedingly critical and emotionally abusive, and it was not difficult to hypothesize a connection between Michael's manner in the present and the emotional climate of his home growing up. In essence, Michael seemed to anticipate from everyone the kind of response to him that he had regularly received at home.

Not surprisingly, he saw me too as critical and unsympathetic. Also not surprisingly, I was only too happy to view that perception as an example of transference. I saw Michael many years ago, at a time when I was in the midst of a transition from a more traditional psychoanalytic point of view to the integrative and relational perspectives that characterize my present thinking. At the time I began working with Michael, I was still inclined to view transference as a relatively direct persistence of earlier modes of perception for which I was just the "trigger": Michael, I thought, was seeing me as like his father *despite the fact that I was not.* I was also inclined to have much more faith in interpretation than I do now. Hence, my comments were largely of the sort that sounded something like, "Isn't it interesting that you see me as being just the way your father was." I cringe as I read this last sentence now. To begin with, it was delivered in the stilted manner that was clinically de rigueur at the time, supposedly neutral, enlisting the patient's "observing ego," attempting to make him *curious* about himself. But in fact, as I have noted in a more extended discussion of the clinical habits of psychotherapists when they speak to patients (Wachtel, 1993), "Isn't it interesting?" is usually not, in this context, either neutral or an expression of interest. It is, very often, a disguised putdown, a way of pointing out to the patient that he is distorting, misperceiving, that what he has said or experienced is not so much interesting as *wrong.* Most of us are only too happy to be told that something we have said is interesting. But this particular version (employed very frequently by therapists at the time my career was in its early stages) would be unlikely to warm the cockles of the patient's heart.

The second aspect of the comment that feels quite alien to the way I approach things now is that the comment leaves me out. It portrays his perception of me as having essentially nothing to do with me, as being the result simply of applying an old schema or representational mapping to a new, *inappropriate* object—namely, poor, innocent, "neutral" me.

I am not suggesting that there was no distortion—or at the very least, an idiosyncratic way of interpreting the data—in Michael's perceptions. Michael's *problem* was that he saw so many people as unsympathetic and out to thwart or demean him. But his problem was more complex than that. It was also that Michael's perceptions had *consequences.* They caused him to *act* in certain ways and those actions in turn evoked responses from others. Those latter responses, reactions to being viewed quite negatively and suspiciously by Michael, were frequently ones of annoyance, of seeing Michael as unpleasant, difficult, paranoid, and a little "off the wall." As a consequence they frequently ended up being responses to Michael that "confirmed" the expectations that led to his behavior in the first place, and hence started the cycle over once again.

At the time I began working with Michael, however, I had not yet developed the more thoroughgoing, two-person, vicious circle perspective that I employ now. I was inclined to focus on the patient's "internal structures" and how those structures played themselves out, almost inexorably, as he went through life. And it must be said that often such a viewpoint can be quite compelling and seem to conform very well to the clinical data. Thus not only did Michael tend to see me as a rather critical and unsympathetic person (a perception that I will vigorously deny later in this account!) but he also had a strikingly jaundiced view of others that seemed at times to verge on the truly paranoid. One particularly striking example had to do with his need, as a student, to take out some rather expensive and complicated equipment in order to complete his assignments. He found that whenever he went to the department office where the equipment was available for students, it was already taken, and he began to feel that the other students in the program were taking out the equipment even when they didn't need it just to thwart his efforts.

The reader will probably not be surprised that I viewed his interpretation of events with some skepticism. It was part of what gave a somewhat paranoid cast to Michael. As a result of the interaction I am about to describe, however, my skepticism about his view of why the equipment was so frequently out became a little less certain. I am still inclined to view Michael's interpretation of events as improbable, but it felt a little *less* improbable after I was forced to look at how unhelpfully I myself could interact with Michael at times.

The turning point occurred after most of the patterns I have been describing had already become quite evident, as had my substantial lack of success in resolving them through the "interpretations" I was making. On one occasion, Michael asked me to change an appointment time. Ordinarily, even at that earlier stage in my career, I was rather easygoing about such requests, rarely engaging in the ritual questioning, as some of my supervisors might have counseled, of why he was asking for this change at this particular moment. But on this occasion what ensued was a reversion to "classical" technique with a vengeance (quite literally, I am afraid). I began to say things like, "What comes to mind about your asking me for an appointment change?" "Why do you think you are asking for this change at this particular point in our work together?" "What do you think it would mean to you if I said yes?"

I don't know how many of these oafish statements I made before I came to my senses, but it certainly went on for much too long. What I meant above by "quite literally" with a vengeance is that what I finally realized was that I was not "exploring" or "analyzing" but simply giving Michael a hard time, and that indeed this way of grilling him on my part was a response to the hard time he frequently gave me. I had thought that I had my feelings under control, that his tensely hostile manner and his constantly accusing me of misunderstanding, of being ungiving, unhelpful, and even cruel were all things that I was "understanding" in light of my knowledge of his past. But, as happens so often, I was in fact more caught up in his interactive web than I had realized.

Fortunately, I *did* come to my senses. I began to feel very uncomfortable with how I was handling the session, and at a certain point I stopped myself and said something like the following: "Wait a minute, Michael. I'm just realizing something I should have realized a lot sooner. You made a simple and straightforward request. You had something you needed to do next Tuesday morning and it was something difficult for you to change. You asked if I could see you a different day. And what I did was to give you a very hard time, to be very difficult and unhelpful in response to your request. So first of all, let me apologize. I'm really sorry I did that. But I want to say something else as well. You have no way to know if what I'm telling you is true, you'll just have to take my word for it, but the way I just behaved is not the way I *usually* behave. Usually, if someone makes a request like you did, I would simply say something like, 'How about Wednesday?' Instead, I responded as if I were an FBI agent grilling you. And when I think of how I responded, it strikes me that it was very much like the way you describe many other people in your life acting toward you. I'm even thinking now about what you told me about the equipment at school. When I think of what *I* just did, that I don't usually do, I'm beginning to think that it's not impossible that your fellow students really did take it out on purpose, that they too got drawn into a pattern that seems to be very characteristic of your life and that leaves you feeling hurt, angry, and misunderstood. So I'm wondering, what goes on that leads people to act toward you the way they do? What was it that led *me* to act in a way that (again you'll just have to take my word for it) is quite untypical of me? I think if we can understand this, if we can understand the kind of tangle we got into, and that seems to happen to you so often, this could really be helpful."

To my significant surprise (and, I must say, relief—he did *not*, after all, have to "take my word for it"), Michael did not come back at me with a complaint about what I had just said. Instead, his posture and facial expression became noticeably more relaxed and open than I could ever recall seeing. He was clearly genuinely interested and intrigued by what I had said.

I think there were several things that contributed to Michael's interest and openness. Certainly part of it is that I was talking about something that had just happened between us that had been vivid and compelling. This is part of the rationale for the traditional emphasis on transference interpretations and the more recent emphasis on the examination of enactments. As Freud (1912b) famously said in discussing the transference, it is difficult to slay the enemy in absentia or in effigy. The transference makes the issues real and alive. But there was, I think, another element that was crucial in Michael's responsiveness to what I said. It was a *two-person* comment about a pattern in which *both* of us were participating, not a one-person observation of what *he* was doing. My including myself in the picture and taking responsibility for my own role in what had transpired enabled Michael to experience my comment from a different vantage point, and to transcend his usual narrative of being treated unfairly. As he expressed to me in a later session, he *experienced* himself in this exchange as being treated fairly, an experience that was quite rare for him.

At the same time, my description also fit within his usual, dominant vantage point as well, because my portrayal of how people consistently treated him badly resonated with his daily subjective experience. Consequently, what I was saying "made sense" to him. This combination of an experience that challenged his usual way of seeing things and, simultaneously, offered an *affirmation* of that way of seeing things, thereby enabling him to feel understood, is a combination of great potency clinically (see Wachtel, 1993, Ch. 8, and Chapter 12, this volume). In this instance, it enabled him to be genuinely open to the question of *how come* this happens again and again in his life, and, perhaps for the first time in an effective manner, interested in the question of what *his own* role was.

What I think was crucial was that my comments depicted Michael as *caught in something*. Rather than his being simply the one at fault, the very real *suffering* that was central in his life was the primary focus of the narrative. And for this very reason, his own role in the pattern could begin to be opened up and explored. What followed was, of course, not an instant resolution of his difficulties. Many repetitions of the earlier patterns, both between the two of us and between Michael and other people in his life, had to be endured and examined. But it was definitely a turning point, a moment of significant nonlinear change (cf. Thelen & Smith, 1994; Stern et al., 1998; Stolorow, 1997a, 1997b) and a foundation on which later important work could be built.

ENACTMENT AND ITS VICISSITUDES

In part, what transpired in this clinical interaction can be understood from the traditional vantage point of insight. I invited Michael to *understand* the pattern we had identified, to see it more clearly. But it can also be understood in relation to what has come to be called enactment (Jacobs, 1986; McLaughlin, 1991; Maroda, 1998; Frank, 2002; Aron, 2003; Black, 2003; Bass, 2003). The term "enactment" has come into increasingly wide use in recent years, but its meaning can differ subtly and even significantly in different usages. At times, the term is little more than a new label for what used to be called "acting out." That is, the patient is seen as "enacting" his conflicts or forbidden desires instead of expressing them verbally. In this meaning, enactment has the same largely pejorative and blaming connotation that acting out had, including the potential for invalidation that accompanies viewing the patient's behavior not as a meaningful effort to give expression to his needs in light of his perceptions, but as the manifestation of pathology or of "something earlier." The substitution of "enactment" for "acting out" is perhaps a bit of an advance because it generally connotes that the patient is (unconsciously) providing "material" that can be analyzed. That is, enactments are part of the "grist for the mill" that characterizes ordinary or normal therapeutic work, in contrast to the frequent way in which acting out is viewed even more pejoratively as something the patient has to be persuaded to *stop* so that the "proper" procedure of interpreting his *words and associations* can proceed. This advance, as it were, parallels the way in which transference, once thought of primarily as a *disruptive* force getting in the way of the "real work" of analysis became, over time, the central *medium for* that real work.

A different meaning of enactment, more compatible with the present point of view but still in important ways problematic, can be thought of as the "one-and-a-half-person" version. In this version, lying between one- and two-person perspectives, there is the *appearance* of a two-person account, in that the therapist or analyst is attending to her own participation in the pattern, the way in which she was drawn in. In that respect, this version accords with the depiction I have offered of my interaction with Michael. But in what I am calling the "one-and-a-half-person" version, the therapist is, in essence, the *innocent victim* of the patient's pathology or conflicts. It is essentially *the patient* who is "enacting," and the therapist is merely a bit player in the drama. This version resembles the way in which the concept of projective identification is often used. The patient "puts something into" the therapist and *for that reason* the therapist enacts her part in the story. (See again the discussion of projective identification in Chapter 6.)

In the version of the concept more fully compatible with the way of thinking being emphasized in this book, the enactment is an event in which the role of *both* parties is taken into account. Thus in my interaction with Michael, my apology to him was not perfunctory or pro forma. Although I believed my behavior to be in good measure a response to the specific experiences I had with Michael (and those experiences became, very centrally, the focus of much later exploration by both of us), *I* behaved in a way that was my own doing, not just "his fault." We got caught *together* in a pattern that, as it turned out (at least in the short run) was problematic for *both* of us: I experienced myself behaving badly and like the caricature of the very kind of therapist I have written about quite critically (Wachtel, 1993), and he experienced himself as once more being *treated* badly (and, perhaps, even at that early stage in the unfolding of the event, as also somehow *bringing about* such treatment). I say it was problematic "in the short run" because from a different vantage point, our both having gotten caught in this tangle turned out to be a useful experience that advanced the therapeutic work.

This last way of thinking about enactments is, essentially, a *systemic* version. It is not the patient's foibles that become the focus but *the pattern*, the repetitive sequence that he gets caught and entangled in again and again with various people. For a time, systems thinking was a *challenge* to psychoanalytic thought, a way of thinking that usually went along with strong criticism of the focus in psychoanalysis on the individual alone. But in recent years, there has been increasing interest in integrating systemic thinking *into* psychoanalysis (e.g., Beebe & Lachmann, 2003; Fosshage, 2003b; Ghent, 2002; Harris, 2005; Stolorow, 1997a, 1997b; Wachtel & Wachtel, 1986), and this synthesis seems to me to hold great promise for improving both our clinical work and our understanding.

Finally, from the vantage point of the concept of the corrective emotional experience, we may see that in almost any successful analysis of enactments, the playing out of the enactment entails two stages. The first (as in the experience with Michael that I described) is a decidedly *non*corrective experience, an instance of getting *caught* in the pattern. But then, with the stepping back and stepping outside, with the *reflection on* what has been transpiring, comes the potential for a *corrective* emotional experience. The enactment and its resolution are not just matters to be "analyzed"; they are processed as an *experience*, in much the way that, as discussed in Chapter 9, direct exposure to stimuli and situations that one fears can yield a therapeutic effect that no amount of "talking about" the experience can accomplish. With Michael, for example, it was not just "analyzing" what had transpired between us, and certainly not analyzing it as an occurrence that reveals something exclusively about him, that was therapeutic. Rather, it was the very way in which we discussed it as something also about me, as something that *I* did to *him,* that made an impact and represented a genuinely new experience for Michael.

Thinking in terms of corrective emotional experiences or new relational experiences does not in itself point to particular ways of being with the patient. For one patient, it may be particularly helpful to be ready to apologize where one has erred in some way or to bring oneself into the picture more generally in discussing what is transpiring. For another, with a different history and a different set of issues (say, someone who was raised in a home in which the parents turned every experience of the patient's into something about them) it may be important, for some period of time, to maintain the focus almost exclusively on the patient's experience and *not* to emphasize one's own experience or behavior. It is important to understand that *either* focus in any particular interaction with the patient can derive from a two-person or contextual viewpoint. As the quotation from Mitchell earlier in the chapter illustrates, such a viewpoint can lead to a wide range of ways of interacting depending on the patient and the particular point in the work. The constant is in understanding that *whatever* choice one makes, one is in fact playing a significant role. If one chooses not to mention or focus on one's own role, that is itself a choice of what role one intends to play at that moment. Being with the patient and focusing only on him *is* a way of interacting with him just as much as mentioning one's own role explicitly. The therapist's task is to understand, as best she can, the potential consequences of her choice.

Not all of what transpires, of course, will be conscious, nor can the therapist always see clearly the options and implications. From a contemporary vantage point, we may see that it is precisely enactments that the concept of the corrective emotional experience is about, and enactments occur with varying degrees of awareness and in ways that vary quite considerably in how able the parties are to reflect on what has been transpiring between them. What the concepts of corrective emotional experience or new relational experience highlight is that these enactments are not simply fodder for interpretations but also consequential instances of lived experience. It is not only in the *understanding* of what is transpiring that change can be generated but in *what is transpiring per se.*

PROCEDURAL LEARNING AND THE PROCESS OF THERAPEUTIC CHANGE

Understanding the range of directly experiential dimensions of the therapeutic process—reflected in concepts such as the corrective emotional experience, enactment, passing the patient's tests (Weiss & Sampson, 1986), or now moments (Stern et al., 1998), as well as in the powerful directly experiential role of *exposure* in helping people to overcome long-held and crippling anxieties—is further aided and clarified by attention to a set of distinctions that derive from seminal research in cognitive science and the study of brain functioning. In a discussion of the role of memory in therapeutic action that draws significantly on this work, Fonagy summarizes its basic thrust as follows:

> Cognitive science makes a key distinction between two kinds of memory system both of which have important functions in psycho-

analytic treatment: a declarative or explicit memory that is involved with the conscious retrieval of information about the past, and the procedural or implicit memory system from which information may be retrieved without the experience of remembering. Declarative memory relates to remembering events and information. . . . Procedural memory is content-free, it is involved in acquiring sequences of actions, the "how" of behaviour; for example skills such as playing the piano (regardless of the specific piece) or driving (independent of destination); changes "that are produced by prior experiences" that do not require any intentional or conscious recollection of those experiences. (1999, p. 216)

Examining the currently dominant psychoanalytic theories of therapeutic change, Fonagy argues that "the modern emphasis on the therapeutic relationship as the primary motor of therapeutic action, for which we are indebted to Winnicott (1956) and Loewald (1960), [has not] succeeded in eliminating the emphasis on the recovery of childhood experiences," despite there being "no evidence" for this emphasis, and he adds that in his view, "to cling to this idea is damaging to the field" (p. 215). In contrast to this traditional view, Fonagy argues that "there is good reason to believe that psychoanalysis works by modifying *procedures* rather than by creating new *ideas*" (p. 219, italics added).

In elaborating on this idea, Fonagy further states,

The therapeutic action of psychoanalysis is unrelated to the "recovery" of memories of childhood, be these traumatic or neutral. In agreement with a group of psychoanalysts working creatively in Boston (Stern et al., 1998), we have proposed that the experiences contributing to representations of object relations will have occurred mostly too early to be remembered, to be remembered that is in the conscious sense of experiencing recovering a past experience in the present. Early experience is, however, formative and is retained in parts of the brain that are separate from those where memories, as we normally think of them (autobiographical memory), are encoded, stored and retrieved. (p. 216)

The distinction between procedural and declarative or implicit and explicit realms of psychological and neural functioning has applicability to our thinking, in the context of therapeutic practice, about more than just memories of early experiences. It applies as well, for example, to how best to address and make therapeutic use of the phenomenon of transference. In working with transference, interpretations, designed to produce explicit verbal insight, are not the only route to change, or even necessarily the most important. Implicit or procedural dimensions are relevant here as well, and overlap in important ways with the concept of the corrective emotional experience and with the other closely related concepts I have been discussing. Much of the way we learn from experience—not just in such realms as driving or playing the piano, but in learning to feel more comfortable being with others, to establish intimacy or friendship, to maintain a conversation, and so forth—proceeds in a similarly "procedural" way rather than through explicit verbal channels.[4] In this connection, Eagle (2003b) has suggested that "changes in procedural 'rules' are not especially susceptible to interpretation, insight, and reflective (symbolized) knowledge, but are mainly accomplished through the noninterpretive and nonverbal means of feeling understood, test-passing, enactments, in general, corrective emotional experiences" (p. 49; see also Frank, 1999, p. 197).

The necessity of a more directly experiential dimension of learning and reworking of internal representations is, as Fonagy noted, especially highlighted in the work of the theorists and researchers of the Boston Process of Change Study Group (e.g., Stern, 2004; Stern et al., 1998; Lyons-Ruth, 1998, 1999). Lyons-Ruth, for example, addresses much the same distinction in modes of processing as Fonagy, but from a broader vantage point than just memory. Describing the explorations of the Boston group regarding the "something more" than interpretation that is required for deep therapeutic change, she notes that in the course of exploring this topic,

> it became clear that two kinds of representation processes needed to be separately conceptualized. The first kind of representation we will call semantic in that it relies on symbolic representation in language. The second kind we will call procedural representation. . . . Procedural representations are rule-based representations of how to proceed, of how to do things. Such procedures may never become symbolically coded, as for example, knowledge of how to ride a

---

[4] Note here that "verbal" can be used in two senses. Conversation, of course, is quintessentially verbal, as is much of establishing intimacy or comfortable and enjoyable relatedness. But we learn *how* to maintain an enlivening conversation or to joke around, initiate intimacy, establish dominance or friendship via experiences that are largely *procedural* learning of implicit rules. The *content* is verbal, but the rules and skills we must master are often unable to be verbalized, even by the person who manifests considerable skill in working within these rules.

bicycle. More important to us than bicycle riding, however, is the domain of *knowing how to do things with others*. Much of this kind of knowledge is also procedural, such as knowing how to joke around, express affection, or get attention in childhood. This procedural knowledge of how to do things with others we have termed "implicit relational knowing." In using this term, we want to differentiate implicit relational knowing from other forms of procedural knowledge and to emphasize that such "knowings" are *as much affective and interactive as they are cognitive.*" (Lyons-Ruth, 1999, p. 284, italics added)

The authors of the Boston Process of Change group note that by and large implicit relational knowing, or procedural knowledge of relationships, operates outside of both focal attention and conscious, verbally expressible experience. Well before infants have the language to express such an idea, for example, they learn complex skills that enable them to know how to approach their parents in a way that evokes an affectionate response, and concomitantly (but again without linguistic representation) they learn what kinds of calls for attention are counterproductive (Lyons-Ruth, 1998). Adults (and older children), of course, integrate this knowledge with the realm of verbal, cognitive, or conscious knowledge of relationships. We do certainly learn many rules of "how to be with someone" in a way that can be articulated and, of course, much of the relating that all humans over the age of one or two engage in is verbal in the sense that words are the *medium*. But the "knowing how" that the concept of implicit relational knowing is concerned with is, so to speak, about the melody rather than the lyrics. To the dismay of adolescents who try to imitate the "lines" of their more successful peers, the same words said in the wrong tone of voice or with the wrong body language, dimensions over which we have much less conscious control, can be mystifyingly unsuccessful. Some people do benefit from "how to" books on shyness or social skills or making conversation, but the robust sales of such books probably attests more to both the pervasiveness of the experience of something problematic or missing in people's capacity to connect with another in a satisfying way and the failure of the *previous* books they have read to accomplish their mission. (Buyers of such books, I suspect, tend to be *serial* buyers.)

Knowing "how to be with someone" (Stern et al., 1998) in a way that enhances the experience both of connection and of self-integrity is a capacity that is largely gained through experience, not explicit instruction. In everyday life, that experience is very largely a gradual matter of trial and error. In the therapy relationship, it is fostered by the skilled therapist, who (both consciously and in an implicit, nonconscious manner, in the moment to moment participation in the therapeutic interaction) promotes experiences that will enable the patient to learn to achieve more comfortable and satisfying relations with others and, as well, to feel more whole, coherent, and genuine as an individual.

The direct, affectively immediate experience with the therapist enables the patient to achieve these changes in a way that is not possible to achieve through insight alone. As I will discuss in Chapter 12, this directly experiential dimension of therapeutic change is best pursued not only via experiences with the therapist but also through attention to the patient's experiences with others in his life who help create the texture of daily living. For now, though, we may simply note Stern et al.'s (1998) point that in contrast with declarative knowledge, which is "gained or acquired through verbal interpretations that alter the patient's intrapsychic understanding," implicit relational knowing occurs "through 'interactional, intersubjective processes' that alter the relational field within the context of what we will call the 'shared implicit relationship' " (p. 905).

Eagle (2003b) has made a similar point, arguing that

> the basic idea that noninterpretive factors play a central role in all psychotherapy and psychoanalysis has gained a new currency and vitality from the recognition, gained from attachment research and theory, as well as developmental and cognitive psychology, that early, overlearned, and nonverbal representations—procedural knowledge and "rules"—are not easily and fully translatable into reflective (symbolized) knowledge, and *are not always susceptible to change via interpretation and insight, but require noninterpretive, interactional, and strong emotional experiences in order for them to change.* (p. 50, italics added)

In this connection, Eagle explicitly endorses the concept of the corrective emotional experience, stating that "changes in procedural 'rules,' such as internal working models, interactional structures, unconscious pathogenic beliefs, and governing fantasies . . . occur mainly through the 'noninterpretive mechanisms' of enactments and corrective emotional experiences in the therapeutic relationship" (p. 49). In illustrating this view through a case example, he argues that "the corrective emotional experience inherent in our interaction could speak for itself and did not need to be made explicit. Indeed, I felt then and continue to feel that making any explicit *interpretation* of what I thought took place would dilute and interfere with the therapeutic value of our interaction" (p. 49, italics added).

Downgrading the role of interpretation or highlighting the procedural dimension of the therapeutic process, it is important to understand, is not a turning away from verbal exchange or the attempt to articulate and verbalize experience. In the therapy relationship, as in most other relationships in our lives, words are obviously the primary medium of exchange. Patient and therapist *talk to* each other. What goes on procedurally or relationally is very largely a matter of *how* the words are used, of the music that accompanies the lyrics, to use the metaphor I introduced earlier. But the analogy to music is in some ways misleading because some of the music resides in the words themselves. Different ways of phrasing things, over and above the impact noted earlier of tone of voice or body language, can make the message—and the experience—quite different. This is in part why I feel no conflict about emphasizing the procedural and directly experiential dimensions of the therapy while having written an entire book about the therapist's use of language and the differing implications of subtly different ways of expressing what can seem to the therapist the same basic idea (Wachtel, 1993).

Moreover, neither I nor any other advocates of the more directly experiential dimension of the therapeutic process reject the role of interpretation as *one part*—indeed, a very important part—of the process. The effort to help the patient better understand himself, to look more closely at himself and his life, to gain new perspectives on his experiences, to find a vocabulary to express the inchoate yearnings that have been sources of nagging dissatisfaction or seemingly inexplicable behavior—all this is a central part of what good therapy entails. But even this process of gaining greater self-understanding is not a process that inheres exclusively (or at times even predominantly) in the semantic content of the interpretation. In therapy, as in everyday life, we move back and forth between experiencing and reflecting on that experience and, of course, we do both simultaneously as well. Indeed, each is infused with the other to such an extent that the distinction itself is somewhat artificial.

Reflective awareness is a powerful survival tool and a unique characteristic of our highly verbal species. But in the course of our evolution we also learned to survive by making adjustments and adaptations that were quicker than words can follow and more complex than words alone can fully capture (see Gladwell, 2005). These subtle and often largely nonverbal forms of learning and adaptation include not just dealing with the physical world—in our species' prehistory, for example, the world of leaping predators or fleeing prey—but also the adaptations we make in the realm of social interaction, in the fostering of cooperation and communication that were essential in the evolution and the very survival of our species.

It is in some ways ironic that psychoanalysis has been so insistent on explicit verbal awareness as the key to therapeutic change. For such an agenda oddly underestimates what psychoanalysis ordinarily highlights—the power of the unconscious. What many of the recent trends in psychoanalysis and in other realms of therapeutic practice point to, in essence, is that healing too may very largely go on unconsciously, that many of the processes that are mobilized in the course of a successful psychotherapeutic experience are likely never to be fully brought to consciousness. This fact does not make the changes achieved less deep or enduring, nor, indeed, does it bypass the engagement of the individual in actively creating meaning in his life. Rather, it reflects that there are more modes of making meaning and more dimensions of learning and processing than psychoanalysis originally conceived. New relational experiences, both with the therapist and with others in the patient's life, provide an opportunity for the kind of procedural learning that is an essential complement to the more explicit, declarative learning that was for so many years the exclusive focus of psychoanalytic practice.

■　■　■　■　■

11

Confusions about
Self-Disclosure

REAL ISSUES, PSEUDO-ISSUES,
AND THE INEVITABILITY OF TRADE-OFFS

Self-disclosure is probably the issue that most plagues and confuses beginning therapists, and is often a source of consternation for experienced therapists as well. It is also the issue that most creates confusion regarding the nature of relational practice. There is a common misperception that to work relationally means to self-disclose relentlessly. It is certainly true that a relational point of view encourages greater self-disclosure than more traditional psychoanalytic approaches. The essence of the relational view on self-disclosure, however, is not that one is *required* to self-disclose but that one is *permitted* to. The differences and implications for clinical practice of these two understandings are very considerable.

The problem of self-disclosure is most illuminatingly considered when it is pursued not as a question of self-disclosure per se but as a subset of the larger and more important issue of trade-offs. *Everything* we do in our role as therapists—and everything we *don't* do as well (for absence has "presence")—has multiple possible meanings and implications. The same choice may have positive implications for one patient and negative for another; may be positive at one moment in the work and negative at another; and, indeed, may be positive in certain respects and negative in others *at the same time.* It may open certain doors and close others, diminish certain anxieties and restrictions and stir or increase others. We have no way around this. We can't not choose or not act, because "not choosing" or "not acting" is itself a choice and an act. This is one of the key implications of the relational or two-person or intersubjective point of view. And it is *this* that is our inevitable dilemma as psychotherapists, not self-disclosure per se.

Self-disclosure has *felt* to many therapists like a special dilemma because there has been a false assumption that there is almost a God-given "frame" to therapy, and that to "violate" that frame is to do serious harm to the therapy. That traditional frame, however—what I have been calling throughout this book the default position—is an arbitrary human invention, a historical accident. It is one of *many* ways to approach the task of helping liberate people from the fears, inhibitions, constrictions, and troubling affective and interpersonal patterns that arise in the course of development and perpetuate themselves through the vicious circles they generate.

This questioning of the traditional frame does not mean that anything goes. Some ways of working do seem to be so preponderantly likely to be harmful that it is appropriate to rule them out altogether. Sex with patients is the most frequently cited example, but similar in their problematic implications are physical aggressiveness and verbal abuse. Over the years, even these extreme examples have had their advocates, from proponents of "love cures," to drug addiction programs that claim that their abusive berating of clients is the only way to break through the hold that their addiction has on them, to "boot camps" for young violent offenders. It would take us too far afield to address here whether there are ever times when such extreme measures are justified, but what is important to understand is that self-disclosure is *not* like these more problematic (and at the very least highly risky) departures from tradition. Rather, self-disclosure is a feature of *all* therapeutic work (see, e.g., Frank, 1997; Singer, 1977; Renik, 1995, 1999b), and questions about how much, when, and how to disclose are not ventures into dangerous new territory, but considerations that require the same sophisticated, reflective, patient-centered attention that is accorded to any other feature of "ordinary" therapeutic work.

There are, to be sure, potential costs and drawbacks to self-disclosure, as there are to any other dimension of the work. In each decision about disclosing or not disclosing, our task is to assess and anticipate, as best we can, what the overall consequences or implications for the work are likely to be. And, paralleling the last chapter's discussion of the corrective emotional experience, we must live with the reality that we *cannot* always anticipate correctly, and that a good part of the process of psychotherapy entails working with the consequences of our anticipating incorrectly and using the experience to therapeutic benefit.

As with every other aspect of psychotherapy, our task is to individualize the treatment and individualize our decisions, thinking not about what is appropriate for all patients at all times, but what is appropriate for *this* patient at *this* time. This again, of course, requires us to anticipate and estimate the likely experience of the patient in response to what we decide—and to deal with the inevitability of the fact that much of the time we will be wrong. Here once again, the guiding assumption is not that the therapist needs to be "correct" in her choices (an impossible goal) but that she must be *attentive to the consequences* of those choices. This close and continually subject-to-revision attention to the patient's experience of what we have done, whether wittingly or unwittingly, is what marks the good therapist, not the correctness of any particular intervention per se.

Nonetheless, prohibitions regarding self-disclosure continue to be expressed in the literature. McWilliams (1994), for example, in her influential textbook, states that, at least with "neurotic-level" patients, they "have subtle and unconscious transferences that surface *only when the therapist is carefully opaque*" (p. 75, italics added). Jacobs (1999), in contrast, speaking from what might be described as a progressive-traditionalist point of view, states that, while in theory (and in some clinical situations) "certain revelations on the part of the analyst can limit or inhibit aspects of the patient's imagination and the free flow of fantasy," in actual practice "nondisclosure and analytic anonymity, especially if rigidly and automatically applied, do not always serve patients' interests." Indeed, he adds, "In certain individuals—for instance, those who have had long experience with secretive, non-responsive parents or whose self-esteem is particularly fragile—the traditional analytic attitude with regard to self-disclosure may be experienced as hostile and *may have an inhibiting effect rather than being liberating.* Instead of functioning to open up communications and to free up the mind, it can shut it down" (p. 164, italics added). Other writers, addressing the issue from the vantage point of the relational tradition (e.g., Aron, Frank, Hoffman, Mitchell, Renik, Stern, Fosshage, Davies,

Slavin, Gerson, Pizer, etc.), have particularly highlighted the potential clinical benefits of appropriately employed self-disclosures and the clinical and theoretical costs of pretending that anything even approaching anonymity is a possibility. I myself, in an earlier publication, also devoted a lengthy chapter to the topic (Wachtel, 1993, Ch. 11). In what follows, therefore, I will not attempt to review this now voluminous literature. The reader interested in a detailed examination of the important literature on the topic is referred to the above-mentioned sources as a very useful point of departure.

INTENTIONAL AND UNINTENTIONAL DISCLOSURES

Part of the confusion regarding self-disclosure derives from the fact that self-disclosure is in fact not one thing but several, and understanding the *different* phenomena and experiences that have been referred to under the rubric or label of self-disclosure is perhaps the most important starting point for discussing the issue or, really, *set* of issues. To begin with, we may note a distinction between those disclosures that happen involuntarily and inevitably (Frank, 1997, calls these "inadvertent" self-revelations)—a reality of the therapeutic situation that is highlighted especially sharply by the two-person perspective of the relational point of view—and those disclosures that are *voluntary*; that is, where the therapist consciously chooses to disclose something that the patient may not have seen or experienced. Many writers have commented on the wide variety of ways in which self-disclosure is inevitable. The location and style of decoration of the therapist's office, his or her gender, age, physical appearance, voice, accent, clothing style, and a host of similar variables all contribute to the way in which the therapist is "known" by the patient. But so too do the ways the therapist chooses to conduct the therapy—for example, when (and how often) she speaks and when (and how often) she is silent. This latter set of choices, reflecting in good part (though certainly not exclusively determined by) the therapist's *theory*, also reveals much about her. Indeed, as Frank (1999) points out, even voluntary or deliberate disclosures inevitably carry along with them a considerable degree of *inadvertent* disclosure as well. The particular *way* the therapist chooses to disclose, the timing of her disclosures, the multiple linguistic and paralinguistic dimensions, far exceed the therapist's capacity to control consciously, and thus every deliberate and conscious disclosure also inevitably contains elements of inadvertent disclosure as well.

VARIETIES OF INTENTIONAL SELF-DISCLOSURE

Beyond the distinction between voluntary and involuntary or intended and unintended disclosures, there are also further important distinctions *among* the various forms of voluntary disclosure. As we move from the more obviously involuntary and often unconscious disclosures to those that are more planned, conscious, and part of the therapist's overall approach to pursuing the work, we encounter still a further set of distinctions that need to be considered. The most immediate and pressing disclosure decisions—and the places where it is most obvious that the therapist is doing something when she *does not* disclose as much as when she does—occur when the patient asks a direct question. Therapists, of course, vary in how they respond to such questions, and at least in part that variation depends on the nature of the question that is asked. It is difficult to imagine a therapist not answering in some way the question, "Next Monday is President's Day, are we having a session?" The therapist may wonder why this question comes up at this point and may relate the patient's uncertainty to some other issues that are in the air—she might, for example, wonder whether the patient hopes he can avoid the next session or whether he feels insecure about whether the therapist will be there when he needs her, and she might include some discussion of these issues as part of her response. But it is hard to imagine a therapist not also responding in a way that makes it clear whether they will be meeting or not.

Next along the continuum, so to speak, are questions such as, when the therapist comes back from a vacation, "Where did you go on your vacation?" There are therapists who actually do respond routinely to such questions with an inquiry into the patient's "fantasy" as to where she went on vacation, but in the 21st century such a response is mercifully relatively rare. More therapists will begin to demur when the next question is, "Did you have a good time?" Among those who answer more or less straightforwardly, some will simply offer a perfunctory yes, while others will find it harmless (and even, depending on their theoretical orientation, the state of the therapeutic relationship, and the patient's particular issues, a therapeutically *valuable* option) to offer some elaboration. For still others, the point at which the caution sign goes up is when the patient asks something like, "Did you go with your whole family, or was it just you and your husband alone?"—although again, depending on a host of dimensions and variables, others will be perfectly comfortable here as well.

For therapists who are inclined to answer questions such as these, their response is usually guided by the *feeling* in the room. That is, for one patient, such a question will feel "innocent" or even like a kind of "coming out" for the patient, a willingness on the patient's part to be more available and related and to permit his curiosity about and interest in the therapist, perhaps previously suppressed, to find expression. In such a context, the therapist may feel that to participate in this give and take, however much it looks like "chit-chat" rather than "therapy," is actually therapeutic in very much the sense that the previous chapter discussed vis-à-vis corrective emotional experiences. In other instances, however, the same kind of question may feel *uncomfortable* to the therapist. She may experience it as intrusive or as an evasion of the issues that they really should be discussing and working on. She may worry where this is going or when it will stop. And in such circumstances (not given in the morphology, so to speak, but in the affective meaning that is experienced), she may respond quite differently, perhaps looking for a therapeutic way of making this experience "grist for the mill."[1]

Here once again, the therapist must make her choices based on her best guess of what is transpiring, and has no assurances that she is "right." Whether she is more struck by the uncomfortable or question-raising dimension of the patient's request, and chooses to respond in a more "exploratory" way, or experiences the patient's question as "innocent" and meriting a more socially conventional response, the potential for error cannot be ruled out. Error can lie in *either* direction. All we can do is to proceed with our best effort and to *pay attention to what happens next*, both overtly and more subtly or unacknowledgedly.

"HOW DO YOU FEEL ABOUT ME?"

The decision about how to respond to a patient's question tends to become increasingly complex and potentially uncomfortable for most

---

[1] I will have more to say below about the therapist's discomfort and its important role in decisions about whether, how, and how much to disclose.

therapists when the question is about the therapist's feelings about the patient or about some other more "personal" feature of the therapist's life, such as about her marriage, her family, her satisfaction or dissatisfaction with her work, and so forth. Here (in contrast to some of the other forms of self-disclosure discussed later in this chapter) we are still in the realm of responding to a direct question, and in that sense the therapist may feel less choice about responding to this situation in *some* way; but the situation may feel less "simple" than the ones discussed thus far. One cannot *ignore* the question, since even to not answer it—not just in the sense of "interpreting" it or turning it back upon the patient, but even just by remaining silent—is to respond, and indeed to respond in some respects "dramatically." In that sense, one is "stuck" with the question.

But not every therapist will feel "mugged" by such questions. Depending on the therapist's theoretical orientation and her assessment of the key issues and conflicts for the patient, questions such as these may be experienced by her more as an *opportunity* or a welcome sign of progress by the patient than as a dilemma or invasion. The considerations that enter into such decisions are much the same as for the more "optional" disclosures discussed next, those in which the immediate stimulus of a direct question by the patient is not a part of the picture. They include tact, concern with not saying things in a form that will leave the patient feeling diminished or damaged, and remaining aware that the full picture is likely to be more complex than any single comment or answer is able to capture. I will discuss these considerations further after turning to the next variant in the spectrum of disclosure decisions that therapists may encounter.

VOLUNTARY DISCLOSURE OF THE THERAPIST'S FEELINGS IN THE SESSION

The immediate stimulus for the therapist's voluntary disclosure need not be a direct question from the patient. For some therapists, either because they operate from a more relational stance within the psychoanalytic spectrum, or because their practice is guided by a broader, integrative mix that is not confined to psychoanalytic thought alone, it is not uncommon to disclose something about themselves even if the patient *has not* asked. The issues raised by these disclosures are somewhat different depending on whether the therapist is disclosing a feeling or thought in relation to what is immediately happening in the room or is sharing with the patient something about her life outside the consulting room.

The former is almost certainly more common than the latter. In part this is because the therapist often has reason to think that the patient has in any event noticed her reaction as they sit together in the room. The immediate back-and-forth between patient and therapist will, inevitably, stir feelings in the therapist (understanding here that, in this context, *indifference* or *lack* of strong feelings is *also* one of the feelings that can be stirred, and indeed, a very important one for understanding what is going on). The patient may or may not pick up all of those feelings, but it is very unlikely that at least some of them are not registered by the patient at some level (cf. Hoffman, 1983; Aron, 1991b; Davies, 1994). The patient's experience of those feelings will, of course, always be *in his fashion*, and what he thinks the therapist is feeling may not comport very well with the therapist's own understanding of what her feelings are. Moreover, the patient may be registering those feelings (however he attributes meaning to them) in a conscious and fairly articulated way or very largely in a way that is unconscious or unformulated. But nonetheless, they are a fact of life in the room, so to speak, something that is there between them whether they choose to discuss it or not.

There are many variants of this situation (which in a sense, in one form or another, is a constant in the therapeutic situation). If the therapist thinks that the patient has not noticed what she is feeling, she may feel that she can "get away with" not saying anything about it. If she thinks that the patient may well have noticed, but has nonetheless not actually said anything about it, she may feel the same temptation to avoid bringing the topic up, but probably with a little less comfort or certainty about that avoidance. The therapist may be sleepy or distracted, for example, and hope to "hide" it, but also be aware that her hiding is unlikely to be successful, or she may be annoyed at the patient and think that it is likely to have been picked up by the patient, even if the patient has not said anything about it. In such circumstances, there is a considerable potential for the therapist's disclosure of what she was feeling to be of therapeutic value. To begin with, as with *all* disclosures, there is new input that enables the patient to examine his experience more closely and to understand better the sequences in his life, the ways in which he repeatedly evokes responses in people that evoke responses in him that perpetuate the problems he has come to therapy to resolve. The interaction with Michael described in the last chapter is an example of this. Additionally, in this specific configuration there is also potentially enormous therapeutic benefit deriving from the way that disclosing can contribute to *demystifying* the patient's experience. Often, in the course of growing up, certain feelings were just not talked about in the home, and as a consequence they were not just rendered forbidden or dangerous but also, quite literally, unthinkable. A lacuna develops in which the patient himself begins to be unclear not only about what *he* feels but about how important *others* in his life feel.

In this situation, the patient is not only unlikely to ask a direct question about what the therapist is feeling, but may well *not* have consciously registered it. That is, there are some times when the patient does not ask but still clearly sees or at least strongly guesses; but perhaps even more important are the times when the patient does in some way register the therapist's feeling, and indeed respond to it (perhaps by inhibiting some of what he himself is feeling or twisting it to fit with what is acceptable), but is not conscious of doing so. In such situations, the therapist's acknowledging her own feelings can be enormously liberating and generative, freeing the patient to see more clearly and openly what she has theretofore both seen and not seen simultaneously. It is remarkable how validating it can be for the patient when the therapist acknowledges *especially* a feeling she "could have gotten away with" not acknowledging, and how clarifying and validating such experiences can be for the patient.

Here too, of course, there are trade-offs, potential negatives as well as positives. The possibility that the therapist's introducing her own reaction could feel intrusive or inattentive to where *the patient* wants to go with the experience is real. So too is the possibility, when the feeling the therapist might disclose is anger or boredom or some other negative or potentially hurtful feeling, that expressing it could be a form of "acting out" the countertransference, a self-indulgence on the therapist's part that is rationalized as for the benefit of the patient. The therapist must be alert to this possibility and examine herself as best she can, knowing that she can never be sure—especially, of course, of the *unconscious* meanings of her behavior—and that even after self-scrutiny, she may be wrong.

But here too, the therapist must understand that, rather than therapist errors necessarily fatally compromising the process, working on the breach or rupture and repairing it by staying with the experience, exploring it together with the patient, and acknowledging the therapist's own participation in what transpired is a significant part of what is therapeutic about psychotherapy (Safran & Muran, 2000). Moreover, it is again essential to be clear that there is also a potential price to *not* acknowledging the feeling the therapist hesitates to express. Being cautious that one may be rationalizing in expressing the feeling to the patient can itself be a rationalization—in this instance for hiding her own not so praiseworthy feelings or actions. The consequence may be the further mystification of the patient's experience, both in the sense that he may be left unable to address his uncomfortable (though perhaps not consciously elaborated) feeling that the therapist *is* angry or bored and in the sense that the therapist's collusion in avoiding this difficult topic makes it harder for the patient to notice or accept *his own* feelings of anger, boredom, or what have you. Here once again, there is no "free lunch" in psychotherapy; every choice has potential costs, whether one chooses to disclose, not to disclose, to answer a question, not to answer, to give advice, not to give advice, and so forth.

DISCLOSURES ABOUT THE THERAPIST'S *OUTSIDE* LIFE

Many therapists who, in the present theoretical climate, are increasingly inclined to openly discuss with patients their feelings and reactions in the session are nonetheless chary about similarly introducing disclosures about their lives and experiences outside the therapy room. In part, this is again a matter of "what they can get away with." When it comes to our reactions in the room, it has become increasingly clear that whether we say something about them or not, they are likely to be registered by the patient. Hence many therapists now believe that the process can be enhanced when the therapist, judiciously and skillfully, brings those reactions out into the open for discussion and helps the patient better understand how they may be related to what has gone on between them. In contrast, many aspects of the therapist's life outside *can*, to a very large extent, be hidden from the patient. Therapists perhaps overestimate how much can be truly unknown to the patient, especially in this age of Google, but clearly, especially when it comes to experiences in one's personal history, the likelihood that the patient "already knows" is considerably less.

The greater reluctance to disclose outside-of-session information about the therapist or her life, of course, is not just a function of what can be kept hidden. Many therapists tend to exclude such types of disclosure for the very reason that they *advocate* in-session disclosures—that is, out of a concern for affective and relational immediacy. Disclosing one's feelings, or even one's associations, as they arise in the room in response to the evolving relational field, entails a focus on the affective ties between the two participants and the tensions and variations in those ties. Disclosing aspects of one's life outside feels to many therapists instead to *divert attention away from* the immediate relational field.

Several considerations are relevant here in thinking through the options regarding this type of disclosure. To begin with, sometimes the therapist is reminded of something about her life outside the session because of something going on *within* the session. In those instances, the therapist may be more likely to share this thought with the patient, anticipating that this might help illuminate what has been transpiring between the two of them or help uncover and clarify a previously submerged or defended against aspect of the patient's affective life. This rationale still is largely rooted in the interpretive, insight-oriented mode. But there can also be other reasons to tell the patient something about oneself, as the following example illustrates.

Sam was a man in his late forties who had felt quite thwarted in many aspects of his life. He was a man of considerable talent and a sharp sense of humor. Were he not his own worst enemy in certain respects, he would probably have been quite impressively successful in his career, and even as things stood he was doing much better than he felt he was. Sam grew up in a home in which both parents were quite fearful and very largely had an attitude toward the world of resentful envy. They disparaged people who were more materially and professionally successful than they were, depicting them as undeserving and hollow frauds. But at the same time, they viewed these people as powerful and capable of keeping people like Sam and his parents in their place. They communicated to Sam, in a variety of ways, that no matter how hard he tried, "they" would get him, that it was not for the likes of him to mix it up with the big shots. At the same time, the messages often included that "we" were really much smarter and more capable than "them," even though they were the ones who held the reins and were in power. This combination of messages left Sam tied in knots. He had moved considerably beyond his bus driver father economically, but lived out, at a higher socioeconomic level, the "civil service" life his parents had conveyed was the only available or safe option. While he expressed considerable resentment and disdain toward his parents, he lived in a way that was loyal to their vision of the world and hence maintained the unconscious attachments that both sustained and constricted him.

Sam saw me as living on the other side of the divide, a "big shot," confident, capable, unhampered by the constraints within which he lived. Although he never quite said it, it was apparent from a number of things he said that he imagined me as having grown up in a home that was far more cultured and worldly than his and as having had parents who helped me to step forth confidently into the world. My aim in the following disclosures was not to quell or mute those feelings—considerable useful work was done prior to these interventions on those feelings of envy and resentment on Sam's part, and it was important not to close off his access to (and sense of safety about expressing) those feelings. But at a certain point, I saw an opportunity to help Sam take some steps to extricate himself from the tangle in which he was caught. All too often, I believe, therapists limit their participation to *pointing out* to the patient how he is stuck, but are hesitant to lend a hand in pulling him out. The assumption seems to be that interpretation alone or insight alone will do the trick, and that actively helping is ultimately counterproductive and undermining of the patient's initiative and autonomy, an attitude that is a holdover from the one-person psychology that characterizes not just versions of psychoanalytic theory but elements of the larger society's individualistic value structure (Cushman, 1990, 1996; Wachtel, 1983).

At one point in the work, when Sam made one of many statements that conveyed wistfully that he was stuck because of the home he grew up in and implied that it was too late now to do anything about it, I told him that I understood very well the experience he was talking about. I said it reminded me of what was perhaps the most important experience in my own therapy. Knowing this would surprise him, I told him that I too grew up in a home in which my parents were fearful and in which they really didn't prepare me very well for going out into the larger world. In fact, I told him, I never even learned to ride a bike as a kid. I told him that this last deficit particularly hurt, and left me feeling both inadequate and resentful. And I said that the most important moment of my analysis came when my analyst, sensing that my *complaining* about what I *hadn't* gotten was right now, in the present, continuing to ensure that I would feel deprived and inadequate for many more years to come, asked me why it was that I couldn't go out and learn to ride a bike *now.* This led, after some period of shocked resistance on my part, to my actually doing just that. At the age of 27, I went with my wife to Central Park, and with her holding up the bike as I pedaled, the way the parent of a 5- or 6-year-old might, I learned to ride a bike. This was one of the most thrilling experiences of my life, and now, so many years later, I suspect I still enjoy riding my bike more than those who learned to ride at the "appropriate" time.

Sharing this experience with Sam offered him a vivid sense that it was possible to change rather than just complain. The impact of my relating this personal story (a story I certainly did not "have to" tell him, in the sense that there was no way he would know it independently) was, of course, mediated by the transference that existed at that time and, particularly, by the idealization of me up to that point that made this disclosure of what had felt to me like a shameful feature of my childhood especially dramatic to him. I certainly was offering myself as a model with whom to identify, but, in the terminology of social learning theory I was a *coping* model. That is, rather than demonstrating how easy it is to achieve mastery, I was modeling how even someone who *found it hard* could reach the goal. Consequently, I was a model, in this instance, with whom he *could* identify.

Here (as in the example of my apologizing to Michael in the last chapter) I was in certain ways diminishing the patient's idealization of me. In some respects, this is in itself of value, since the tendency to idealize others who are seen as authorities is one part of what keeps many patients locked into the experience that they are not up to par. This was in fact the case for Sam. But there are also ways in which idealizing the therapist is a *positive* thing, as Kohut (1971, 1977) in particular has pointed out. Most of us, in essence, need a *mix* of attitudes toward those we admire or depend on, a combination of idealization, readiness to learn from them, freedom to compete with them, freedom to see their flaws without the danger of toppling or losing them, and so on. It is not one attitude that is essential to achieve—though one may predominate at any particular moment or period in one's life history—but rather the capacity to contain them all within the fullness of the self.

Had Sam shown signs of being troubled by the potentially diminished picture of me resulting from my disclosure, I would have had to address that experience, much as the side effects and multiple meanings of any interpretation or intervention need to be addressed. It was amply evident, however, that the self-disclosure that I just described, although in certain respects humbling, did not significantly impede Sam's capacity to idealize or admire or identify in a positive sense with me. Emotional attitudes are not necessarily logical or intellectually consistent. We feel and believe what we need to feel and believe at any given moment, largely dissociating what does not fit. Moreover, the way any particular experience is constructed and given meaning can vary quite considerably. Indeed, one of the "dangers" of a self-disclosure such as this (bearing in mind the point I have been repeatedly making in this chapter that alongside every opportunity lies a danger and vice versa) is that there can be a kind of infinite regress of admiration if the patient is so inclined—*I* am so admirable for overcoming what he now sees were significant handicaps; or *I* am so courageous for revealing this, since he would have hidden it. And every deconstruction on my part of this relentless admiration creates but one more opportunity, if the patient is so inclined, for my modesty, my honesty, my courage, and so forth, to be evident. The best I could do—and the most honest version of it with which I was in touch—was to acknowledge that yes, I *was* proud of having overcome this, and yes, I *am* offering myself as a kind of model in that respect, but that it misses something crucially important to leave out how genuinely thwarted and genuinely ashamed I felt *before* I took the step of going to Central Park with my wife and that it is the possibility of *moving beyond* shame and stasis that he and I share.

The bicycle disclosure had, as its main aim, promoting Sam's identification with me as a coping model. I sought to enable him to see me as someone who has been in the same kind of quagmire as he was in order to bolster his belief that he too could move beyond his current state of shame and stasis. His perception of me as someone for whom everything comes easily was impeding not only that identification but his progress more generally, because it was feeding into his perception that there are only top dogs and bottom dogs in the world and that he has been assigned, almost inexorably, to the latter category. Another self-disclosure I made in the course of the work with Sam similarly revealed a less than heroic picture of my growing-up years, but its implications for the work were somewhat different. It did have some of the same meaning for Sam as the first disclosure, but it also evoked in Sam a sense of *feeling understood.* Sam had often described aspects of his mother's intrusiveness, and I had been emphasizing in the weeks before the next example the impact on Sam of the feeling of being constantly scrutinized and the self-conscious inhibition that that scrutiny had instilled. On one occasion he was telling me about an experience in which he was talking on the phone and, intuiting that his mother was listening with her ear to the door in their small apartment, he opened the door and his mother fell into the room. After we laughed together over this story,[2] I told him I knew very well what it felt like to be scrutinized that way. I said that my mother too was a listener at the door, and that as a teenager, whenever I wanted to call a girl for a date, I went down to the corner candy store and called from a phone booth rather than expose my fumblings to the sympathetic but overly involved ears of my mother.

In the next session, and on numerous occasions over the ensuing months, Sam made a point of how important to him this particular revelation on my part was. It left him feeling that I could really understand him in a way that especially stood out for him, and thus was an important foundation for much else that it was possible to accomplish in the work. (Curtis, Field, Knaan-Kostman, & Mannix, 2004, among others, have reported research that indicates that it is often moments such as this that patients remember as among the key events in their psychotherapy experience.)

It is important to be clear that therapeutically useful disclosures are not limited to embarrassing personal details, as in the two examples just discussed. Some patients, for example, have great difficulty in acknowledging or frankly displaying their strengths and accomplishments. It is not likely to be helpful to such patients if the therapist's self-disclosures are exclusively about vulnerabilities. Rather, where the appropriate occasion arises, it can be helpful either to acknowledge something the patient says or knows about you, or even spontaneously to introduce something you feel good about, saying something like, "Yes, I feel very proud of having accomplished that. I wonder why it's so hard for you to similarly feel proud of your own achievements."

---

[2] My laughing with him too was a departure from the strictures of the default position. Apropos trade-offs, I suppose that my laughing may have impeded the expression or elaboration of any fantasy Sam had that I would disapprove of his action toward his mother. But at the same time, the demonstration of my *positive* response to the story had a conscious therapeutic aim—to *support* the more rebellious side of Sam, to stand side by side with this anger and his sense of outrage. Here again, there is no free lunch. One must, in essence, decide *which* "opportunity cost" is higher, the loss (or at least reduction) of the opportunity to analyze a possible fantasy that I disapproved of his behavior or the loss of the opportunity to side with and strengthen an emerging new capacity and aspect of self on his part.

It must also be emphasized that, as in so many other interventions and choices, the therapist's genuineness is of central importance. If my laughter was forced or artificial, just a "technique," it would be unlikely to be of therapeutic value. What made it part of an experience that Sam found therapeutic was that I simply *permitted* something that was spontaneously occurring but which could have been inhibited if I had decided to "act more like a therapist."

One important point in these various examples, which I will elaborate on further in the next chapter, is that the aim of the work from the vantage point of the particular version of relational thinking I am describing here is not just to promote the patient's insight but to help him to *move*, to take action that will change his life and his experience of himself. Discussions of self-disclosure have tended to be dominated by considerations of whether it interferes with "analyzing" the patient, and not concerned enough with whether it *helps* the patient. Notwithstanding the very real and considerable value of self-awareness both as a value in its own right and as one important element in the larger process of therapeutic change, there is more to helping people achieve deep and fundamental change than just promoting greater self-awareness. Among these additional dimensions are the positive effects of the patient's identification with the therapist and the ways that that can contribute to the likelihood that the patient will take the risk of acting in new ways and/or will feel more capable of doing so. The therapeutic value derives not just from whatever contribution this makes to getting the patient moving in a new direction, but also from the further consequences of the actions that then follow. The process of therapeutic change, like the process of neurotic stasis, is not a purely intrapsychic process but a process of continuing transaction between the individual's predispositions and the experiences in the world that both reflect and maintain those predispositions.

SELF-DISCLOSURE AND THE COURAGE TO EXPLORE

It is not only *the patient* who has defenses or who has learned that certain experiences, certain ways of thinking and feeling, are dangerous and potentially disorganizing. Although all therapists should have had the experience of being in therapy themselves, that does not "clear" them of conflicts and inhibitions. One of the important functions of the therapist's traditional anonymity is to protect the therapist from too much exposure and, hence, too much anxiety. If we are to encourage the patient to venture into territory that he has devoted his life to avoiding, we must feel safe enough *ourselves* to go there. If every time we inquired about the patient's sexual experiences or his *avoidance* of talking about his sexual experiences; if every time we inquired into the subtly angry and nasty dimensions of a seemingly benign interaction (a necessary preliminary to *making room* for the patient's less agreeable side); if every time we explored his hidden fears, avoidances, and bad feelings about himself, we were required to, or even vulnerable to, exposing and opening up further exploration of our own sexual preferences or inhibitions, our own nastier or sneakier side, our own fears, avoidances, and secret bad feelings about ourselves, it would make it much more likely that we would jointly engage in an unacknowledged conspiracy of avoidance that would severely restrict the therapeutic work and what it could accomplish. Our courage to explore is not a function of our sterling character but of the structure of the situation. It is not in the patient's interest for us to be too vulnerable.

Of course, if we attempt to render ourselves *totally* invulnerable, we do just as great a disservice to the patient, putting ourselves on a different path to the same arid end. *Some* vulnerability is essential to face if we are to go into the forbidden realm at all. Even if the therapist completely rules out explicit self-disclosure as an element in her work, she is subject to her own associations and subjective experiences. Simply asking about certain things, *paying attention* to certain things, even if one says nothing about oneself out loud, will stir thoughts and feelings that avoiding the topic will not. And the deeper one goes into the patient's experience, the more one explores the hidden recesses that have been left to operate in the dark, the more likely one will come upon material that stirs *one's own* hidden recesses. Consequently, as I have discussed in more detail elsewhere (Wachtel, 1993, Ch. 11), self-protection on the therapist's part is actually a more legitimate rationale for limiting self-disclosures than is the illusory goal of anonymity supposedly necessary for "uncontaminated" exploration. Finding the proper balance between the necessary self-protection to promote the patient's own fullest self-exploration and the equally necessary willingness to take risks and enter realms of uncertainty is a challenge not dissimilar to that posed by any of the other trade-offs that are at the heart of clinical work.

THE PERSISTING (BUT NOW MORE SUBTLE) OPPOSITION TO SELF-DISCLOSURE

I began this chapter by noting that the question of self-disclosure has been one of the most vexing for many therapists, especially beginning therapists. At the same time, there are ways in which the once almost forbidden topic of self-disclosure may seem to have been tamed. Even from the vantage point of contemporary ego psychology—a theoretical perspective that was once a bastion of warning that disclosure will obstruct, and perhaps even permanently impair, the necessary process of exploration—there is increasing acknowledgment that both disclosure and *non*disclosure entail trade-offs, that silence can be as provocative, and even distracting, as disclosure. Busch (1998), for example, states that "just as the analyst's silence can represent powerful listening or hostile withdrawal, the analyst's self-disclosure is inherently neither better nor worse than silence, and in fact can represent a myriad of attitudes toward the analysand" (Busch, 1998, p. 518). Here, the ego psychological conclusion converges very largely with that reached by most relational thinkers: Self-disclosure is neither better nor worse than silence or refusal to disclose; each choice must be examined for the attitude on the therapist's part that it may be unconsciously expressing and for its meaning for the patient and for the dyad.

In fact, however, the issue of self-disclosure remains a continuing source of unease for many traditional analysts. Beneath apparent expressions of openness and ecumenicism often lie persisting conservative biases, reflecting a more sophisticated version of what I have called the default position. Thus while Busch's comment might seem to place the burden of proof equally on silence or disclosure, close examination of his paper (interestingly titled "Self-Disclosure Ain't What It's Cracked Up to Be, at Least Not Yet") makes it clear that it is not quite that evenhanded. The not-very-difficult-to-discern aim is to correct for what he views as an *over*evaluation of self-disclosure by contemporary relationalists and a self-satisfied assumption on their part that the therapist who discloses her thoughts or feelings is more humane and less authoritarian than the therapist who does not. He states, for example, that "what on the surface may seem to be a humane gesture can in fact be a sadistic reenactment, while what seems like sterile listening can be a most humane gesture" (p. 518). Any reasonably sensitive clinician should have little trouble discerning from the tone of this statement which of the "falsely perceived" alternatives he prefers, the "humane gesture" (i.e., self-disclosure) that is actually sadistic or the humane *silence* that is falsely believed to be sterile. In presenting what seems clearly a stand against what he views as a tide of compulsive self-disclosers, Busch states:

> A not uncommon scenario for certain types of patients is to grow up believing that in order to survive, they need to be a narcissistic

object for a parent. These patients become experts at reading the unconscious needs of those around them, including their analyst. Unconsciously sensing the analyst's need for attention at certain key times, they strategically ask questions of the analyst's activities. In such a situation, the analyst's answering could be a subtle enactment of a narcissistically enhancing, authoritarian relationship, in which the patient's sense of self is being destroyed. It is anything but an interactive collaboration. In short, one cannot determine a priori that self-disclosure is a manifestation of anything in the psychoanalytic moment. The more meaningful question is: self-disclosure by whom, with whom, at what time, for what purpose. (1998, pp. 518–519)

The last two sentences of this quotation are unobjectionably even-handed, and indeed converge almost totally with the views of almost all relational thinkers. But one does not need years of psychoanalytic training to read the meaning in the paragraph as a whole: Self-disclosure is a *danger*, a danger that those inclined to disclose have not sufficiently considered and that can be harmful to the patient and to the therapeutic process.

In fact, however, the main difference between the more traditional analytic stance and the relational stance is not that proponents of the latter have not considered sufficiently the potential consequences of self-disclosure. It is of the very essence of the relational viewpoint that *everything* that transpires in the session has meanings—indeed, *multiple* meanings—and that those meanings must be a central concern of the therapist in everything she decides to say and not to say. Rather, the difference is that the more traditional view—although reworked versions such as Busch's acknowledge the trade-offs in the abstract—includes a very strong *presumption* that the pros of nondisclosure are likely to be greater than the cons, and vice versa for disclosure. For most relational thinkers, in contrast, the question is not so predecided. Rather, each instance requires an examination of the choices in a balanced and evenhanded way. In that sense, it is actually the relationalists who are more "neutral" in this respect, not prejudging but listening to the patient and the dialogue to determine—or, to be more accurate, to guess—what the best choice might be.

It is almost certainly true that the relational literature has focused more on the departures from standard strictures than on their affirmation (cf. Greenberg, 2001). In part this is simply a reflection of the fact that here is where the innovations lie. Just as we don't write papers in which the point is that the therapist was sitting during the session, since that can be more or less taken for granted, but would be much more likely to write a paper about a session in which for some reason we were standing or walking around, so too with any departure from the usual. It is simply more interesting *to write about.* There is no presumption that what we have written about is what is more useful to do *most of the time.* But there *is* a presumption that writing about these variations helps one to think about the range of options in a more open and creative way—including thinking in a more sophisticated and differentiated fashion about the value of the more traditional stance as well.

Relational writers have also concentrated particularly on departures from the default position because for so many years those departures were strongly proscribed in the psychoanalytic community. When there is a very strong conservative *presumption* that dominates a field—and when that conservative presumption is bolstered by the structures of authority and transference I discussed in Chapter 3—it is not surprising that when a movement of alternative views finally coalesces, there is a strong tendency to emphasize the departures.

There are conservative writers (e.g., Michels, 2001) who maintain that relational challenges to the traditional analytic stance entail the absurd idea that "there are no principles of technique" at all (p. 409). This is a tendentious misrepresentation of the relational position, which rather than rejecting all principles, simply rejects as the most useful principles those that have guided analysts such as Michels. The relational principles may be more complex, perhaps they are even harder to learn, but they are neither absent nor arbitrary. Among the principles that I have discussed already in this book, for example—principles that most definitely guide and channel my interventions—are discerning/diagnosing the vicious circles in the patient's life and working to help him overcome them; tracing the ways in which he evokes experiences that keep the pattern going; attempting to help the patient overcome the anxiety, guilt, and shame that have constricted his life and impeded access to some of his most vital and enlivening desires and experiences; emphasizing not just insight in this latter aim but the promotion of direct exposure to the experience that he has been fearfully avoiding (and avoiding awareness of avoiding); attending to the potential ways in which the therapist's comments can be subtle rebukes or can undermine the patient's self-esteem, and emphasizing instead the patient's greater *acceptance* of his own thoughts and feelings; promoting new relational experiences with the therapists that can help him further to overcome those anxieties and to change the problematic and constricting patterns in his life; and working to extend that change pattern into the patient's *daily life*, not just in the consulting room.

Some of these principles and guidelines parallel the views of other relational writers; some represent a departure from the thinking and practice of at least some influential relational thinkers. But neither in the cyclical–contextual version of relational thought emphasized in this book nor in any other relational approach of which I am aware is there anything like the absence of principles or guidelines alluded to in Michels's caricature. In the next and concluding chapter, I will elaborate on some of the further clinical implications of the principles I have just mentioned and will consider further the way in which the particular relational approach described in this book differs from and converges with the range of other relational perspectives that are a prominent part of the contemporary therapeutic scene.

12

The "Inner" World, the "Outer" World, and the *Lived-In* World

MOBILIZING FOR CHANGE IN THE PATIENT'S DAILY LIFE

In this last chapter, my aim is to pull together a variety of themes that have been introduced throughout this book in order to give a fuller sense of how I work clinically and how the various parts of the argument I have been developing throughout the book fit together. I do not agree with those who contend that the theories we hold bear little or no relationship to practice (cf. Wallerstein & Richards, 1984; Fonagy, 2003); it will be evident to the reader that much of what is presented in this chapter reflects the cyclical–contextual vision of relational thinking that is at the heart of this book But it will also be clear that the relation between theory and practice is not a one-to-one matter. It should not be at all surprising to anyone who thinks relationally that some, if not much, of what I describe in this chapter (as in this entire book) reflects not just my theory but who I am as a person. This is *my* way of working with people. It bears a significant relationship to what my theory is, but it is partly simply me.[1] One could do or say many of the things I describe in this chapter without holding my particular theory, and one could hold my theory and, at least to some degree, do things differently. I do believe there is a connection, indeed a significant connection. But the connection is a loosely coupled one.

One consideration that has shaped a good deal of how I work derives from an experience that I have had on surprisingly numerous occasions. As a teacher and therapist, I regularly get into conversations with people (apart from my own patients) about their therapy experiences. In these conversations—with acquaintances, colleagues, students—I have noticed with some frequency a pattern that has troubled me. The person describes how wonderful his therapist is, while it seems to me, from all I hear or know about the person, that he is still *living his life* in the same painful and self-defeating way. From what I can discern, the relationship to the therapist *has* improved. There is a vitality, aliveness, and genuine connection in the room that perhaps was not there when they began. Consequently, the therapist too has probably felt that good work was being done. But the patient's life *outside* the sessions is not nearly as different. He continues to live in a way that is painful or constricted. The therapist becomes a wonderful oasis, but the patient still lives in the desert.[2]

Sometimes, ironically, the very qualities that have made the therapeutic relationship so enlivening and meaningful to the patient are related to the failure of the therapy to help him change his life. It is not that there is any *intrinsic* connection between these positive attributes and inattention to the quality of the patient's daily life. Indeed, much of the focus of this chapter will be precisely on how to bring the two together in an integrated and coherent way. Rather, the issue is that therapists who are concerned with understanding people in depth, who attempt to make contact with the rejected and warded-off parts of the personality, often tend to think about people in terms of an "inner world," a sequestered realm that is thought to exist quite apart from the self of social adaptation. Within this highly boundaried vision of the dynamics of personality, the inner world is sharply contrasted with

---

[1] As Stolorow and Atwood (1979) have pointed out, one's theory too is a reflection of one's personality and subjectivity, though it reflects these characteristics, one might say, at a different level of abstraction and in a way that is tempered by a different set of constraints.

[2] Obviously, I am discussing here people who have been in therapy for a substantial period, not people who are in the early stages of the work, where it might be objected that there has simply not been sufficient time for the changes to be evident yet in the rest of their lives.

the more superficial patterns that are directed toward adaptation to the outer world, and too much attention to these latter patterns is thought to lead to the loss of vital connection with the person's inner being. Therapists of this persuasion may, drawing inspiration from Winnicott (1975), think in terms of a "true self" that is buried and vulnerable while a "false self" presents itself to the world, or may conceptualize a "one-person" self of profound and uniquely individual experience as a necessary complement to the two-person self conceived of as exclusively manifested in direct interaction with others (e.g., Ghent, 1989).

Such accounts have strong intuitive appeal. They seem to reflect commitment to the deepest valuing of the individual and to directing oneself to the difficult task of attending to and nurturing the vulnerable but vital core of the personality. Often, moreover, these accounts articulate in valuable ways a hard to express sense of emptiness or meaninglessness that plagues many people in our society, providing a vocabulary for a pain and an absence that had theretofore gone unnamed. But in the process, these "inner world" focused accounts often place at the periphery of their concerns the patient's day-to-day life, treating patients' accounts of their conscious aspirations, their daily activities, their interactions with friends and coworkers, as a distraction from the encounter with the depths. It is only when the patient talks of his childhood or his feelings about the therapist that the "real" work can proceed.

I am very much in tune with the commitments and aspirations that animate these therapists' work. But I regard the pursuit of admirable *aims* by many therapists to be combined with problematic *theories*, theories that excessively compartmentalize and dissociate inner and outer, true and false selves, the individual and the social, yielding a misleading vision of the relation between deep subjectivity and the interactions with the world that characterize our lives and express our character. When offered by relationalists, such accounts have the ironic consequence of *diminishing* attention to the relational matrix, confining the therapist's interest to only a limited portion of the web of relationships that are the vital context for experience, namely those stored in memory from the earliest years of life.

The cyclical psychodynamic model, with its emphasis on the pervasively reciprocal and circular nature of human psychological experience and dynamics, leads to a therapy that engages the individual at the deepest experiential levels, but does so not as a foray into a separate and isolated inner realm, but as a process of engaging *the experience of living*, the multiple ways in which our deepest aspirations are expressed in (or frustrated by) not only the way we interact with those who are close to us, but also in our experiences in our work lives, in our communities, and in the larger society and culture in which they are embedded. From a cyclical psychodynamic vantage point, the *interconnectedness* of our "inner" world and the events of daily living is of the essence. Our innermost thoughts, feelings, desires, fantasies, or representations of self and other do not exist in some separate realm, sealed off from the "superficial" world of daily life. These dynamic psychological structures and processes shape the ways we act in the world and contribute to the qualities—for example, of vibrancy or deadness, confidence or hesitancy, relatedness or withdrawnness—that give a particular color, texture, and impact to those acts. In turn, these ways of interacting with the world evoke responses from others, which feed back either to change or to further maintain the thoughts, feelings, desires, expectations, and representations of self and other that originally gave rise to the action. And in so doing, they set the stage for the *next* moment's actions in the world and for the affective tone that will accompany them. The process is continuous, and the causal arrows flow in all directions simultaneously—self shapes social context as social context shapes self; feelings shape behavior as behavior (and its consequences) shape feelings; motives imbue our representations, as our representations shape our motives; affects instigate thoughts as thoughts stir affects. The interconnections and feedback loops are virtually limitless. No realm is more real or fundamental or "deep" than any other.

Such a view points us to look not just at the patient's subjective experience or at his unconscious motives or fantasies—though these remain a crucial concern—but also at the ways in which that subjective experience and those motives and fantasies are manifested and embedded in *a way of life*. And it calls for interventions that do more than *name* or *describe* or *explain* in the traditional fashion of "interpretations." It calls for interventions that will *disrupt* the vicious circles and create virtuous circles in their place, new patterns that expand rather than constrict the person's experience and that create their own self-perpetuating consequences. From this vantage point, then, the therapist's interventions are designed not just to help clarify the patient's subjective experience or enable him to feel understood—as essential as both are—but also *to help him to move*, to make it possible for him to interact differently with the world. Changes in *either* subjective experience or concrete interactions with the world about us help to amplify and solidify changes in the other, and the absence of change in either makes change in the other unlikely to be enduring.

RETHINKING INTERPRETATION: EXPLANATORY NARRATIVES, NARRATIVES OF POSSIBILITY, AND THE NEED TO PROMOTE NEW ACTIONS IN THE WORLD

I have at various points in this book raised questions about the prominence given to the concept of interpretation in understanding the therapeutic process, and have pointed to serious limits to a primarily interpretive approach to the work. In this, my thinking converges considerably with Renik's (1993), who notes that "the term interpretation dates from a conception of the psychoanalytic process that is now generally criticized, a conception in which the analyst decodes the patient's thoughts to reveal the unconscious, decides what hidden meanings lie beneath the manifest content of the patient's verbalizations—like the well-traveled railway conductor of Freud's famous analogy who tells the ignorant passenger where he is" (p. 560). Renik notes that one serious problem with this approach to the work is that "the interpreter is always better informed than the recipient of the interpretation."

Aron (1996), like many relationalists, endorses rather thoroughly this critique of the false assumption of the therapist's or analyst's objectivity and the implication that the patient is the passive recipient of enlightenment from the analyst. He opts, however, *not* to reject the term interpretation, which is by now very strongly ingrained in psychoanalytic discourse, but to give it a different meaning or emphasis:

> I like the term interpretation because it can also be used to mean the expression of a person's conception of a work of art or subject, as for example, the pianist's interpretation of a sonata or an actor's interpretation of a role. This use of the word interpretation emphasizes the individual's unique, personal expressiveness. I like to think of an analyst's interpretation as a creative expression of his or her conception of some aspect of the patient. (p. 94)

Here Renik and Aron come to different conclusions about the utility of the term "interpretation," but they do so *from almost exactly the same premises.* Both emphasize, in essence, the *epistemological* dimension of the process, the consequences of a false assumption of objectivity. This epistemological challenge to traditional analytic assumptions has, to be sure, very substantial implications for therapeutic technique, both for Renik and for Aron. For both authors, for example, it opens up the field of therapeutic interaction for considerably greater self-disclosure and considerably greater therapist *presence* and affective engagement in the process. Their critique is thus very far from an empty intellectual exercise.

But I believe it is nonetheless important for us to move beyond this particular dimension of critique, which has dominated the focus of relational theorists thus far, and to consider more thoroughly and focally the implications for clinical practice of the pervasive self-perpetuating processes that I have been emphasizing in the last few chapters. Regarding the specific term "interpretation," I tend to lean more toward Renik's position, mainly because, as I discussed in Chapter 8, the idea that what the therapist does is to "interpret" has historically had a problematically constricting effect on the way many therapists relate to and interact with their patients. But—to introduce here a perspective that agrees with *both* Renik's and Aron's main point, but applies it to the word "interpretation" itself—the meaning of the term "interpretation" too is in the eyes of the beholder. There is no canonical, God-given meaning or connotation to the term. Renik rejects it in its connotation of offering objective truth to a benighted patient, and so does Aron. Aron embraces the term in its connotation that the very idea that a pianist "interprets" a piece of music means that she is offering *her* understanding of the music, not "the" meaning of it. And this is a view thoroughly consonant with Renik's way of thinking.

The important point, then, is not whether one is "pro-interpretation" or "anti-interpretation," that is, whether one supports or challenges the term "interpretation" per se, but rather *what kind* of interpretations one engages in or *what one means by* interpreting. If one's main aim is "explaining" the person to himself—as Aron (1996) notes it was for most analysts over the years and continues to be for many—then a primarily interpretive approach is likely to be arid and ineffective. If, on the other hand, one means by interpreting something more like the analogy Aron draws to the seeking of meaning from a work of art with which one is seriously engaged, then interpreting is not only acceptable but salutary. Especially is this the case if one draws out a further meaning from what is implicit in Aron's analogy to the interpretation of a work of art—such interpretations, generally, are *appreciations*. That is, what I find important about the analogy Aron draws (quite apart from the question of whether the word "interpretation" per se is useful or problematic) is not simply the epistemological lesson—that the therapist's interpretation is *her* interpretation, her individual take on an experience that can be seen in other ways by other interpreters. Equally important is that one approaches a work of art with interest, pleasure, respect. One is *engaged with* the work, eager to find meaning in it, interested in experiencing it again and again with the expectation that one will learn something new each time. This is indeed an attitude that befits the psychotherapist, and the attentive reader will readily see how it reflects and parallels the attitude described in Chapter 8 and, indeed, in all the clinical portions of this book.

But even this expansion of the traditional meaning of "interpreting" takes us only so far toward the goal of enabling the patient to change his life for the better. Identifying, illuminating, even appreciating, *what is* constitutes only part of the story. The patient comes to us seeking to be affirmed and understood; but he also comes to us seeking to *change* what is. Most interpretations in psychotherapy, even those pursued from the vantage point so interestingly introduced by Aron, are rooted in the past and in the present. They seek to help the patient to see more fully who he is and what he feels and to enable him to better understand how he came to be that way, how his life history has led to the present moment. But the patient also needs to understand *what could be,* to imagine and dare to pursue greater possibilities, to see the path toward an *alternative* way of experiencing himself and an alternative way of living. And he needs as well experiences that help him develop the *wherewithal* to live differently in the ways he is beginning to envision.

There are a variety of ways to conceive of and to approach this future-oriented, change-oriented pole of the therapeutic process. In previous publications (e.g., Wachtel, 1977a, 1987a, 1997; Wachtel & Wachtel, 1986) I have highlighted how the traditional insight-oriented approaches to psychotherapy can be valuably complemented by a range of methods and ideas deriving from alternative systems of therapeutic thought and intervention, particularly those deriving from behavior therapy and from family therapy. In those writings, I have spelled out in some detail why the inclusion of such methods not only enhances the therapeutic effectiveness of the work but also comports, much more than is generally appreciated, with the most vital and fundamental essence of psychoanalytic thought. Many of the objections to such active-intervention methods, and to the theoretical assumptions on which they rest, it turns out, are rooted in misconceptions of both behavior therapy *and* psychoanalysis.[3]

In further amplifying the clinical implications of this way of thinking, I have also attempted to show how this integration of ideas and methods from different schools of thought can be made more "seamless" (e.g., Wachtel, 1991). My aim, further pursued here, has been to illuminate how the action-oriented, future-oriented dimension of therapeutic work can be incorporated into and can infuse the interpretive effort itself, yielding a therapeutic approach in which the effort to understand the person in depth and the effort to help him to move more effectively toward a way of life that feels more whole, genuine, and gratifying are essentially inseparable (Wachtel, 1993).

In certain respects, this approach, which relies considerably on the artful use of language, converges with a range of other approaches to therapy that share an emphasis on *narrative* as a central theme. We are all powerfully influenced by the narratives we create for ourselves about our lives, our history, the nature of those we interact with, and our own characteristics, motives, and feelings. The narrative emphasis has been especially strong both in the realm of psychoanalysis (e.g., Aron, 1989; Schafer, 1992; Spence, 1982) and in systemic or strategic approaches (e.g., White & Epston, 1990; Molnar & de Shazer, 1987; de Shazer, 1997; O'Hanlon & Weiner-Davis, 2003; Zeig, 1985; Angus & McLeod, 2004). But it is implicit in cognitive therapy as well, in its assumption that *what we tell ourselves* about an experience is crucial to its impact and psychological implications. The cognitive therapy approach, however, often limits itself to critiquing the "rationality" of what we tell ourselves.[4] Psychoanalytic and systemic/narrative therapies, in contrast, approach the reconstruction of narratives in a much more comprehensive and open-ended fashion. Their emphasis is on facilitating a different version of the patient's story of his life, a story

---

[3] For further elucidation of these issues, see also the excellent discussions by Frank (e.g., 1990, 1992, 1993, 2001).

[4] *Constructivist* cognitive therapy (e.g., Neimeyer & Mahoney, 1999; Guidano, 1991; Feixas & Botella, 2004; Fernandez-Alvarez & Opazo, 2004) represents a noteworthy exception to this limitation.

that enables the patient to make sense of what has previously felt confused or incomprehensible and that gives his life story new meanings and new possibilities.

Often, however, especially in psychoanalytic narratives, these have been primarily *explanatory* or descriptive narratives, narratives that explain how the patient got to be the way he is or explain elements of his present experience and motivations that have been unclear or have been understood in a problematic way. What has been more characteristic of the narrative approaches that have derived from more systemic or strategic perspectives, in contrast, has been what might be called "narratives of possibility," narratives that enable the patient to envision a different *future* and to take action to achieve that future.

From the vantage point of this distinction, it might be said that thus far in this book I have primarily been highlighting the limits of a therapeutic approach that is excessively rooted in narratives of explanation and description. But an approach that is too exclusively rooted in the narrative of possibility carries its own dangers and limitations, especially that of devolving to a form of *manipulation*. Narrative and strategic approaches are sometimes a bit too clever for their own (or the patient's) good. Deep, enduring, and genuinely satisfying change must be rooted in the patient's sense that he is understood and appreciated for who he is and that the therapist's understanding is capacious enough to embrace all of the complexly intersecting and conflicting facets of his makeup. When either pole of the dialectic between the narrative of description and the narrative of possibility is missing or deficient, the therapy is likely to be significantly limited in its value to the patient.

THE DIALECTICAL RELATION
BETWEEN ACCEPTANCE AND CHANGE

Viewed from a slightly different vantage point, we may say that the key to effective therapeutic practice lies in embracing and working with the dialectical tensions between the patient's need for affirmation and his need for change. He needs to be deeply appreciated and understood for who he is, but he needs as well to see (and to know that the therapist sees) that he can be *different* from who he has been, and in important ways *more* than he has been. This dialectical tension can fail to be held by therapists from either direction. My discussion in previous chapters of the "attitude of suspicion" and of theoretical positions that emphasize the patient's "primitive" and "archaic" fantasies points to what is an often unappreciated failure to be sufficiently accepting of the patient as he is. These viewpoints embody a covertly critical attitude that, as Aron (1991a) has pointed out, has the implicit agenda of requiring the patient to "grow up," as well as to *give* up his infantile aims and defenses. But the dialectical tension between the patient's need for affirmation and his desire for change may be flattened from the opposite direction as well, when the therapist insists in such a single-minded manner on seeing things through the patient's eyes, on attending to his "psychical reality," that the patient's need to find a way to see things *differently* is given short shrift. This equal and opposite failing can be seen among therapists of a variety of persuasions, including some who have contributed substantially to the emergence of the relational tradition. Kohut (1984), for example, in describing a key case, states:

> The patient, as I finally grasped, insisted—and had a right to insist—
> that I learn to see things *exclusively* in his way and *not at all* in my
> way. . . . To hammer away at the analysand's transference distortions
> brings no results; it only confirms the analysand's conviction that
> the analyst is as dogmatic, as utterly sure of himself, as walled off in
> the self-righteousness of a distorted view as the pathogenic parents
> (or other self-object) had been. (p. 182, italics added)

Here Kohut is offering a very important corrective to the "attitude of suspicion" I discussed in Chapter 8. His aim to understand the patient empathically, sympathetically, and in a way that affirms the patient's experience and point of view converges very strongly with an essential feature of the clinical approach I am advocating in this book. But the either–or attitude that is evident in this example—which is taken not from a publication early in Kohut's struggle to emerge from the strictures of the classical model, but from the posthumous publication of his last mature work—reflects how difficult that struggle with orthodoxy was and how reactively single-minded it could leave those who attempted to emerge from it. Kohut does not just advocate seeing things from the patient's point of view, but "exclusively" from the patient's point of view and "not at all" from his own. Such a view of the clinical process reflects a still insufficient integration of the two-person point of view, from whose vantage point it is utterly impossible to even come close to seeing things "not at all" from one's own perspective. But at least as important, Kohut's comment in this quotation reflects the vision of interpretation that was prevalent in the psychoanalytic milieu from which Kohut emerged and against which he eventually rebelled, a conception of interpretation in which the analyst "hammer[s] away at the analysand's transference distortions."

This crude form of "interpretation" is indeed best left behind as the practice of psychotherapy advances. But "hammering away" at "distortions" is by no means the only way to provide the patient with an alternative to the way of seeing things that is at the heart of his deprivations and suffering. However much the patient seeks affirmation for the way he sees and experiences things now, he also is seeking to *extricate* himself from that very way of seeing things, or at least from those aspects that contribute to his pain and difficulties. Kohut, armed (and I use the word advisedly) only with the traditional idea of what an interpretation entailed, could see no alternative to "hammering" the patient other than to eschew interpretation altogether for a long period of time and to see things *only* from the perspective that the patient has come to therapy not only to have affirmed but *also* to have questioned.

In contrast to the flattened, either–or thinking I have just been describing, other writers in the relational tradition have offered much more complexly dialectical accounts, in which acceptance of the patient as he is and explicit efforts to help him to see things differently and to change are pursued in concert. Bromberg (1993), for example, notes that "the ability of an individual to allow his self-truth to be altered by the impact of an 'other' . . . depends on the existence of a relationship in which the other can be experienced as someone who, paradoxically, both *accepts the validity* of the patient's inner reality and participates in the here-and-now act of constructing a negotiated reality discrepant with it" (p. 160, italics added). Similarly, Ghent (1995), attending to the simultaneous and sometimes opposite needs of the patient for affirmation of the old and recognition of the new and potentially different, states that "mixed in with the apparent need to repeat, another (and opposing) motivational system, or need, is operating as well, one that is usually much weaker and less developed; it is an expansive rather than a conservative system, one whose tendency or need is either to seek out a new quality of experience or to destabilize the smooth functioning of the old, constrictive system" (p. 485). Commenting further on the multiple perspectives needed for effective therapeutic work,

Ghent adds, in a way that parallels the emphasis in this book on the multiple levels of intervention needed to address the patient's self-replicating vicious circle dynamics, that

> we tend to overlook the plurality of routes by which psychic change occurs, both within and outside of analysis. Some types of intervention focus on the perceptual pole of an interactive circle, others on the effector or response end. A change in either may, and often does, result in a change in the entire system. Classically, psychoanalysis has concentrated on the perceptual end of the loop. Interpretation is aimed at helping the patient see, or perceive, things differently, that is, from a new perspective. The implicit assumption was that changed perception would result in changes in ways of being and doing in the world, that is, that changes at the effector or response end will result. Insight will lead to change. That this has, by no means, been the universal result has caused great problems for psychoanalysis, problems often spoken of under the rubric of the uselessness, even counterproductiveness, of "intellectual insight." . . . Even in those instances where it seems that insight has made for change, one is often left with the lingering suspicion that substantial, perhaps critical, change had already occurred and that the insight was made possible as the concluding step in the long buildup of change, much like the sudden precipitation of crystals in a supersaturated solution. One might reasonably conclude that change in the system, however it is brought about, may result in insight. (pp. 485–486)[5]

There are many ways to promote the "effector end" of the multifaceted change process Ghent describes or—to state it in a way that more clearly highlights the connection of these ideas to the frame of reference I have been emphasizing in this book—to interrupt the vicious circles that maintain the patient's suffering or deprivation. The kind of dialectical thinking that enables the simultaneous pursuit of understanding and acceptance of the person as he is, on the one hand, and promotion of *change* in how he experiences and lives in the world, on the other, is evident, for example, in a range of systemic and narrative approaches in which paradox is often a key element (e.g., White & Epston, 1990; de Shazer, 1985; O'Hanlon & Weiner-Davis, 1989; Zeig, 1985; Angus & McLeod, 2004; Selvini-Palazzoli, Boscolo, Cecchin, &

---

[5] Note in this last portion of the quotation the similarities to the views of Alexander discussed in Chapter 10.

Prata, 1990; Weeks, 1991). It is evident as well in Linehan's dialectical behavior therapy (e.g., Linehan, 1993; Hayes, Follette, & Linehan, 2004; Dimeff & Koerner, 2007), which has been one of the most influential therapeutic innovations of recent decades.[6] Since I have extensively discussed elsewhere the use of explicit behavioral interventions in the context of a psychoanalytically informed therapy (e.g., Wachtel, 1997), I will not go into that topic in much detail here. The influence of that earlier integrative work certainly will be evident in the way that I attempt to go beyond the limits of the traditionally interpretive focus and incorporate elements of the narrative of possibility into the therapeutic dialogue. But my focus here will be on that dialogue itself, on the ways in which the specific qualities of the therapeutic dialogue can enhance (or detract from) the ways in which that dialogue is helpfully therapeutic.

My lack of focus here on explicitly behavioral interventions by no means implies a shift in my view that such interventions are both clinically valuable and compatible with the essential core of psychoanalytic understanding. What I am exploring here, however, is the nature of therapeutic dialogue in virtually *all* therapies; behavioral interventions too are almost always conveyed in the context of dialogue or discourse. Ensuring that one is intervening appropriately and helpfully in introducing an explicit behavioral intervention requires the same attention to the two-way communications between patient and therapist as in a more avowedly relational therapy. In either case, the same sensitivity to feedback from the patient is required so that the therapist proceeds not according to her own agenda but in accordance with the patient's own experience and desires.

The feedback the patient offers is not always explicit, and he may not even be aware he is offering feedback at all. But sensitivity to subtle cues that the patient is feeling misunderstood or pushed in a direction he is not comfortable with—even if he may not yet be able to formulate or express it in words—is perhaps even more important if one is employing explicit behavioral interventions than it is generally (and it is *very* important generally). Conversely, whether one uses explicit behavioral measures or the more "seamless" integration of different approaches I referred to above—in which the behavioral element may

---

[6] Interestingly, Linehan, whose roots lie in behavior therapy, shares with Ghent's more psychoanalytic vision a profound interest in the implications of Buddhist thought for therapeutic change. Her approach, however, clearly differs considerably from more psychoanalytic applications of either Buddhist thought (see, e.g., Safran, 2003) or dialectical thinking (e.g., Hoffman, 1998).

be implicit and woven into the overall dialogue between patient and therapist rather than specifically identified as an "intervention"—it should be our aim to ensure that the patient learns effective ways of dealing with the circumstances he encounters in his life. Some therapists may not *call* such efforts behavioral, and may address via other forms of therapeutic dialogue the need for the patient to monitor and in some respects change his actual behavior in the world. But in one way or another, the therapist who is alert to the pervasive presence of vicious circles, in which actions in the world continuously feed back either to maintain or to change internal psychic structures, must address the consequences of the inhibitions and restrictions that have inevitably been a part of the patient's developmental history and its ongoing but always evolving legacy.

We *all* in one way or another have gaps in our emotional and behavioral development that result from the anxieties that inevitably arise in the course of growing up dependent and small for so many years (see again Chapter 9). Virtually no one emerges from the long years of dependency that characterize becoming human without some peaks and valleys in his or her ability to cope effectively with life's challenges. For each person there are different situations, different emotional or relational configurations that are implicated in the vicious circles in his or her life. However socially skilled or cognitively or emotionally competent we may be *in general,* for each of us there are certain situations that reveal the emotional stigmata of our upbringing and the odd and surprising gaps in our social and emotional skill set. What is revealed in these situations is the compounding effects of avoidance—the ways in which the need to avoid pain and humiliation can impede the trial and error process through which, over developmental time, we develop our capacity to handle a wide range of emotional and social challenges; the ways in which, as a consequence, the situation continues to feel dangerous or potentially humiliating; the ways in which this then leads us to further avoid the situation, thereby again foreclosing opportunities to develop the emotional and behavioral repertoire needed to feel comfortable in that realm; and so on through the life cycle.

Because many situations cannot be avoided in their entirety in the course of daily living, the avoidance often comes in the form of perceptually reinterpreting the situation in order to protect ourselves from having to manifest the behavior about which we feel insecure. Both the reinterpretation and the insecurity are likely to be largely out of awareness, but they are certainly no less impactful for that. Thus someone who is insecure about his capacity to express anger or assertiveness in a way that is either strong enough or modulated enough may respond to an interaction that might consensually be seen as a confrontation, and thus as requiring an assertive response, as instead an occasion for nervous laughter and ingratiation. He thereby gains the immediate experience of feeling safer, but is again deprived of the opportunity to develop the skills and experiences that would enable him to respond to the next similar situation more confidently.

Another person may be perfectly comfortable with and good at being confrontational and effectively aggressive, but may persistently avoid seeing *softer* overtures. In contrast to the first person, he will consistently turn situations that could be perceived as opportunities for reconciliation or as friendly or affectionate overtures into situations of confrontation. And in the process, his capacity to respond to such overtures remains undeveloped. His unacknowledged but powerful fear that he would turn to mush, be "too much," or just "not get it right" if he opened himself to responding positively keeps him from going through the experiences that would enable him to *learn how* to deal with this different set of challenges more effectively. When he turns the situation into one of confrontation, he can feel strong and masterful, but as a consequence, he continues to feel inadequate in the realm of "softer" feelings.[7] If he is "good at" his defensive style, he will barely be aware of his avoidances or feelings of inadequacy (and certainly not of his depriving himself of opportunities to practice what is in fact as much a skill as dominating is). Instead, he may enter therapy with depressed affect that makes no sense to him since he is "doing so well" in life, or perhaps with some awareness that he misses love and friendship in his life but little understanding of how the very ways he goes about feeling more secure or better about himself *moment-by-moment* contribute to the chronic sense of dissatisfaction that plagues him so mysteriously.

It is certainly true that for some people the realms in which they do not function well are pervasive and for others they are quite limited and specific; but the very nature of human childhood is such that essentially everyone has some areas of surprising inaptitude, and it is almost certain that for everyone who finds some aspect of his or her

---

[7] Horney (e.g., 1945, 1950) has valuably described these different life strategies in terms of the "moving toward" and "moving against" neurotic trends. She has noted as well that a third strategy, which she calls "moving away," can offer a pseudo-resolution through avoiding real engagement with others altogether. But as she notes, this strategy too usually collapses under the weight of the contradictions it is designed to obscure and of the essential human needs it causes to go unmet.

life troubling enough to consult a psychotherapist, part of the pattern the person is coming to address will include a need to learn to handle certain situations differently. For healthier looking people, their high functioning is in large measure a reflection of their placing themselves mostly in the situations that they have the capacity to handle reasonably well. Often, what brings them into therapy is encountering a situation that reveals previously unrevealed vulnerabilities—vulnerabilities that become evident when the person is brought face-to-face— whether through a promotion, a marriage, or some unforeseen set of contingencies—with the emotional and relational configurations that, over the years, they have avoided so skillfully that they were not even required to recognize they were avoiding them at all.

It is not easy for the therapist to address the ways in which the patient's concrete actions or subtle incongruities in his social and emotional repertoire have contributed to perpetuating the difficulties he has come to therapy to resolve. It is much easier to feel empathic and in tune with the patient when one is attending solely to what he is feeling or to how he sees things. When we inquire into what the patient actually did and the consequences it brought about, he can readily feel criticized or second-guessed. Yet as Ghent (1995) pointed out, the response or effector end of the patient's way of living is as important to attend to as the perceptual end. What is required in doing so is both skill in using language therapeutically and a genuine humility in areas where we do not know. As is frequently emphasized in writings on therapy, much of what we do is to help the patient find *his own* solution, to clarify his aims and examine more closely the consequences of his actions; aiding people in this kind of exploration is one of the most important parts of the good therapist's skills. But it must also be acknowledged and understood that sometimes we *do* see certain possibilities and solutions more clearly than the patient does. We are able to do so not because we are necessarily emotionally healthier than the patient (a tempting assumption we should be hesitant to make), but in part simply because we are not as immersed in the problem as he is; that is, because it is *his* problem. We are also able to be helpful in this way because any reasonably intelligent person cannot spend much of her day listening to people's stories of their lives without hearing how some things tend to work better than others. We do become experts in human relations, and it is a kind of hubristic antihubris, if you will, when we refuse to offer what we know or pretend that we do not know it. We must, to be sure, keep inquiring and listening for whether our input is consonant with the patient's own values and his subjective sense of who he is, but an excessive concern with letting the patient "do it on his own" reflects the rather extreme individualistic bias of our culture (Cushman, 1990; Wachtel, 1983) much more than the genuine interests and needs of the patient.

BUILDING ON STRENGTHS

One key element both in helping the patient to achieve new behavior in his daily life and in reconciling the seeming contradiction between his need for affirmation and his desire for change is attention to the patient's strengths and to the buds or kernels of new ways of being that are *already evident* in his makeup. One of the great obstacles to effective psychotherapy is the tendency for therapists to focus so preponderantly on pathology that neither patient nor therapist sees clearly enough the strengths and alternative potentials on which meaningful change can be constructed. When this happens, the patient's experience of feeling *seen* often amounts to feeling *exposed*, leading either to resistance to the therapist's messages and perceptions or to an acceptance of them that only deepens his discouragement and self-disparagement. Successful psychotherapy, I believe, very largely entails enhancing, developing, building upon trends and capacities that already exist in the patient but that have been impeded and constrained by the ironic circular dynamics of the patient's life. The beginning of the process of building on those alternative kernels of different ways of being, of course, is *seeing* them—something that therapists (whose education is usually primarily directed to signs of psychopathology) are often poorly trained to do.

Part of why the patient may insist, à la Kohut's account discussed earlier, on being seen *only* from his own already existing point of view, however much it is also the foundation for the very miseries he is coming to therapy to alleviate, is that therapists' comments so often have an implicitly negative or critical focus.[8] When the therapist's efforts to examine the problematic features of the patient's view of the world are invalidating or pathologizing, it is not surprising that the patient— especially the narcissistically vulnerable patient—may find them unwelcome. A good part of the patient's difficulty lies in *his own* inability to see his real strengths and assets, and this holds even (and perhaps especially) for patients who may seem, on the surface, to be

---

[8] In this regard, see again Chapter 8.

full of bluster and *excessive* self-regard. Self-regard of this type is, by and large, *defensive* self-regard, and it stems from the person's inability to value himself *as he is,* an inability that creates a need to *exaggerate* his strengths in order to ward off the secret fear that they are actually minuscule or nonexistent. He does not need a therapist to demonstrate to him that underneath his surface presentation of self lies pathology. His problem is that *he* believes this.

Certainly the patient needs a way of understanding himself, and of feeling understood by the other, that *does not leave out* the uncomfortable or unpretty parts, for that will simply leave him feeling they are too unacceptable to acknowledge. But he also needs a way of framing and contextualizing these tendencies that aids him in extricating himself from the painful patterns of living and feeling in which he has become entangled. The constructivist perspective that is closely associated with the relational point of view teaches us that there are many equally valid ways to depict the patterns of thought, feeling, and behavior that trouble the patient, and it points us to consider which of the multiple possible depictions and understandings is most helpful to the therapeutic aim. But one of the ironies of the way that relational thinking has evolved thus far is that the relational literature remains so laden with references to patients' "preoedipal" levels of organization or to "primitive" or "archaic" or destructive or schizoid characteristics. It is not that these ways of thinking about the patient are "wrong" per se. A constructivist or perspectival position certainly permits such constructions, among others. But a constructivist approach valuably opens up the possibility of *other* understandings as well, understandings that are more likely to enable the patient to liberate himself from the life patterns that are the source of his pain.

Reflecting the continuing legacy of the medical origins of psychoanalysis, many psychoanalytic writers and therapists continue to focus on diagnosing pathology, and it is not an exaggeration to suggest that much of psychoanalytic discourse is pathocentric.[9] Think of the fre-

---

[9] I do not mean by this to imply that it is only psychoanalysts who think of psychological difficulties through such a lens. Behavior therapists have long criticized psychoanalysis for being immersed in such a "medical model," but ironically, there are ways in which the thinking of behavioral and cognitive-behavioral therapists tends even more than that of psychoanalysts to follow an essentially medical model. Often even their very notions of what is required for proper "empirical validation" are linked to the diagnostic categories of the psychiatric manuals (see Wachtel, 2006, for a critique of this mode of thinking) and their emphasis on specific techniques for specific symptoms is also much closer to a medical model than is the approach of most psychoanalytic therapists, with their emphasis on understanding and treating the whole person.

quent references to such concepts as paranoid/schizoid and depressive positions, psychotic cores, or arrested development, and the ways in which these ideas shape many analysts' vision of the fundamental building blocks of personality development or the sources of the psychological distress our patients bring to our offices. Some might argue that terms such as *paranoid, schizoid,* and *depressive* are merely technical names for phenomena that do not necessarily have a pejorative connotation. But psychoanalysts, of all people, should take seriously the overtones of the language people use, including themselves. Certainly there are other ways of pointing to and conceptualizing the experiences to which these pathology-soaked terms allude, and *it matters* that the field continues to use these terms so widely.

Substituting different terminology for the pathocentric terms so pervasive in clinical theory and discourse is not a mere translation, simply another way of saying "the same thing." Nor is it a euphemistic cleaning up of messy truths. Different ways of *saying* things yield different ways of *seeing* things. The way our brains are wired, every word or image or concept, represented by a pattern of neuronal firings, has a somewhat different set of links to other neuronal networks, tripping off a different set of further associations, actions, and affects, which in turn set off still further associational networks. Subtle differences can thus, at times, lead to large effects. By framing things differently we actually *make* things different.

These alternative ways of conceptualizing the phenomena are constrained, not arbitrary. The versions that will work well enough in accounting for the observed phenomena that they will be maintained are not unlimited. It is for good reason that Hamlet said, "There are more things in heaven and earth. . . . Than are dreamt of in your philosophy," not "Anything goes." But the differences in different framings can be significant, which is indeed why psychotherapy—or conversation in general for that matter—is a valuable human activity. Skill in reframing and redescribing—when combined with clear-eyed perception of the patient's ways of being in the world rather than euphemistic avoidance of what is problematic or unpleasant—can help the patient to initiate new ways of interacting with others that break the cycle of self-defeat that for so long seemed to function inexorably.

The therapist's challenge is to communicate a vision of who the patient is that *feels to the patient himself* like an accurate appreciation of his experience; but it includes as well being able to see the strengths that the patient has been too demoralized or too self-loathing to appreciate, and hence to further develop. What is communicated must include an acknowledgment of the patient's "darker" side, but it must be approached in a fashion that does not exacerbate the patient's already fragile self-esteem. If one is working, for example, with a patient who struggles with feelings of rage toward those he loves, one could say something like, "I think it scares you that sometimes you get so furious that you have the thought that you'd like to really hurt the person you love, and you wonder if anyone can know that about you without finding you loathsome. It feels like if anyone knew that you have those feelings, they would have contempt for you, that they could not possibly understand them, and I guess you wonder about me too in that regard."

But if effective clinical work entails finding creative ways to address the patient's most subjectively unacceptable feelings and behavior, it also includes helping the person to see the *kernels of strength* in a realistic way. Thus, with the same patient, one might also comment, "Sometimes you get so furious at your son that you actually have the thought you would like to punch him. That feels so terrible, so shameful, to you that it feels like you have to hide it from everyone, even yourself. But what that leaves out is, first, what's going on between you and him that *stirs* that frightening feeling, and second, what is it within you that *enables you not to act on it*? Those are pretty terrifying feelings, I agree, and I also understand very well why you wish you didn't have them, and even why you feel ashamed of them. But I think it's really important for our work for us to understand much better what you draw upon that keeps them as scary *feelings,* while—almost without noticing that you're doing so— you actually *treat* your son in a rather appropriate fatherly way most of the time."

If his angry feelings lead some or much of the time to actual behavior that is hostile or unsupportive or disparaging, I would address that frankly, but I would also inquire into what enables him to be *differ-ent* from this on *other* occasions. The point would not be a simple "you're not so bad; see, you're nice to him sometimes." Rather, it is that the less-than-admirable behavior is not a simple expression of his *essence*; the *different* ways of being with his child (or his spouse, his friends, his subordinates at work, whomever) are *also* part of who he is, and our task is to understand when and why one side comes out and when and why the other does.

The question then becomes, "How can we help *the side of you that you admire more* to come to the fore more often?" At the same time, we need to be open to exploring whether there are ways in which the patient may in fact *not* value more highly the more conventionally admirable behavior. We may find, for example, that he has a longstanding preoccupation, rooted in both his childhood and his ongoing life interactions, with not being taken advantage of, not being a patsy or a sucker, and that as a consequence he feels better about himself when he is strong and tough, even to the point of being insensitive or hurtful—a dynamic well described by Horney (1945, 1950) in her discussions of the moving-against neurotic trend. When that is the case, then clearly we must address it, not ignore it.

But here again, it is important not to hold to a monolithic vision of the person's dynamics. I am a great admirer of Horney's conceptualizations, and believe her to be one of the most unjustly ignored and underrated figures in the history of our field (at least in the years since her death, since she was clearly very influential, if also controversial, during her lifetime). But one place in which I view her formulations as limited and problematic is in the overly generalized, insufficiently contextual nature of her understanding of personality. Horney's theory has been described as a holistic theory, and that is both its strength and its weakness. She creatively illuminates how the conflicts and issues she describes pervade the personality, but, like so many psychoanalytic theorists, especially of her day, she is insufficiently attentive to the ways in which the balance of forces, and even the *very nature* of the forces that are contending, shifts quite significantly from context to context.

Alongside the dominant dynamics that occupy our attention, there are *almost always* at least buds of alternative tendencies already existing. Attending to those alternative, if still largely undeveloped, modes of experience and behavior, is a crucial element in enhancing the patient's possibilities for change. To be sure, the patient will not feel understood if the news from the therapist is all upbeat. He comes to therapy because he feels stuck, confused, in pain, and perhaps experiences even a good measure of self-contempt. Yet at the same time, he *does* come for hope, and at some level, even if he has great difficulty in consciously accessing it, he comes knowing better than anyone else the hidden resources that have been buried beneath the avalanche of despair and the self-defeating patterns that plague him. Those resources are crucial to access if the therapy is to succeed.

ATTENDING TO VARIATIONS AND TO THE CONTEXT IN WHICH THEY ARE MANIFESTED

It should be clear from what I have already said that a key link to finding the kernels of strength and of new patterns of living lies in attention to the variability in the patient's behavior and experience from context to context. As I noted in Chapter 7, this attention to variability has been an important element in the evolution of the relational point of view, addressed largely through the concept of multiple self-states. This self-state conceptualization has the advantage of referring to *complex configurations* of psychological experience and organization. Self-states are not simply tendencies toward particular ways of acting, but rather organizations of experience characterized by particular affects, by inclinations to perceive events in certain ways and to respond to them in certain ways, by the evocation of and focus on certain memories and not others, by particular ways of experiencing the individuals with whom one is directly interacting and of experiencing resonances with interactions with prior individuals, and so forth. In that sense, the idea of multiple self-states is a more powerful and comprehensive idea than simply acknowledging that behavior and experience vary from situation to situation. At the same time, however, there is often an inclination to attend to the self-state per se, rather than to the way it is evoked by, and in turn evokes, particular contexts—contexts that are a crucial part of the self-state itself. Conceptualizations of multiple self-states are also at times primarily employed to represent the varying kinds of *pathology* manifested by the individual or the varying ways in which "primitive" or "archaic" organizations of experience can be manifested. When the concept is used in this fashion, self-states often are depicted from an almost purely "internal" vantage point: They arise or alternate almost by whim, rather than in response to ongoing experiences in the world.

Although none of these limitations are *intrinsic* to the concept of multiple self-states, and although, as I noted, the complexly configurational nature of the self-state concept represents an enormous strength of this way of thinking, in my own thinking about these phenomena I prefer to emphasize the idea of *variability*. For me, this emphasis has two advantages. First, when I refer to variability I am always thinking of variability *from context to context*. Consequently, this conceptualization provides a constant reminder of the need to contextualize our thinking about psychological matters. It alerts us to our vulnerability to remaining immersed in the one-person depiction of what the "internal structure" of an experience is without placing that structure in the context of the person's life course, life trajectory, and immediate circumstances. Second, thinking in terms of the prominence and pervasiveness of variability reminds me, apropos the discussion above, to pay attention to (and to call the patient's attention to) the fact that "you are not *always* like that." This emphasis has given a particular cast to my clinical work.

For example, in calling attention to a patient's silence, or tense, sparse communication, or hesitancy to open up a topic that seems clearly in the air, I might, instead of saying, "You seem to be having difficulty talking today," say something like, "Sometimes you seem to be able to talk to me about what you are feeling more easily than others." I am especially inclined to put it in this fashion if the patient seems, either today or more chronically, to be *feeling bad about* his noncommunicativeness.

The difference between the two versions of calling attention to essentially the same observation is that the latter version highlights that the patient is not always that way, that there are times that he is more communicative than this. It may also be noted that even the *less* preferred version, "You seem to be having difficulty talking today," partakes to some degree of the principles I am elaborating here—calling attention to and building on the patient's strengths and attending to the *variations* in his functioning and in his experience. That is, in saying that he is having trouble talking *today*, the message implicitly includes the idea that on other days it is not necessarily the same. Moreover, by referring to this behavior as *having difficulty* talking, it presents the observation in a less critical fashion than that I have frequently heard in supervision sessions or practica—comments, often thought of as "defense interpretations," that call attention to his avoidance rather than to the *difficulty* he is having. It should be evident that this relates to the discussion in Chapter 8 of being alert to implicitly *accusatory* elements in therapists' comments, as well as to the discussion in Chapter 9 of the ways that attention to the *anxiety* that drives the patient's defenses helps create more empathic and supportive communications.

I might also add—to further illustrate how the emphasis on attending to variations and building on the patient's strengths go together—that with some patients, who are especially vulnerable and prone to self-criticism or discouragement at any sign they are "failing," I would be inclined, unless there was a very strong reason to proceed otherwise, to *not* call attention to the variability by noting when they are having more difficulty. Rather, I would wait until the patient is being at least a little bit *more* communicative than he ordinarily is (even if he is still being less communicative than most people are) and then say something like, "I notice that you are able to elaborate a little more than usual today on what your experience was like. I wonder what enabled you to do that this time." In so doing, I am avoiding "hitting him when he is down," while at the same time still calling attention to and exploring the pattern of relative uncommunicativeness. At a moment when his self-esteem is likely to be higher, I am attending implicitly to the fact that at *other* times he is *less* communicative; but I am doing so in a context in which the message also includes that he is *capable* of communicating more fully, that he does not simply have a "deficit."

Such ways of communicating have the advantage of being *dynamic* formulations, in contrast to the static formulations that are all too common in our field. They imply that this is not simply "the way the patient is" but the way he *sometimes* can be, and they therefore make it clear that he also can be different. I have been struck by how frequently I have heard therapists—including quite seasoned and respected ones—say things like, "This patient *is not capable of* intimate relationships," or "This patient's inner emptiness makes it impossible for him to relate to others in any but a superficial way," or "This man's unintegrated omnipotence and aggression make him incapable of intimacy and mutuality."

At times, such static, essentialist ways of thinking are tied to particular diagnostic formulations. When a patient is described as borderline, or narcissistic, or hysteric, there is often an implicit (though not necessarily acknowledged or examined) assumption that *everything about him* is borderline, or narcissistic, or hysteric. Sometimes, this is tied to formulations about patients in at least some of these categories being "primitively organized" or at a certain "developmental level," and therefore incapable of genuinely transcending those structural limits. In other instances, it is more that the diagnosis becomes the filter through which the patient is seen, rendering exceptions to the expected mode of functioning either largely invisible or dismissed *as* exceptions. Challenging this all too common clinical tendency does not require ignoring or downplaying these patients' difficulties and limitations. Some people clearly do have quite severe and pervasive problems. But the tragedy in the lives of people with diagnoses such as borderline or narcissistic personality disorder does not lie in a complete absence of "higher level" functioning (see Westen, 1989), but in their terrible *vulnerability* to more problematic modes of functioning. Attending to the variations in their behavior and experience, finding the upward reaches, so to speak, of their personal capacities and modes of relating is not to engage in denial but to find the rungs in the ladder they need to climb.

The static descriptions that often characterize clinical theorizing and therapeutic practice, however astute they may be in some respects, are also impediments to change. The patient is acutely *described,* but the description does not have a trajectory. In the terms introduced earlier in this chapter, there is a narrative of description or explanation, but no narrative of possibility. Especially if we are attentive to the reciprocal, co-constructed nature of what transpires in the session, we may see that such static, essentialist descriptions of patients can yield self-fulfilling observations of the patient's lack of movement. The therapist, relating to the patient as someone who is "arrested" at a particular developmental level, who is "borderline" or "narcissistic," or even (in the everyday language of trait descriptions) who is "angry," or "passive–aggressive," or "dependent," or "manipulative," *brings out* and perpetuates those qualities and inclinations. When, in contrast, the focus is on *when* the patient is hostile or dependent or passive–aggressive, and on when the exceptions to these tendencies come to the fore, the patient is not as locked into the pattern and both parties in the room can begin to relate in new ways and to explore the synergies that such changes from both sides make possible.

Much of the time, such synergies will seem a distant dream. The pull of the patient's dominant pattern is likely to be very strong. If it were not, he would be unlikely to be in the therapist's office in the first place. But understanding that even when an identified pattern is pervasive, there are subthemes and variations that are also part of who the patient is, and examining the circumstances that enable that aspect of the person to be expressed and brought to the fore can be a powerful contributor to the therapeutic process and to the prospects for change.

ATTENDING TO CONFLICT

What I have been discussing under the rubric of variability is closely related to another important dimension of clinical work that addresses the patient's most troubling concerns while also attending to the unnoticed or as yet only partially developed strengths and countertendencies. I am referring here to the concern with *conflict* that has traditionally been at the core of the psychoanalytic point of view. One of the critiques that is sometimes offered of relational thinking, a critique that overlooks a huge number of counterexamples but that indeed does address some versions and dimensions of relational thought, is that the centrality of conflict in psychological development can be lost. This is most evident in theoretical positions that emphasize developmental arrest or the need for the therapist to offer emotional provisions that were not provided by the parents (see Mitchell, 1988a, 1993a, 1997, for good discussions of how these assumptions may be manifested in various versions of object relations and self psychological theories and the limitations they impose).

Downplaying of conflict has also at times been evident in the literature on multiple self-states, including some of the most seminal and illuminating contributions to our understanding of this phenomenon. Bromberg, for example (e.g., 1998a), in certain respects introduces the concept of multiple self-states as an *alternative* to an understanding in terms of conflict. While not denying the relevance of conflict altogether, Bromberg presents the shift from one to another self-state as an *alternative* to conflict, and he sees as one crucial therapeutic task bringing the patient to the point where he *can* experience conflict rather than shift to an alternative, incompatible self-state.

What Bromberg is pointing to, I believe, is the way that particular states of mind can be called forth to *foreclose* conflict. These self-states, we might say, are "purifying" self-states, states in which the experience of self-abnegation, for example, momentarily obliterates inclinations toward grandiosity or experiences of grandiosity obliterate self-doubts, or anger obliterates painful longing for a loved object, or what have you. When the patient is in such a seemingly monolithic state, the challenge is to be able to "stand in the spaces" and recognize that there are other states of mind and states of feeling that are also part of him.

Such a state of affairs, however, may be understood not as the *absence* of conflict but rather as reflecting a particular way of *dealing* with it. People do not, in my view, get into self-states that are radically dissociated from their other states of being *unless* they are deeply in conflict, unless they are inclined to experience things in ways that are so painfully incompatible that when one side of the conflict is at the fore the other seems to disappear. Put differently, the dissociative phenomena to which Bromberg and others have so importantly called our attention, are *preceded* by conflict; they *arise because* the person feels painfully pulled in competing directions and needs, as a consequence, to separate one state of feeling or desire or perception from another in radical fashion.[10]

The clinical importance of this way of seeing things is that it permits one to say something along the lines of, "You feel so angry right now that *you don't even want to think about* the part of you that cares about her and would miss her" or "When you're feeling so totally isolated, the way your do now, it feels dangerous *even to think* about the times when you've felt close to people, even to imagine that you could connect with anyone or remember when you have" or "When you're feeling so intensely self-blaming, the way you are now, and the only thing that feels right is to berate yourself, it's very hard to keep in mind how betrayed you felt, how much you yourself have felt at other times that you were the vulnerable one and he took advantage of you." The intent of such statements is to help the person build a bridge between the different aspects of his experience and of his overall makeup, to help him to stand firmly within the experience he is having even while beginning to see another side to that very experience. This may be seen as a version, approached from the vantage point of conflict, of what Bromberg (1998a), thinking in terms of dissociated self-states, calls "standing in the spaces."

The aim in what I am describing here is not to "interpret" the conflict in order to promote insight (though something like insight is likely to develop if the effort is successful). Rather, the most central aim is to facilitate the patient's *acceptance* of the painfully conflicting experiences, to enable him somehow to experience them all as part of him. As Bromberg describes, the most likely source of therapist comments that are likely to be helpful in facilitating this bridge between experiences is not the therapist's verbal awareness or hermeneutic cleverness. Rather, it is her attention to her own subjective experience, to the subtle state shifts that are part of her side of the enactments that are often the prime medium for expressing dissociated tendencies (Bromberg, 1998a; Stern, 2003, 2004).

---

[10] This understanding does not contravene the frequent role of *trauma* in contributing to severely dissociated self-states. Detailed discussion of the role of trauma would take us too far afield here. But it can be noted that traumas are usually not just a quantitative overwhelming of the individual's resources but generators of intense conflict—for example, between feelings of love and attachment and feelings of rage and betrayal, or between feelings of helplessness and pervasive danger and defensively grandiose feelings of invulnerability.

Our challenge in pursuing this work of bridge building is to find a way to honor the patient's need to have his immediate experience understood and affirmed and his simultaneous (even if submerged) wish for help in moving beyond the splits and constraints that have contributed to that very experience. I use the word "honor" here advisedly. Especially when there are radically dissociated self-states in the room, we are dealing with feelings that are often both desperate and fervent and that *do* conflict. To attend to *either* side alone, I believe, is to betray the patient, though of course, given the linear nature of time and language and the limitations of human discourse and understanding, at any given moment we may be (and may even need to be) rather overweighted in one direction or the other. Our task, however, is to keep our vision fixed most of all on the *conflicts* that lie behind the alternating experiences. Our job as psychotherapists, we might say, is that we are converters of either–or to both–and. That is the work we do, and, to a significant degree, the measure of whether we are doing our work well.

Consider, by way of illustration, the following dilemma described by a student therapist. She frequently felt that her patient was experiencing more distress and sadness than she was able or willing to acknowledge, and the patient's rejection of any comments about her dysphoric affect left her feeling "unreachable" to the therapist. We discussed how this tendency on the patient's part could be addressed without getting into what could seem to the patient like a debate or an effort to *persuade* her that she was feeling sadder and more upset than she had acknowledged—an approach that the therapist understood clearly would be unlikely to help. I suggested, as an approach that was simultaneously rooted in the elements of affirmation discussed earlier and of attending to the *conflict* the patient was struggling with, two potential points of entry that the therapist could try as a way of addressing the patient's experience without *arguing* with the patient. One was to say something like, "I can see that it's *really important to you* not to be sad." Such a comment approaches the sadness from a different angle. It does call attention to the sadness and make some potential room for it, but it does so in a way that acknowledges the importance to the patient of *not* being sad. It implicitly invites her to reconsider, but it does not dismiss or disparage the patient's resolve.

A somewhat more explicit approach rooted in much the same overall perspective was embodied in the second, slightly more elaborate suggestion I offered regarding how to deal with this clinical dilemma: "Not allowing yourself to be submerged in sadness or overwhelmed by sadness has been a real strength of yours. In your life, you've *needed* to keep on keeping on. But on the other hand, you end up getting *cheated* when you're feeling sad and deserve to have someone understand that and respond to it." One could add to this, depending on the nonverbal cues one is receiving from the patient, simply "It's a real dilemma." Saying this indicates that you are not expecting her to change instantly, and that you don't see it as a one-sided "You're making a mistake by not talking about your sadness." There *is* a good reason she has felt it is not a good idea to open the sluice gates or to reveal her vulnerability. But there is also a good reason why breaking the pattern could prove helpful as well, and the therapist's comment here opens up the possibility of perhaps finding a way to do so.

THE ATTRIBUTIONAL DIMENSION

Notice that in the foregoing example, the therapist does not directly challenge the patient's defenses. The reference to sadness is almost incidental, introduced not as something the therapist is *pointing out* to the patient, but as something the patient *already knows*. It thus attributes to the patient knowledge and understanding of the sadness and of the conflict over it. In essence, it addresses the situation, so common in clinical discourse, of the patient both knowing and not knowing something, and leads the patient to the insight by giving her credit for already having it. In so doing, the therapist does not challenge or confront the patient's defenses. Rather, she stands *side by side* with the patient, acknowledging something they both already know.

Comments of this sort are part of a larger category I have called attributional, because in one way or another they share the quality of attributing to the patient an insight, a capacity, an attainment that he does not yet have or does not yet know he has. And in the process, by attributing to him the particular quality, we aid him in coming closer to actually achieving it. As Loewald earlier put it from a somewhat different frame of reference, "The patient, being recognized by the analyst as something more than he is at present, can attempt to reach this something more" (1960, p. 27).

A common thread in what I am calling attributional comments is that they do not have the form of an interpretation but of an acknowledgment. That is, the therapist takes the role not of bringing news (or insight) to the patient, but rather of simply acknowledging what the patient *already* knows, or sees, or feels, or has begun to do. The therapist's comment is in fact an important element in the patient's actually getting there, but it is silent assistance, so to speak. Thus in one case, described in *Therapeutic Communication* (Wachtel, 1993), the patient had struggled for a long time with the burden of having to deny how seriously disturbed her mother was and with (unconsciously) having to take on the role of the sick one to distract attention from the mother's own illness. She was the object of her mother's relentless criticism, and, increasingly, was being told by her mother that she (the patient) was crazy and needed medication. Although she was unable to acknowledge it, it seemed apparent that she feared that to challenge these accusations and demands by her mother could lead to a breakdown in the mother's very precarious mental balance. Thus, under this pressure from her mother, the patient began to put pressure on her therapist to prescribe medication for her.

The therapist, who had consulted me for some recommendations on how to handle the case, did not think that medication was appropriate, and in fact felt that it was really the mother who needed strong psychoactive medication. But her efforts to point out to the patient the mother's psychological difficulties, or what was going on between her and her mother, met with considerable resistance. She had been making comments such as "There's no pleasing your mother," or "Whatever you do, your mother finds fault with it," or "It sounds to me like your mother is the one who needs medication more than you do. You take on the burden of her disturbance."

These comments sounded accurate to me on the basis of what I had been hearing, but it was also apparent that the response to them was usually the patient's even more vigorous defense of her mother. They created an adversarial interaction between patient and therapist, in which the therapist was trying to persuade the patient of something which the patient then felt compelled to rebut. As we discussed the case, and the therapist's increasing concern about the patient's insistence on medication, I suggested a change in therapeutic approach in a more attributional direction: Instead of trying to *persuade* the patient that her previous view of her mother was wrong, I suggested, focus on what she *already knows* about her mother. She has been living with her mother much longer than you, and in some way knows more about the mother's disturbance than either you or I ever will. Approach the task of illuminating what is going on by *giving the patient credit* for knowing this (the essence of an attributional interpretation).

Thus over a period of several weeks, the therapist began to offer the patient the following kinds of comments (presented in roughly their sequential order, with the last one understandably being the most difficult, and hence requiring the assimilation of the earlier ones before it could be usefully offered): The first attributional comment was, "It must be hard to know that no matter what you do you can't please her." Here, the content was very similar to what the therapist had been trying to say for quite some time, but the response to it was quite different. The comment, instead of taking the form of telling the patient what she somehow didn't know, essentially *assumed she did* know. It didn't *tell* her that her mother was impossible to please, it sympathized with how hard it was to be in that situation and how hard it was *to know* this.

A bit later, again with my guidance, the therapist said to her, "It must be hard to have to pretend that you can please her, knowing that that's not really possible." Here the focus extended to the patient's having to pretend that she *could* please her mother, and then led to a whole variety of other ways in which she had had to pretend, and then had to further bolster the pretending by *not acknowledging to herself* that she was pretending. The impossibility of pleasing the mother was further stated here as well, again not as "news" to be conveyed to the benighted patient by the all-seeing therapist (think of Renik's discussion, noted earlier in this chapter, of Freud's metaphor of the railway conductor who tells the ignorant passenger where he is) but as a simple acknowledgment of what the patient already knows.

Finally, after some more work on making room for the patient's perceptions to become acceptable to her, the therapist eventually said, "It must be very hard to know that your mother is crazy." By the time the therapist said this (the first time since the attributional strategy had been introduced that she directly approached this particular reality), the patient was more ready to acknowledge it; but again, it was conveyed not as "news," but as a sympathetic acknowledgment of how difficult and painful it was to know this about her mother. This then was followed by comments such as, "I can easily understand why it felt necessary for so long not to let yourself see what you were actually seeing every day, and why it even felt necessary to sacrifice yourself, to pretend to yourself that *you* were the crazy one." Here the same general line of approach was followed, with the further emphasis on the patient's response being *understandable*, not something odd or pathological.

ATTRIBUTIONAL INTERPRETATIONS AND COMMENTS: A MORE EXTENDED CLINICAL ILLUSTRATION

In further elaborating on the nature and implications of attributional interpretations, I want to present a somewhat more detailed discussion of a clinical case in which attributional comments played a significant role. An experienced therapist consulted me about a case he was having some difficulty with. The patient, Tim, was in his mid-20s, a sensitive, artistic man from a family in which such characteristics were not valued in a man. The parents were Portuguese immigrants who had achieved a measure of success running a small grocery store in a suburb of Providence. Tim was the youngest in the family, 8 years younger than his next oldest sibling, a sister. He had three older brothers, all of whom were very stereotypically male. They liked to play and watch football, get their hands dirty fixing cars, have a few beers with their buddies. Tim, in contrast, enjoyed reading poetry, went to the opera, and aspired to be an actor. He had, however, a symptom that was rather inconvenient, given his career choice—he was prone to break out in hives and a cold sweat while on stage or even anticipating being on stage.

As I explored with the therapist the sources of this symptom—which, interestingly, was limited only to these two situations (being on stage or anticipating or thinking about being on stage)—there were numerous indications that Tim was very conflicted about, and consciously denied and rejected, wishes for attention and admiration (what clinicians often call *exhibitionistic* wishes). One feature of Tim's psychological life that seemed related to this conflict was an intensely preoccupying fantasy, which he expressed frequently to his therapist, in which he was so strikingly handsome that he would not need to go up to women to make their acquaintance or connect with them but would find that they just naturally approached him. Tim's therapist referred to this as his "passive wish" or "passive fantasy," and apparently this terminology was a shared one between them; Tim too thought of it this way. I suggested that this way of viewing it cast Tim's wish in a rather critical light, and that it failed to address the *conflict* Tim experienced, in which the wish both expressed *and* defended against the same forbidden desire that plagued him on the stage, the desire to be looked at and admired. While in one sense Tim's fantasy was a direct expression of that wish (women looked at him and were immediately smitten), in another sense it helped to ward off the uncomfortable awareness, because it placed him in the position of not *trying* to get people's attention, of just being the recipient of approaches he had not sought. I suggested that the next time this came up the therapist take a different tack, saying something like, "I can understand how you'd wish that. Everyone probably does to some degree. But for *you* to wish it also means accepting an idea that you've been working so hard at overcoming—the idea that somehow it's not all right for you to *try* to get people's attention, for you to *want* it. It's only okay if it *happens* to you."

Several features of this comment are worth noting. First, the opening comment, "I can understand how you'd wish that," is a kind of explicit reassurance or support that many therapists think they should eschew. It felt to me especially important in this context, where the therapist had been implicitly disparaging the patient's wish, but it is a kind of explicit acceptance and affirmation that therapists are often too sparing with. To be sure, on its own, offered with nothing more substantial along with it, it can be an empty reassurance; but as part of a more complex intervention, it sets a tone that can be useful. The next sentence, "Everyone probably does to some degree," is similarly reassuring and normalizing. Indeed, its implicit message includes implicating the therapist himself, since he is a part of "everyone." Thus, this further contributes to the normalizing, noncritical dimension of the comment.

But this part of the comment, while I believe it to be a useful element of the overall message, is hardly the most interesting. It is in the rest of the comment that the approach I am spelling out here becomes more evident. This latter part of the message addresses quite directly the patient's conflicted wish to get people's attention, his *wanting* this. That wish, of course, is evident in the patient's expressed fantasy as well—he is, after all, imagining himself being so striking looking that he gets *loads* of attention. But in the form he has permitted himself to express up till now, the attention is not something he is actively seeking, something he is *doing*. It just happens to him. The comment I suggested the therapist make addresses the *active wish* for others' attention, and it endorses and accepts it. It does so, however, in the fashion I have called attributional. It does not directly "interpret" it, *tell* the patient he has it, implying that before being told he *didn't know* he did. Rather, it *assumes* he has this wish, and assumes as well that he knows it. The therapist's tone is not one of informing the patient about something but of *acknowledging* something the patient already knows.

The comment also has an additional—and different—attributional element that I also want to call the reader's attention to. Included in the suggested comment is the phrase, "an idea that you've been working so hard at overcoming," a phrase that underlines the patient's movement and momentum and which, by depicting him as "working hard" at overcoming it, also counters the vision of himself as passive that both he and the therapist had been immersed in. It is essential, of course, that the other side of the patient's experience, the ways in which he feels stuck, *not* moving, passive, *also* be acknowledged, or else that side will begin to be experienced as forbidden, and will be less accessible to examine and work with. The discussion immediately below about Tim's dream will illustrate this. But, apropos much that I have discussed in this chapter, it is also crucial to highlight and underline movement. The illustrative comment being discussed here does this, and it does it in a way that reflects additional elements of attributional communications as well. To begin with, the acknowledgment is presented in an incidental, "we both already know this" way. Just saying to the patient, "You've been working very hard at overcoming this tendency," can easily result in a kind of (explicit or implicit) debate. Tim could say, "No, I'm not. I've been avoiding doing that," and the therapist is then likely to either feel checkmated or tempted to argue with him. In contrast, the comment as stated refers to Tim's working hard on the problem, as a kind of incidental background observation. Tim *could* still say, "Wait a minute, what do you mean an idea I've been working so hard at overcoming? I haven't been working hard on it at all," but it is much less likely that he would. The message slips in under the radar of the defenses, so to speak, and becomes more likely to be assimilated.

A second feature of the comment that makes it attributional in the sense that I am discussing here is that it gives the patient credit for movement that perhaps has hardly begun, but by depicting the patient's progress and determination, the comment contributes to developing and enhancing those very qualities. In a slightly different context, my wife (E. Wachtel, 1994, 2001) has described a very similar process in work with children. She calls this "the language of becoming" and encourages parents to say things to kids like, "I see you're becoming more able to be patient with your little brother," or "you're becoming more able to get your studying done first when you want to play with your computer." Such comments—which, to be effective, can't just be "made up," but must be rooted in careful attention to the incipient (but not yet emergent) trends in the child—help to support, amplify, accelerate these changes. They help parent and child not to get locked into a static vision of the child that becomes a self-fulfilling prophecy. Attributional comments serve much the same function.

An interesting opportunity to apply the principles of attributional interpretations arose in the course of responding to one of Tim's dreams. The dream was a very interesting one. He is in elementary school (but, as can happen in the world of dreams, he is simultaneously his current age—25). All the other students are writing letters (A, B, C, D), and he is writing numbers. The patient notices this and he cheats, copying their answers. The teacher sees this and takes his paper away from him. He says to her something like, "I won't take this, you can't do this to me" (but he tells his therapist this last part almost in passing).

The therapist was inclined to see the dream as a reflection of Tim's self-defeating tendencies and to comment on it to Tim in that connection. What he was focusing on was that (1) Tim was writing numbers when everyone else was writing letters, which was in a certain sense doing things in a way that caused him trouble—indeed, that seemed almost to *be going out of his way* to cause himself trouble; and (2) that he then cheated and got caught, getting him into still further trouble. My emphasis on a different approach to the dream was not because the therapist's view was "wrong." Viewed from a constructivist perspective, there are multiple ways of understanding the dream. But each way of understanding it has implications, and my concern was that the implication for Tim of highlighting his being self-defeating would not be therapeutic. Tim was already feeling demoralized and inclined to blame himself and had already received considerable emotional rejection in his family for "writing numbers instead of letters," in the sense that he was pursuing a course quite different from the family's macho vision of what it meant to be a man. I therefore suggested to the therapist two alternative ways of approaching the dream. Both had significant attributional elements. The first was to say to Tim, "Part of what I hear in the dream is your announcing (to me and to yourself) that you *can* stand up for yourself, and that you're tired of submitting." In this, the therapist would point to the part of the dream that Tim presented almost incidentally: "I won't take this, you can't do this to me." This framing of the dream highlights Tim's active assertiveness (*and*, interestingly, his "masculine" standing up to authorities; in essence, "being a man" precisely through *not* "being a man" in the stereotyped way that the other men in his family pursued it). It also, by *attributing* to Tim the feeling of being "tired of" submitting, encourages whatever nascent wishes he has to stand up for himself.

The second attributional approach to the dream that I suggested to the therapist elaborated further on some of the themes alluded to in the first comment. "It sounds like what you're **struggling with** in the dream is that on the one hand, **you sense** that you have your own unique way of seeing things (numbers instead of letters), but on the other, you're **tempted** to assume that your own way is wrong, and to try to copy what the majority does. That's what your parents wanted. But this is a dream about the **stirring** of your wish to stand up for *your own* view **and about the fear that still makes that hard.**"

This somewhat more complicated version had several elements, highlighted in bold type, which further utilize and illustrate an attributional approach. The use of the term "struggling with" casts Tim (who has so often been accused—and has so often accused himself—of being "passive") in a light that highlights his activity. For someone like Tim, saying "what you're struggling with in the dream" can have a quite different emotional impact than saying "what the dream is about." Both are roughly equivalent in denotation but quite different in connotation, in what elsewhere (Wachtel, 1993) I have called the meta-message, in contrast to the focal message. Using language in such fashion, incidentally highlighting important connotative messages that can, one might say, "get in" without having to pass through the censor, can be a very important element of effective therapeutic practice.

The second feature of the way the comment is cast that I wish to call attention to is the *pair* of phrases "you sense" and "you're tempted." The former implicitly conveys that what the patient "senses" is both real and accurate. The latter implies that assuming his way is wrong is a temptation *to be resisted.* That is, the structure of the comment clearly aligns on the side of affirming his unique way of seeing things and opposing the ever-present temptation to see himself as wrong. The significance of this choice of words becomes especially apparent if one imagines reversing the two terms: *you're tempted* to think that you have your own unique way of seeing things, but *you sense* that your own way is wrong. This "reversed" version is clearly highly antitherapeutic, implying that the patient should disparage his own perceptions and go along with how others see things. And in its very egregiousness, it highlights why the version I did suggest can help to liberate him from his tendency to devalue and retreat from the qualities that make him unique and original, a tendency that contributed both to his conflict about displaying his creativity on stage and to his difficulties socially. The use of phrases such as "you sense" and "you are tempted" can make a potentially powerful and therapeutically important point, yet do so in such an incidental way that it does not have to pass through a gauntlet of defenses to be heard.

Finally, I want to call attention to two more features of this illustrative comment which in different ways address a similar issue and challenge. The first is the reference to the "stirring" of Tim's wish to stand up for himself. The second is the reference to "the fear that still makes it hard." Both acknowledge that the patient still remains afraid and hesitant. Glossing over this part of his experience, attributing to him a degree of courage or resolve that he feels he does not have, will not be useful and may indeed leave him feeling worse, because it leaves him feeling misunderstood or not truly seen. The fear, the hesitancy to stand up for himself *is* still a part of him, and unless that part of him is acknowledged and respected, the therapist is unlikely to be able to reach him. Thus, the fear is acknowledged very explicitly at the end of the statement. But it is acknowledged as an additional part of his experience, not as the essence. Moreover, by referring to the fear as something that "makes it hard," the comment offers a *sympathetic* casting (it's not something bad about him, something cowardly, a sign of failure; *it's hard* to move ahead when one is afraid). Additionally, referring to the fear as making it "hard" implies that he is doing it anyway. It is not fear that makes it *impossible,* or that *prevents* him or dissuades him from proceeding. It is "hard" precisely because he is continuing to push on in the face of it.[11]

Relatedly, referring to the "stirring" of his wish to stand up for his own view has several important implications. First, the "stirring" of a wish suggests a *beginning.* It does not require Tim to pretend that he has been doing this or aware of this for a long time. He can hear this new, encouraging rendering without having to deny his previous experience. "Stirring" is also an *active* word; it links up with the other aspects of this approach to Tim that counter the framing of him as "passive." Finally, returning to the implication of stirring as a *beginning,* it has a connotation of "I'm just getting started. Wait till you see me in full throttle." Think of phrases such as "the beast is stirring." It may have been safe to treat him lightly while he was sleeping, but he will be someone to be reckoned with now.

It should be apparent that the considerations introduced in my discussion of attributional comments and interpretations are closely related to my previous discussions of addressing conflict and alternat-

---

[11] The additional resonances of the word "hard" to a man who is seeking to find his path to feeling masculine need not be pointed out to a readership of psychotherapists.

ing self-states, of attending to variability, of highlighting strengths while acknowledging the other side of the patient's experience, and of attending to and holding the dialectic between affirmation and change. One of the important characteristics of attributional comments is that they often serve as a way of weaving together and integrating these various dimensions.

CONCLUDING COMMENTS

In this book I have offered not just analysis of theoretical positions and examination of empirical findings. I have also offered my personal convictions about what is most essential in helping people achieve the changes in their lives that they come to us to pursue. I remain deeply committed to those convictions, but I wish to end with one final conviction that may seem to clash with the passionate presentation and defense of the others. This final conviction is that there is no single right way to conduct psychotherapy. When I think of the many different ways in which I have engaged with my patients over the years, I am struck by the incredible variety of things that I have done or said in the name of psychotherapy and by the ways that different patients have seemed to need or to be helped by different ways of being with them and interacting with them. Whatever "rules" may guide our work, perhaps the most important rule is not to take those rules too seriously (cf. Hoffman, 1998). By this I do not mean to take them lightly. The responsibility we assume as psychotherapists is a weighty one. But every patient teaches us something new about what people need. The day we think we know all we need to know in order to help people is probably the day we cease to be able to help at all.

We have much to teach our patients. One of the ways that I differ from some therapists, indeed, is in my comfort with acknowledging and embracing this dimension of the therapeutic encounter. But our patients have much to teach us as well. If we can listen—not just listen to "interpret," but listen to learn—then our chance for success is greatly increased. I have had my share of failures as a psychotherapist, as anyone who has been in practice for a long time has had. But I have also on many occasions been successfully taught by my patients what they need in order to achieve the changes they seek. That is one of life's great pleasures, and it is a pleasure that I hope both the readers of this book and their patients will enjoy in abundance.

References

Ainsworth, M. D. S., Blehar, M. C., Waters, E., & Wall, S. (1978). *Patterns of attachment: A psychological study of the Strange Situation.* Hillsdale, NJ: Erlbaum.

Alexander, F. (1950). Analysis of the therapeutic factors in psychoanalytic treatment. *Psychoanalytic Quarterly, 19,* 482–500.

Alexander, F. (1953). Current views on psychotherapy. *Psychiatry, 16,* 113–122.

Alexander, F. (1954). Some quantitative aspects of psychoanalytic technique. *Journal of the American Psychoanalytic Association, 2,* 685–701.

Alexander, F. (1956). *Psychoanalysis and psychotherapy: Developments in theory, technique, and training.* New York: Norton.

Alexander, F. (1961). *The scope of psychoanalysis.* New York: Basic Books.

Alexander, F., & French, T. M. (1946). *Psychoanalytic therapy: Principles and application.* New York: Ronald Press.

Angus, L. E., & McLeod, J. (Eds.). (2004). *The handbook of narrative and psychotherapy: Practice, theory, and research.* Thousand Oaks, CA: Sage.

Arlow, J., & Brenner, C. (1964). *Psychoanalytic concepts and the structural theory.* New York: International Universities Press.

Aron, L. (1989). Dreams, narrative and the psychoanalytic method. *Contemporary Psychoanalysis, 25,* 108–126.

Aron, L. (1991a). Working through the past—working toward the future. *Contemporary Psychoanalysis, 27,* 81–108.

Aron, L. (1991b). The patient's experience of the analyst's subjectivity. *Psychoanalytic Dialogues, 1,* 29–51.

Aron, L. (1996). *A meeting of minds: Mutuality in psychoanalysis.* Hillsdale, NJ: Analytic Press.

Aron, L. (2003). The paradoxical place of enactment in psychoanalysis: Introduction. *Psychoanalytic Dialogues, 13,* 623–631.

Aron, L. (2006). Analytic impasse and the third: Clinical implications of intersubjectivity. *International Journal of Psycho-Analysis, 87,* 349–368.

Aron, L., & Harris, A. (1993). *The legacy of Sandor Ferenczi.* Hillsdale, NJ: Analytic Press.

Aron, L., & Anderson, F. S. (Eds.). (1998). *Relational perspectives on the body.*

Atwood, G. E., & Stolorow, R. D. (1984), Structures of subjectivity: Explorations in psychoanalytic phenomenology. Hillsdale, NJ: The Analytic Press.

Bacal, H. A. (Ed.). (1998). *Optimal responsiveness: How therapists heal their patients.* Northvale, NJ: Aronson.

Bacal, H. A., & Herzog, B. (2003). Specificity theory and optimal responsiveness: An outline. *Psychoanalytic Psychology, 20,* 635–648.

Balint, M. (1950). Changing therapeutical aims and techniques in psycho–analysis. *International Journal of Psycho-Analysis, 31,* 117–124.

Balint, M. (1965). *Primary love and psycho-analytic technique.* New York: Liveright.

Balint, M. (1968). *The basic fault: Therapeutic aspects of regression.* London: Tavistock.

Basch, M. F. (1995). Kohut's contribution. *Psychoanalytic dialogues, 5,* 367–373.

Basescu, S. (1972). Existence and experience. In G. D. Goldman & D. S. Milman (Eds.), *Innovations in psychotherapy.* Oxford, UK: Thomas.

Bass, A. (2003). "E" enactments in psychoanalysis: Another medium, another message. *Psychoanalytic Dialogues, 13,* 657–676.

Beebe, B., & Lachmann, F. (2002). *Infant research and adult treatment: co-constructing interactions.* Hillsdale, NJ: Analytic Press.

Beebe, B., & Lachmann, F. (2003). The relational turn in psychoanalysis: A dyadic systems view from infant research. *Contemporary Psychoanalysis, 39,* 379–409.

Benjamin, J. F. (1988). *The bonds of love: Psychoanalysis, feminism, and the problem of domination.* New York: Pantheon.

Benjamin, J. (1990). An outline of intersubjectivity. *Psychoanalytic Psychology, 7*(Suppl.), 33–46.

Benjamin, J. (1996). *Like subjects, love objects: Essays on recognition and sexual difference.* New Haven, CT: Yale University Press.

Benjamin, J. (1997). *The shadow of the other: Intersubjectivity and gender in psychoanalysis.* New York: Routledge.

Benjamin, J. (2004). Beyond doer and done to: An intersubjective view of thirdness. *Psychoanalytic Quarterly, 73,* 5–46.

Bergmann, M. S. (1993). Reflections on the History of Psychoanalysis. *Journal of the American Psychoanalytic Association, 41,* 929–955.

Berlin, I. (1958). *Two concepts of liberty.* Oxford, UK: Clarendon Press.

Berman, E. (1981). Multiple personality: Psychoanalytic perspectives. *International Journal of Psycho-Analysis, 62,* 283–300.

Bibring, E. (1954). Psychoanalysis and the dynamic psychotherapies. *Journal of the American Psychoanalytic Association, 2,* 745–770.

Bion, W. (1959a). *Experiences in groups.* New York: Basic Books.

Bion, W. (1959b). Attacks on linking. *International Journal of Psychoanalysis, 40,* 308–315.

Bion, W. R. (1970). *Attention and interpretation.* London: Tavistock.

Black, M. (2003). Enactment: Analytic musings on energy, language, and personal growth. *Psychoanalytic Dialogues, 13,* 633–656.

Blum, H. P. (1999). The reconstruction of reminiscence. *Journal of the American Psychoanalytic Association, 47,* 1125–1143.

Bollas, C. (1987). *The shadow of the object: Psychoanalysis of the unthought known.* New York: Columbia University Press.

Bonomi, C. (1998). Jones's allegation of Ferenczi's mental deterioration. *International Forum of Psychoanalysis, 7,* 201–206.

Bowers, K. S. (1973). Situationism in psychology: An analysis and a critique. *Psychological Review, 80,* 307–336.

Bowlby, J. (1973). *Attachment and loss: Vol. 2. Separation.* New York: Basic Books.

Bromberg, P. M. (1993). Shadow and substance. *Psychoanalytic Psychology, 10,* 147–168.

Bromberg, P. M. (1996a). Standing in the spaces: The multiplicity of self and the psychoanalytic relationship. *Contemporary Psychoanalysis, 32,* 509–535.

Bromberg, P. M. (1996b). Hysteria, dissociation, and cure: Emmy von N revisited. *Psychoanalytic Dialogues, 6,* 55–71.

Bromberg, P. M. (1998a). *Standing in the spaces: Essays on clinical process, trauma, and dissociation.* Hillsdale, NJ: Analytic Press.

Bromberg,, P. M. (1998b). Staying the same while changing: Reflections on clinical judgment. *Psychoanalytic Dialogues, 8,* 225–236.

Bucci, W. (2000). The need for a "psychoanalytic psychology" in the cognitive science field. *Psychoanalytic Psychology, 17,* 203–244.

Busch, F. (1998). Self-disclosure ain't what it's cracked up to be, at least not yet. *Psychoanalytic Inquiry, 18,* 518–529.

Cassidy, J., & Shaver, P. R. (Eds). (1999). *Handbook of attachment: Theory, research, and clinical applications.* New York: Guilford Press.

Cohen, J., & Tronick, E. (1988). Mother–infant face-to-face interaction: Influence is bidirectional and unrelated to periodic cycles in either partner's behavior. *Developmental Psychology, 24,* 386–392.

Crastnopol, M. (2001). Commentaries. *Journal of the American Psychoanalytic Association, 49,* 386–398.

Curtis, R., Field, C., Knaan-Kostman, I., & Mannix, K. (2004). What 75 psychoanalysts found helpful and hurtful in their own analyses. *Psychoanalytic Psychology, 21,*183–202.

Cushman, P. (1990). Why the self is empty: Toward a historically situated psychology. *American Psychologist, 45,* 599–611.

Cushman, P. (1996). *Constructing the self, constructing America: A cultural history of psychotherapy.* Reading, MA: Addison-Wesley/Addison Wesley Longman.

Davies, J. M. (1994). Love in the afternoon: A relational reconsideration of desire and dread in the countertransference. *Psychoanalytic Dialogues, 4,* 153–170.

Davies, J. M. (1996). Linking the "Pre-Analytic" with the postclassical: Integration, dissociation, and the multiplicity of unconscious process. *Contemporary Psychoanalysis, 32,* 553–576.

Davies, J. M. (1998). Between the disclosure and foreclosure of erotic transference–countertransference: Can psychoanalysis find a place for adult sexuality? *Psychoanalytic Dialogues, 8,* 747–766.

Davies, J. M., & Frawley, M. G. (1994). *Treating the adult survivor of childhood sexual abuse: A psychoanalytic perspective.* New York: Basic Books.

Deacon, B. J., & Abromowitz, J. S. (2004). Cognitive and behavioral treatments for anxiety disorders: A review of meta–analytic findings. *Journal of Clinical Psychology, 60,* 429–441.

de Shazer, S. (1997). Some thoughts on language use in therapy. *Contemporary Family Therapy: An International Journal, 19,* 133–141.

Dewald, P. (1972). *The psychoanalytic process.* New York: Basic Books.

Dimeff, L. A., & Koerner, K. (Eds.). (2007). *Dialectical behavior therapy in clinical practice: Applications across disorders and settings.* New York: Guilford Press.

Dimen, M. (1991). Deconstructing difference: Gender, splitting, and transitional space. *Psychoanalytic Dialogues, 1,* 335–352.

Dimen, M. (2003). *Sexuality, intimacy, power.* Hillsdale, NJ: Analytic Press.

Dimen, M., & Goldner, V. (Eds). (2002). *Gender in psychoanalytic space: Between clinic and culture.* New York: Other Press.

Dimen, M., & Harris, A. (Eds.). (2001). *Storms in her head: Freud and the construction of hysteria.* New York: Other Press.

Dollard, J., Doob, L. W., Miller, N. E., Mowrer, O. H., & Sears, R. R. (1939). *Frustration and aggression.* New Haven, CT: Yale University Press.

Dupont, I. (1988). Fereczi's "madness." *Contemporary Psychoanalysis, 24,* 250–261.

Eagle, M. N. (1987). The psychoanalytic and the cognitive unconscious. In R. Stern (Ed.), *Theories of the unconscious and theories of the self* (pp. 155–189). Hillsdale, NJ: Analytic Press.

Eagle, M. (1993). Enactments, transference, and symptomatic cure: A case history. *Psychoanalytic Dialogues, 3,* 93–110.

Eagle, M. N. (2000). A critical evaluation of current conceptions of transference and countertransference. *Psychoanalytic Psychology, 17,* 24–37.

Eagle, M. N. (2003a). Clinical implications of attachment theory. *Psychoanalytic Inquiry, 23*, 27–53.

Eagle, M. N. (2003b). The postmodern turn in psychoanalysis: A critique. *Psychoanalytic Psychology, 20*, 411–424.

Eagle, M. N., Wolitzky, D. L., & Wakefield, J. C. (2001). The analyst's knowledge and authority. *Journal of the American Psychoanalytic Association, 49*, 457–488.

Ehrenberg, D. B. (1992). *The intimate edge: Extending the reach of psychoanalytic interaction.* New York: Norton.

Eissler, K. R. (1953). The effect of the structure of the ego on psychoanalytic technique. *Journal of the American Psychoanalytic Association, 1*, 104–143.

Erikson, E. H. (1954). The dream specimen of psychoanalysis. *Journal of the American Psychoanalytic Association, 2*, 5–56.

Erikson, E. H. (1959). Identity and the life cycle: Selected papers. *Psychological Issues, 1*, 1–171.

Erikson, E. H. (1963). *Childhood and society* (2nd ed.). New York: Norton.

Fairbairn, W. R. D. (1952). *An object relations theory of the personality.* New York: Basic Books.

Fairbairn, W. D. (1958). On the nature and aims of psycho-analytical treatment. *International Journal of the Psycho-Analysis, 39*, 374–385.

Fast, I. (1992). The embodied mind: Toward a relational perspective. *Psychoanalytic Dialogues, 2*, 389–409.

Feixas, G., & Botella, L. (2004). Psychotherapy integration: Reflections and contributions from a constructivist epistemology. *Journal of Psychotherapy Integration, 14*, 192–222.

Fenichel, O. (1941). *Problems of psychoanalytic technique.* New York: Psychoanalytic Quarterly Press.

Ferenczi, S. (1926). *Further contributions to the theory and technique of psychoanalysis.* London: Hogarth Press and the Institute of Psycho-analysis.

Ferenczi, S. (1952). *First contributions to psycho-analysis.* London: Hogarth Press.

Ferenczi, S. (1955). *Final contributions to the problems and methods of psychoanalysis.* London: Hogarth Press.

Ferenczi, S., & Rank, O. (1925). *The development of psychoanalysis.* New York: Nervous and Mental Disease Publishing.

Fernández-Álvarez, H., & Opazo, R. (Eds.). (2004). *La integración en psicoterapia.* Buenos Aires: Paidos.

Flavell, J. H. (1963). *The developmental psychology of Jean Piaget.* Princeton, NJ: Van Nostrand.

Flavell, J. H. (1977). *Cognitive development.* Englewood Cliffs, NJ: Prentice Hall.

Foa, E. B., Huppert, J. D., & Cahill, S. P. (2006). Emotional processing theory: An update. In B. O. Rothbaum (Ed.), *Pathological anxiety: Emotional processing in etiology and treatment* (pp. 3–24). New York: Guilford Press.

Foa, E. B., & Kozak, M. J. (1986) Emotional processing of fear: Exposure to corrective information. *Psychological Bulletin, 99,* 20–35.

Foa, E. B., & Meadows, E. A. (1997) Psychosocial treatments for post-traumatic stress disorder: A critical review. *Annual Review of Psychology, 48,* 449–80.

Fonagy, P. (1999). Memory and therapeutic action. *International Journal of Psycho-Analysis, 80,* 215–223.

Fonagy, P. (2000). Attachment and borderline personality disorder. *Journal of the American Psychoanalytic Association. 48,* 1129–1146.

Fonagy, P. (2002). Understanding of mental states, mother–infant interaction, and the development of the self. In J. M. Maldonado-Durán (Ed.), *Infant and toddler mental health: Models of clinical intervention with infants and their families* (pp. 57–74). Washington, DC: American Psychiatric Press.

Fonagy, P. (2003). Some complexities in the relationship of psychoanalytic theory to technique. *Psychoanalytic Quarterly, 72,* 13–47.

Fonagy, P., Gergely, G., Jurist, E., & Target, M. (2002). *Affect regulation, mentalization, and the development of the self.* New York: Other Press.

Fonagy, P., & Target, M. (1997). Attachment and reflective function: Their role in self-organization. *Development and Psychopathology, 9,* 679–700.

Fonagy, P., & Target, M. (1998). Mentalization and the changing aims of child psychoanalysis. *Psychoanalytic Dialogues. 8,* 87–114.

Fonagy, P., Target, M., Gergely, G., Allen, J., & Bateman, A. W. (2003). The developmental roots of borderline personality disorder in early attachment relationships: A theory and some evidence [Special issue: Infant research]. *Psychoanalytic Inquiry, 23*(3), 412–459.

Fosshage, J. L. (2003a). Fundamental pathways to change: Illuminating old and creating new relational experience. *International Forum of Psychoanalysis, 12,* 244–251.

Fosshage, J. L. (2003b). Contextualizing self psychology and relational psychoanalysis. *Contemporary Psychoanalysis, 39,* 411–448.

Fosshage, J. L. (2004). The explicit and implicit dance in psychoanalytic change. *Journal of Analytical Psychology, 49,* 49–65.

Fosshage, J. L. (2005). The explicit and implicit domains in psychoanalytic change. *Psychoanalytic Inquiry, 25,* 516–539.

Francis, D., Szegda, K., Campbell, G., Martin, W., & Insel, T. (2003). Epigenetic sources of behavioral differences in mice. *Nature Neuroscience, 6,* 445.

Frank, K. A. (1990). Action techniques in psychoanalysis: Background and introduction. *Contemporary Psychoanalysis, 26,* 732–756.

Frank, K. A. (1992). Combining action techniques with psychoanalytic therapy. *International Review of Psycho-Analysis, 19,* 57–79.

Frank, K. A. (1993). Action, insight, and working through outlines of an integrative approach. *Psychoanalytic Dialogues, 3,* 535–577.

Frank, K. A. (1997). The role of the analyst's inadvertent self-revelations. *Psychoanalytic Dialogues, 7,* 281–314.

Frank, K. A. (1999). *Psychoanalytic participation.* Hillsdale, NJ: Analytic Press.

Frank, K. A. (2001). Extending the field of psychoanalytic change: Exploratory-assertive motivation, self-efficacy, and the new analytic role for action. *Psychoanalytic Inquiry, 21,* 620–639.

Frank, K. A. (2002). The "ins and outs" of enactment: A relational bridge for psychotherapy integration. *Journal of Psychotherapy Integration, 12,* 267–286.

Frank, K. A. (2005). Toward conceptualizing the personal relationship in therapeutic action: Beyond the "real" relationship. *Psychoanalytic Perspectives, 3,* 15–56.

Frankl, V. E. (1959). *From death-camp to existentialism: A psychiatrist's path to a new therapy.* Boston: Beacon Press.

Freud, S. (1905). Fragment of an analysis of a case of hysteria (1905 [1901]). In *The standard edition of the complete psychological works of Sigmund Freud: Vol. 7. A case of hysteria, three essays on sexuality and other works* (pp. 1–122). London: Hogarth Press.

Freud, A. (1936). *The ego and the mechanisms of defense.* New York: International Universities Press.

Freud, A. (1954). The widening scope of indications for psychoanalysis: Discussion. *Journal of the American Psychoanalytic Association, 2,* 607–620.

Freud, E. (Ed.). (1960). *The letters of Sigmund Freud.* New York: Basic Books.

Freud, S. (1912a). Recommendations to physicians practising psycho-analysis. *Standard Edition, 12,* 109–120. London: Hogarth Press, 1958.

Freud, S. (1912b). The Dynamics of transference. *Standard Edition, 12,* 97–108, London: Hogarth Press, 1958.

Freud, S. (1914a). Remembering, repeating and working through. *Standard Edition, 12,* 145–156. London: Hogarth Press, 1958.

Freud, S. (1914b). On the history of the psycho-analytic movement. *Standard Edition, 14,* 1–66. London: Hogarth Press, 1963.

Freud, S. (1915a). The unconscious. *Standard Edition, 14,* 159–215. London: Hogarth Press, 1963.

Freud, S. (1915b). Repression. *Standard Edition, 14,* 141–158. London: Hogarth Press, 1963.

Freud, S. (1916). Introductory lectures on psycho-analysis. *Standard Edition, 15,* 13–79, 81–239. London: Hogarth Press, 1961.

Freud, S. (1919). Lines of advance in psycho-analytic therapy. *Standard Edition, 17,* 157–168. London: Hogarth Press, 1955.

Freud, S. (1920). Beyond the pleasure principle. *Standard Edition, 18,* 1–64. London: Hogarth Press, 1955.

Freud, S. (1921). Group psychology and the analysis of the ego. *Standard Edition, 18,* 65–143. London: Hogarth Press, 1955.

Freud, S. (1923). The ego and the id. *Standard Edition, 19,* 1–66. London: Hogarth Press, 1961.

Freud, S. (1926). Inhibitions, symptoms and anxiety. *Standard Edition, 20,* 75–175. London: Hogarth Press, 1959.

Freud, S. (1931). Letter to Stefan Zweig, 7 February 1931. In E. L. Freud (Ed.), *Letters of Sigmund Freud* (p. 403). New York: Basic Books, 1960.

Freud, S. (1933). New introductory lectures on psycho-analysis. *Standard Edition, 22,* 1–182. London: Hogarth Press, 1964.

Freud, S. (1961). Civilization and its discontents. In *The standard edition of the complete psychological works of Sigmund Freud* (Vol. 21, pp. 57–146). London: Hogarth Press. (Original work published 1930)

Freud, S. (1963). Introductory lectures on psycho-analysis, Part III. In *Standard edition of the complete psychological works of Sigmund Freud* (Vol. 16, pp. 241–463). London: Hogarth Press. (Original work published 1917)

Friedman, L. (1978). Trends in the psychoanalytic theory of treatment. *Psychoanalytic Quarterly, 47,* 524–567.

Friedman, L. (1986). Kohut's Testament. *Psychoanalytic Inquiry, 6,* 321–347.

Friedman, L. (1988). *The anatomy of psychotherapy.* Hillsdale, NJ: Analytic Press.

Friedman, L. (1997). Introduction to panels: Does the face of analytic treatment show its character? *Journal of the American Psychoanalytic Association, 45,* 1225–1229.

Friedman, L. (2002). What lies beyond interpretation, and is that the right question. *Psychoanalytic Psychology, 19,* 540–551.

Gabbard, G. O. (1995). Countertransference: The emerging common ground. *International Journal of Psycho-Analysis, 76,* 475–485.

Gendlin, E. T. (1996). *Focusing-oriented psychotherapy: A manual of the experiential method.* New York: Guilford Press.

Ghent, E. (1989). Credo: The dialectics of one-person and two-person psychologies. *Contemporary Psychoanalysis, 25,* 169–211.

Ghent, E. (1992a). Foreword. In N. Skolnick & S. Warshaw (Eds.), *Relational perspectives in psychoanalysis.* Hillsdale, NJ: Analytic Press.

Ghent, E. (1992b). Paradox and process. *Psychoanalytic Dialogues, 2,* 135–159.

Ghent, E. (1995). Interaction in the psychoanalytic situation. *Psychoanalytic Dialogues, 5,* 479–491.

Ghent, E. (2002). Wish, need, drive: Motive in the light of dynamic systems theory and Edelman's selectionist theory. *Psychoanalytic Dialogues, 12,* 763–808.

Gill, M. M. (1954). Psychoanalysis and exploratory psychotherapy. *Journal of the American Psychoanalytic Association, 2,* 771–797.

Gill, M. M. (1979). The analysis of the transference. *Journal of the American Psychoanalytic Association, 27*(Suppl.), 263–288.

Gill, M. M. (1982). *Analysis of transference.* New York: International Universities Press.

Gill, M. M. (1982). *Analysis of transference: Vol. 1. Theory and technique.* New York: International Universities Press.

Gill, M. M. (1983). The interpersonal paradigm and the degree of the therapist's involvement. *Contemporary Psychoanalysis, 19,* 200–237.

Gill, M. M. (1984). Psychoanalysis and psychotherapy: A revision. *International Review of Psycho-Analysis, 11,* 161–179.

Gill, M. M. (1991). Indirect suggestion: A response to Oremland's *Interpretation and Interaction.* In J. D. Oremland, *Interpretation and interaction* (pp. 137–164). Hillsdale, NJ: Analytic Press.

Gill, M. M. (1993). Interaction and interpretation: Commentary on Morris Eagle's "Enactments, transference, and symptomatic cure." *Psychoanalytic Dialogues, 3,* 111.

Gill, M. M. (1994). *Psychoanalysis in transition.* Hillsdale, NJ: Analytic Press.

Gill, M. M., & Hoffman, I. Z. (1982) *Analysis of transference: II. Studies of nine audio-recorded psychoanalytic sessions.* New York: International Universities Press.

Gillman, D. A. (2006). *An exploration of the influence of relational and contemporary Freudian paradigms on the thinking and practice of beginning clinicians: A Q-methodological study.* Unpublished doctoral dissertation, City University of New York.

Gladwell, M. (2005). *Blink: The power of thinking without thinking.* New York: Little, Brown.

Glover, E. (1931). The therapeutic effect of inexact interpretation: A contribution to the theory of suggestion. *International Journal of Psycho-Analysis, 12,* 397–411.

Goldberg, A. (1986). Reply. *Contemporary Psychoanalysis, 22,* 387–388.

Goldner, V. (1991). Toward a critical relational theory of gender. *Psychoanalytic Dialogues, 1,* 249–272.

Greenberg, J. R. (1986). Theoretical models and the analyst's neutrality. *Contemporary Psychoanalysis, 22,* 87–106.

Greenberg, J. (1996). Psychoanalytic words and psychoanalytic acts—a brief history. *Contemporary Psychoanalysis, 32,* 195.

Greenberg, J. R., & Mitchell, S. A. (1983). *Object relations in psychoanalytic theory.* Cambridge, MA: Harvard University Press.

Greenberg, J. (2001). The analyst's participation: A new look. *Journal of the American Psychoanalytic Association, 49,* 359–381.

Greenson, R. (1965). The working alliance and transference neurosis. *Psychoanalytic Quarterly, 34,* 155–181.

Greenson, R. (1967). *The technique and practice of psychoanalysis.* New York: International Universities Press.

Greenson, R. (1971). The "real" relationship between the patient and the psychoanalyst. In M. Kanzer (Ed.), *The unconscious today.* New York: International Universities Press.

Grossman, K. E., Grossman, K., & Waters, E. (Eds.). (2005). *Attachment from infancy to adulthood: The major longitudinal studies.* New York: Guilford Press.

Guidano, V. E. (1991). *The self in process: Toward a post-rationalist cognitive therapy.* New York: Guilford Press.

Guntrip, H. (1971). *Psychoanalytic theory, therapy, and the self.* New York: Basic Books.

Harris, A. (1996). The conceptual power of multiplicity. *Contemporary Psychoanalysis, 32,* 537–552.

Harris, A. (2005). *Gender as soft assembly.* Hillsdale, NJ: Analytic Press.

Hartman, H. (1939). *Ego psychology and the problem of adaptation.* New York: International Universities Press.

Hassin, R., Ulemann, J., & Bargh, J. (2006). *The new unconscious: Social cognition and social neuroscience.* New York: Oxford University Press.

Havens, L. (1986). *Making contact: Uses of language in psychotherapy.* Cambridge, MA: Harvard University Press.

Hayes, S. C., Follette, V. M., & Linehan, M. M. (2004). *Mindfulness and acceptance: Expanding the cognitive-behavioral tradition.* New York: Guilford Press.

Herman, J. L. (1997). *Trauma and recovery* (Rev. ed.). New York: Basic Books.

Hoffman, I. Z. (1983). The patient as interpreter of the analyst's experience. *Contemporary Psychoanalysis, 19,* 389–422.

Hoffman, I. Z. (1991). Discussion: Toward a social-constructivist view of the psychoanalytic situation. *Psychoanalytic Dialogues, 1,* 74–105.

Hoffman, I. Z. (1992). Some practical implications of a social–constructivist view of the psychoanalytic situation. *Psychoanalytic Dialogues, 2,* 287–304.

Hoffman, I. Z. (1996). Merton M. Gill: A study in theory development in psychoanalysis. *Psychoanalytic Dialogues, 6,* 5–53.

Hoffman, I. Z. (1998). *Ritual and spontaneity in psychoanalysis: A dialectical-constructivist view.* Hillsdale, NJ: Analytic Press.

Hoffman, I. Z. (2006). Forging difference out of similarity: The multiplicity of corrective experience. *Psychoanalytic Quarterly, 75,* 715–751.

Hoffman, I. Z. (2007, April 22). *Therapeutic passion in the countertransference.* Keynote address presented at the meeting of the Division of Psychoanalysis, American Psychological Association, Toronto, Canada.

Horney, K. (1939). *New ways in psychoanalysis.* New York: Norton.

Horney, K. (1945). *Our inner conflicts.* New York: Norton.

Horney, K. (1950). *Neurosis and human growth: The struggle toward self-realization.* New York: Norton.

Howell, E. (2006). *The dissociative mind.* Hillsdale, NJ: Analytic Press.

Jacobs, T. J. (1986). On countertransference enactments. *Journal of the American Psychoanalytic Association, 34,* 289–307.

Jacobs, T. (1999). On the question of self-disclosure by the analyst: Error or advance in technique? *Psychoanalytic Quarterly, 68,* 159–183.

Jaffe, J., Beebe, B., Feldstein, S., Crown, C. L., & Jasnow, M. (2001). Rhythms of dialogue in infancy. *Monographs of the Society for Research in Child Development, 66* (2, Serial No. 264).

Jencks, C. (1987, February 12). Genes and crime. *New York Review of Books,* pp. 33–41.

Jones, E. (1953). *The life and work of Sigmund Freud* (Vol. 1). New York: Basic Books.

Jordan, J. V. (1997). *Women's growth in diversity: More writings from the Stone Center.* New York: Guilford Press.

Jordan, J. V., Kaplan, A. G., Stiver, I. P., & Surrey, J. L. (1991). *Women's growth in connection: Writings from the Stone Center.* New York: Guilford Press.

Keane, T. M. (1995). The role of exposure therapy in the psychological treatment of PTSD. *Clinical Quarterly, 5*(4), 3–6.

Keane, T. M. (1998). Psychological and behavioral treatments of post-traumatic stress disorder. In P. E. Nathan & J. M. Gorman (Eds.), *A guide to treatments that work* (pp. 398–407). New York: Oxford University Press.

Keyes, C. L. (2007). Promoting and protecting mental health as flourishing: A complementary strategy for improving national mental health. *American Psychologist, 62,* 95–108.

Kihlstrom, J. F. (1984). Conscious, subconscious, unconscious: A cognitive view. In K. S. Bowers & D. Meichenbaum (Eds.), *The unconscious reconsidered* (pp. 149–211). New York: Wiley.

Kihlstrom, J. F. (1987). The cognitive unconscious. *Science, 237,* 1445–1452.

Kohut, H. (1971). *The analysis of the self.* New York: International Universities Press.

Kohut, H. (1977). *The restoration of the self.* New York: International Universities Press.

Kohut, H. (1979). The two analyses of Mr Z. *International Journal of Psycho-Analysis, 60,* 3–27.

Kohut, H. (1984). *How does analysis cure?* Chicago: University of Chicago Press.

Kosslyn, S., & Sussman, A. (1995). Roles of imagery in perception: Or, there is no such thing as immaculate perception. In M. Gazzaniga (Ed), *The cognitive neurosciences* (pp. 1035–1042). Cambridge, MA: MIT Press.

Kuhn, T. S. (1962). *The structure of scientific revolutions.* Chicago: University of Chicago Press.

Lachmann, F. M. (1996a). How many selves make a person? *Contemporary Psychoanalysis, 32,* 595–614.

Lachmann, F. M. (1996b). Yes, one self is enough! *Contemporary Psychoanalysis, 32,* 627–630.

Lachmann, F. M., & Beebe, B. (1992). Reformulations of early development and transference: Implications for psychic structure formation. In J. W.

Barron, M. N. Eagle, & D. L. Wolitzky (Eds.), *Interface of psychoanalysis and psychology* (pp. 133–153). Washington, DC: American Psychological Association.

Lakoff, G., & Johnson, M. (1980). *Metaphors we live by.* Chicago: University of Chicago Press.

Lambert, M. (2004). The efficacy and effectiveness of psychotherapy. In M. J. Lambert (Ed.), *Bergin and Garfield's handbook of psychotherapy and behavior change* (5th ed.; pp. 139–193). New York: Wiley.

Langs, R. (1973). The patient's view of the therapist: Reality or fantasy? *International Journal of Psychoanalytic Psychotherapy, 2,* 411–431.

Laplanche, J., & Pontalis, J. B. (1973). *The language of psycho-analysis.* New York: Norton.

Levenson, E. (1983). *The ambiguity of change.* New York: Basic Books.

Linehan, M. M. (1993). *Skills training manual for treating borderline personality disorder.* New York: Guilford Press.

Lipton, S. D. (1977). The advantages of Freud's technique as shown in his analysis of the rat man. *International Journal of Psycho-Analysis, 58,* 255–273.

Loewald, H. (1960). On the therapeutic action of psycho–analysis. *International Journal of Psycho-Analysis, 41,* 16–33.

Loewenstein, R. J., and Ross, D. R. (1992). Multiple personality and psychoanalysis: An introduction. *Psychoanalytic Inquiry, 12,* 3–48.

Lohser, B., & Newton, P. M. (1996). *Unorthodox Freud: The view from the couch.* New York: Guilford Press.

Lynn, D. J., & Vaillant, G. E. (1998). Anonymity, neutrality, and confidentiality in the actual methods of Sigmund Freud: A review of 43 cases. *American Journal of Psychiatry, 155,* 163–171.

Lyons-Ruth, K. (1998). Implicit relational knowing: Its role in development and psychoanalytic treatment. *Infant Mental Health Journal, 19,* 282–289.

Lyons-Ruth, K. (1999). The two-person unconscious. *Psychoanalytic Inquiry, 19,* 576–617.

Main, M. (1995). Recent studies in attachment: Overview, with selected implications for clinical work. In S. Goldberg, R. Muir, & J. Kerr (Eds.), *Attachment theory: Social, developmental, and clinical perspectives,* pp. 407–475). Hillsdale, NJ: Analytic Press.

Main, M., Kaplan, N., & Cassidy, J. (1985). Security in infancy, childhood and adulthood: A move to the level of representation. In I. Bretherton & E. Waters (Eds.), Growing points of attachment theory and research (pp. 66–107). (Monographs of the Society for Research in Child Development, 50 (1–2), Serial no. 209). Chicago: University of Chicago Press.

Maroda, K. J. (1998). Enactment: When the patient's and analyst's pasts converge. *Psychoanalytic Psychology, 15,* 517–535.

Maroda, K. J. (1999). *Seduction, surrender, and transformation: Emotional engagement in the analytic process.* Hillsdale, NJ: Analytic Press.

Maroda, K. J. (2002). No place to hide. *Contemporary Psychoanalysis, 38,* 101–120.

Maroda, K. J. (2004). *The power of countertransference: Innovations in analytic technique* (2nd ed.). Hillsdale, NJ: Analytic Press.

Masling, J. (2003). Stephen A. Mitchell, relational psychoanalysis, and empirical data. *Psychoanalytic Psychology, 20,* 587–608.

May, R. (1990). The idea of history in psychoanalysis. *Psychoanalytic Psychology, 7,* 163–183.

McLaughlin, J. T. (1991). Clinical and theoretical aspects of enactment. *Journal of the American Psychoanalysis Association, 39,* 595–614.

McWilliams, N. (1994). *Psychoanalytic diagnosis.* New York: Guilford Press.

McWilliams, N. (2004). *Psychoanalytic psychotherapy.* New York: Guilford Press.

Meissner, W. W. (1998). Neutrality, abstinence, and the therapeutic alliance. *Journal of the American Psychoanalytic Association, 46,* 1089–1128.

Merton, R. K. (1948). The self-fulfilling prophecy. *Antioch Review, 8,* 193–210.

Messer, S. B. (2000). Applying the visions of reality to a case of brief therapy. *Journal of Psychotherapy Integration, 10,* 55–70.

Michels, R. (2001). Commentaries. *Journal of the American Psychoanalytic Association, 49,* 406–410.

Miller, J. B. (1973). *Psychoanalysis and women: Contributions to new theory and therapy.* New York: Brunner/Mazel.

Miller, J. B., & Stiver, I. P. (1997). *The healing connection: How women form relationships in therapy and in life.* Boston: Beacon Press.

Mills, J. (2005). A critique of relational psychoanalysis. *Psychoanalytic Psychology, 22,* 155–188.

Mischel, W. (1968). *Personality and assessment.* New York: Wiley.

Mischel, W. (1973). On the empirical dilemmas of psychodynamic approaches: Issues and alternatives. *Journal of Abnormal Psychology, 82,* 335–344.

Mitchell, S. A. (1986). The wings of Icarus: Illusion and the problem of narcissism. *Contemporary Psychoanalysis, 22,* 107–132.

Mitchell, S. A. (1988a). *Relational concepts in psychoanalysis.* Cambridge, MA: Harvard University Press.

Mitchell, S. A. (1988b). The intrapsychic and the interpersonal: Different theories, different domains, or historical artifacts? *Psychoanalytic Inquiry, 8,* 472–496.

Mitchell, S. A. (1992a). Introduction. *Psychoanalytic Dialogues, 2,* 279–285.

Mitchell, S. A. (1993a). *Hope and dread in psychoanalysis.* New York: Basic Books.

Mitchell, S. A. (1993b). Reply to Bachant and Richards. *Psychoanalytic Dialogues, 3,* 461–480.

Mitchell, S. A. (1997). *Influence and autonomy in psychoanalysis.* Hillsdale, NJ: The Analytic Press.

Mitchell, S. A., & Aron, L. (1999). *Relational psychoanalysis: The emergence of a tradition.* Hillsdale, NJ: Analytic Press.

Modell, A. H. (1984). *Psychoanalysis in a new context.* New York: International Universities Press.

Modell, A. (1988). The centrality of the psychoanalytic setting and the changing aims of treatment: A perspective from a theory of object relations. *Psychoanalytic Quarterly, 57,* 577–596.

Molnar, E., & de Shazer, S. (1987). Solution-focused therapy: Toward the identification of therapeutic tasks. *Journal of Marital and Family Therapy, 13,* 359–363.

Moore, D. (1999). *The dependent gene: The fallacy of "nature versus nurture."* New York: Owl Books.

Moore, B. E., & Fine, B. D. (Eds.). (1990). *Psychoanalytic terms and concepts.* New Haven, CT: Yale University Press.

Neimeyer, R. A., & Mahoney, M. J. (Eds.). (1999). *Constructivism in psychotherapy.* Washington, DC: American Psychological Association.

Neisser, U. (1976). *Cognition and reality: Principles and implications of cognitive psychology.* New York: Freeman.

Nemeroff, C. B., Bremner, J. D., Foa, E. B., Mayberg, H. S., North, C. S., & Stein, M. B. (2006). Posttraumatic stress disorder: A state-of-the-science review. *Journal of Psychiatric Research, 40,*1–21.

Nichols, M., & Paolino, T. (Eds.). (1986). *Basic techniques of psychodynamic psychotherapy: Foundations of clinical practice.* New York: Gardner Press.

Nietzsche, F. W. (1885/1978). *Thus spoke Zarathustra.* New York: Penguin.

Norcross, J. C. (Ed.). (2002). *Psychotherapy relationships that work: Therapist contributions and responsiveness to patient needs.* New York: Oxford University Press.

O'Brien, G., & Jureidini, J. (2002). Dispensing with the dynamic unconscious. *Philosophy, Psychiatry, and Psychology, 9,* 141–153.

Ogden, T. H. (1979). On projective identification. *International Journal of Psycho-Analysis, 60,* 357–373.

Ogden, T. H. (1982). *Projective identification and psychotherapeutic technique.* New York: Aronson.

Ogden, T. H. (1994). The analytic third: Working with intersubjective clinical facts. *International Journal of Psycho-Analysis, 75,* 3–19.

Ogden, T. H. (2004). The analytic third: Implications for psychoanalytic theory and technique. *Psychoanalytic Quarterly, 73,* 167–195.

O'Hanlon, W. H., & Weiner-Davis, M. (1989). *In search of solutions: A new direction in psychotherapy.* New York: Norton.

Orange, D. M., Atwood, G. E., & Stolorow, R. D. (1997). *Working intersubjectively: Contextualism in psychoanalytic practice.* Hillsdale, NJ: Analytic Press.

Orange, D. M., Stolorow, R. D., & Atwood, G. E. (1998). Hermeneutics, intersubjectivity theory, and psychoanalysis. *Journal of the American Psychoanalytic Association, 46,* 568–571.

Orbach, S. (2004). Beyond the fear of intimacy. *Psychoanalytic Dialogues, 14,* 397–404.

Philipson, I. (1993). *On the shoulders of women: The feminization of psychotherapy.* New York: Guilford Press.

Pizer, S. A. (1992). The negotiation of paradox in the analytic process. *Psychoanalytic Dialogues, 2,* 215–240.

Pizer, S. A. (1996). The distributed self: Introduction to symposium on "The multiplicity of self and analytic technique." *Contemporary Psychoanalysis, 32,* 499–507.

Planck, M. (1936). *The philosophy of physics.* New York: Norton.

Rapaport, D. (1951). *Organization and pathology of thought.* New York: Columbia University Press.

Rapaport, D. (1959). A historical survey of psychoanalytic ego psychology. *Psychological Issues,* Monograph 1 (pp. 5–17). New York: International Universities Press.

Renik, O. (1993a). Analytic interaction: Conceptualizing technique in light of the analyst's irreducible subjectivity. *Psychoanalytic Quarterly, 62,* 553–571.

Renik, O. (1993b). Countertransference enactment and the psychoanalytic process. In M. Horowitz, O. Kernberg, & E. Weinshel (Eds.), *Psychic structure and psychic change* (pp. 137–160). Madison, CT: International Universities Press.

Renik, O. (1995). The ideal of the anonymous analyst and the problem of self-disclosure. *Psychoanalytic Quarterly, 64,* 466–495.

Renik, O. (1999a). Discussion of Roy Schafer's (1999) article. *Psychoanalytic Psychology, 16,* 514–521.

Renik, O. (1999b). Playing one's cards face up in analysis: An approach to the problem of self-disclosure. *Psychoanalytic Quarterly, 68,* 521–539.

Richard, D., & Lauterbach, D. (2006). *Handbook of exposure therapies.* New York: Academic Press.

Rickman, J. (1957). *Selected contributions to psycho-analysis.* Oxford, UK: Basic Books.

Ricoeur, P. (1970). *Freud and philosophy.* New Haven, CT: Yale University Press.

Ridley, M. (2003). *Nature via nurture: Genes, experience, and what makes us human.* New York: HarperCollins.

Rieff, P. (1979). *Freud: The mind of the moralist* (3rd ed.). Chicago: University of Chicago Press.

Robins, C. J., Schmidt, H., & Linehan, M. M. (2004). Dialectical behavior therapy: Synthesizing radical acceptance with skillful means. In S. C.

Hayes, V. M. Follette, & M. M. Linehan (Eds), *Mindfulness and acceptance: Expanding the cognitive-behavioral tradition* (pp. 30–44). New York: Guilford Press.

Rockland, L. H. (1989). *Supportive therapy: A psychodynamic approach.* New York: Basic Books.

Rogers, C. R. (1957). The necessary and sufficient conditions of therapeutic personality change. *Journal of Consulting Psychology, 21,* 95–103.

Safran, J. D. (Ed.). (2003). *Psychoanalysis and Buddhism: An unfolding dialogue.* New York: Wisdom.

Safran, J. D., & Muran, J. C. (2000). *Negotiating the therapeutic alliance: A relational treatment guide.* New York: Guilford Press.

Samuels, A. (2000). Post-Jungian dialogues. *Psychoanalytic Dialogues, 10,* 403–426.

Sapolsky, R. M. (2000, March/April). Genetic hyping. *The Sciences: Annals of the New York Academy of Sciences, 12.*

Schacter, D. L. (1996). *Searching for memory: The brain, the mind, and the past.* New York: Basic Books.

Schacter, D. L. (2001). *The seven sins of memory: How the mind forgets and remembers.* Boston: Houghton Mifflin.

Schafer, R. (1976). *A new language for psychoanalysis.* New Haven, CT: Yale University Press.

Schafer, R. (1977). The interpretation of transference and the conditions for loving. *Journal of the American Psychoanalytic Association, 25,* 335–362.

Schafer, R. (1983). *The analytic attitude.* New York: Basic Books.

Schafer, R. (1992). *Retelling a life: Narration and dialogue in psychoanalysis.* New York: Basic Books.

Schafer, R. (1997). *The contemporary Kleinians of London.* Madison, CT: International Universities Press.

Schimek, J. G. (1975a). The interpretations of the past: Childhood trauma, psychical reality, and historical truth. *Journal of the American Psychoanalytic Association, 23,* 845–865.

Schimek, J. G. (1975b). A critical re-examination of Freud's concept of unconscious mental representation. *International Review of Psycho-Analysis, 2,* 171–187.

Selvini-Palizzoli, M., Boscolo, L., Cecchin, G., & Prata, G. (1990). *Paradox and counterparadox.* New York: Aronson.

Shapiro, D. (1965). *Neurotic styles.* New York: Basic Books.

Shapiro, D. (1981). *Autonomy and rigid character.* New York: Basic Books.

Shapiro, D. (1989). *Psychotherapy of neurotic character.* New York: Basic Books.

Shapiro, D. (2000). *Dynamics of character.* New York: Basic Books.

Shevrin, H. (1992). The Freudian unconscious and the cognitive unconscious: Identical or fraternal twins? In J. Barron, M. Eagle, and D. Wolitzky (Eds.), *Interface of psychoanalysis and psychology* (pp. 313–326). Washington, DC: American Psychological Association.

Silberschatz, G. (2005). *Transformative relationships: The control mastery theory of psychotherapy.* New York: Routledge.

Silverman, D. K. (2000). An interrogation of the relational turn: A discussion with Stephen Mitchell. *Psychoanalytic Psychology, 17,* 146–152.

Silverman, D. K., & Wolitzky, D. L. (Eds.). (2000). *Changing conceptions of psychoanalysis: The legacy of Merton M. Gill.* Hillsdale, NJ: Analytic Press.

Simonds, S. L. (2001). *Depression and women: An integrative treatment approach.* New York: Springer.

Singer, E. (1977). The fiction of analytic anonymity. In K. A. Frank (Ed.), The human dimension in psychoanalytic practice (pp. 181–192). New York: Grune & Stratton.

Skolnick, N. J., & Warshaw, S. C. (1992). *Relational perspectives in psychoanalysis.* Hillsdale, NJ: Analytic Press.

Slade, A. (2000). The development and organization of attachment: Implications for psychoanalysis. *Journal of the American Psychoanalytic Association, 48,* 1147–1174.

Slavin, M. O. (1996). Is one self enough? Multiplicity in self-organization and the capacity to negotiate relational conflict. *Contemporary Psychoanalysis, 32,* 615–625.

Spence, D. P. (1982). *Narrative truth and historical truth.* New York: Norton.

Spezzano, C. (1996). The three faces of two-person psychology: Development, ontology, and epistemology. *Psychoanalytic Dialogues, 6,* 599–622.

Sroufe, L. A., Egeland, B., Carlson, E., & Collins, A. (2005). *The development of the person.* New York: Guilford Press.

Stein, M. H. (1979). Review of H. Kohut, The Restoration of the Self. *Journal of the American Psychoanalytic Association, 27,* 665–680.

Stern, D. B. (1996). The social construction of therapeutic action. *Psychoanalytic Inquiry, 16,* 265–293.

Stern, D. B. (1997). *Unformulated experience: From dissociation to imagination in psychoanalysis.* Hillsdale, NJ: Analytic Press.

Stern, D. B. (2002). Words and wordlessness in the psychoanalytic situation. *Journal of the American Psychoanalytic Association, 50,* 221–247.

Stern, D. B. (2003). The fusion of horizons: Dissociation, enactment, and understanding. *Psychoanalytic Dialogues, 13,* 843–873.

Stern, D. B. (2004). The eye sees itself: Dissociation, enactment, and the achievement of conflict. *Contemporary Psychoanalysis, 40,* 197–237.

Stern, D. N. (1985). *The interpersonal world of the infant.* New York: Basic Books.

Stern, D. N. (2004). *The present moment: In psychotherapy and everyday life.* New York: Norton.

Stern, D. N., Sander, L. W., Nahum, J. P., Harrison, A. M., Lyons-Ruth, K., Morgan, A. C., et al. (1998). Non-interpretive mechanisms in psychoanalytic therapy: The "something more" than interpretation. *International Journal of Psycho-Analysis, 79,* 903–921.

Stolorow, R. D. (1997a). A dynamic systems approach to the development of cognition and action. *International Journal of Psycho-Analysis, 78,* 620–622.

Stolorow, R. D. (1997b). Dynamic, dyadic, intersubjective systems. *Psychoanalytic Psychology, 14,* 337–346.

Stolorow, R. D. (1997c). Principles of dynamic systems, intersubjectivity, and the obsolete distinction between one-person and two-person psychologies. *Psychoanalytic Dialogues, 7,* 859–868.

Stolorow, R. D., & Atwood, G. E. (1979). *Faces in a cloud: Subjectivity in personality theory.* New York: Aronson.

Stolorow, R. D., & Atwood, G. E. (1984). Psychoanalytic phenomenology: Toward a science of human experience. *Psychoanalytic Inquiry, 4,* 87–105.

Stolorow, R. D., & Atwood, G. E. (1989). The unconscious and unconscious fantasy: An intersubjective-developmental perspective. *Psychoanalytic Inquiry, 9,* 364–374.

Stolorow, R. D., & Atwood, G. E. (1992). *Contexts of being: The intersubjective foundations of psychological life.* Hillsdale, NJ: Analytic Press.

Stolorow, R. D., & Atwood, G. E. (1997). Deconstructing the myth of the neutral analyst: An alternative from intersubjective systems theory. *Psychoanalytic Quarterly, 66,* 431–449.

Stolorow, R. D., Atwood, G. E., and Orange, D. M. (1999). Kohut and contextualism. *Psychoanalytic Psychology, 16,* 380–388.

Stolorow, R. D., Brandchaft, B., & Atwood, G. E. (1987). *Psychoanalytic treatment: An intersubjective approach.* Hillsdale, NJ: Analytic Press.

Stolorow, R. D., Orange, D. M., & Atwood, G. E. (2001a). Cartesian and post-cartesian trends in relational psychoanalysis. *Psychoanalytic Psychology, 18,* 468–484.

Stolorow, R. D., Orange, D. M., and Atwood, G. E. (2001b). World horizons: A post-Cartesian alternative to the Freudian unconscious. *Contemporary Psychoanalysis., 37,* 43–61.

Stone, L. (1961). *The psychoanalytic situation.* New York: International Universities Press.

Strachey, J. (1934). The nature of the therapeutic action of psycho-analysis. *International Journal of Psycho-Analysis, 15,* 127–159.

Sullivan, H. S. (1953). *The interpersonal theory of psychiatry.* New York: Norton.

Swann, W. B. (1997). The trouble with change: Self-verification and. allegiance to the self. *Psychological Science, 8,* 177–180.

Thelen, E., & Smith, L. B. (1994). *A dynamic systems approach to the development of cognition and action.* Cambridge, MA: MIT Press.

Tronick, E. (1989). Emotions and emotional communication in infants. *American Psychologist, 44,* 112–119.

van der Kolk, B., McFarlane, A., & Weisaeth, L. (Eds.). (1996). *Traumatic stress: The effects of overwhelming experience on mind, body, and society.* New York: Guilford Press.

Wachtel, E. F. (1994). *Treating troubled children and their families.* New York: Guilford Press.

Wachtel, E. F. (2001). The language of becoming: Helping children change how they think about themselves. *Family Process, 40,* 369–383.

Wachtel, E. F., & Wachtel, P. L. (1986). *Family dynamics in individual psychotherapy.* New York: Guilford Press.

Wachtel, P. L. (1973). Psychodynamics, behavior therapy, and the implacable experimenter: An inquiry into the consistency of personality. *Journal of Abnormal Psychology, 82,* 324–334.

Wachtel, P. L. (1977a). *Psychoanalysis and behavior therapy.* New York: Basic Books.

Wachtel, P. L. (1977b). Interaction cycles, unconscious processes, and the person situation issue. In D. Magnusson & N. Endler (Eds.), *Personality at the crossroads: Issues in interactional psychology* (pp. 317–331). Hillsdale, NJ: Erlbaum.

Wachtel, P. L. (1979). Karen Horney's ironic vision. *The New Republic, 106*(1), 22–25.

Wachtel, P. L. (1980). What should we say to our patients?: On the wording of therapists' comments to patients. *Psychotherapy: Theory, Research, and Practice, 17,* 183–188.

Wachtel, P. L. (1981). Transference, schema, and assimilation: The relevance of Piaget to the psychoanalytic theory of transference. *The annual of psychoanalysis* (Vol. 8, pp. 59–76). New York: International Universities Press.

Wachtel, P. L. (1982a). Vicious circles: The self and the rhetoric of emerging and unfolding. *Contemporary Psychoanalysis, 18,* 273–295.

Wachtel, P. L. (1982b). Phenomenological virtuoso: A review of David Shapiro's autonomy and rigid character. *Contemporary Psychology, 27,* 681–682.

Wachtel, P. L. (1983). *The poverty of affluence.* New York: The Free Press.

Wachtel, P. L. (1987a). *Action and insight.* New York: Guilford Press.

Wachtel, P. L. (1987b). Are we prisoners of the past?: Rethinking Freud. *Tikkun, 2*(3), 24–27, 90–92.

Wachtel, P. L. (1987c). You can't go far in neutral. In *Action and insight.* (pp. 176–184). New York: Guilford Press.

Wachtel, P. L. (1991). The role of accomplices in preventing and facilitating change. In R. Curtis & G. Stricker (Eds.), *How people change: Inside and outside therapy* (pp. 21–28). New York: Plenum Press.

Wachtel, P. L. (1993). *Therapeutic communication.* New York: Guilford Press.

Wachtel, P. L. (1994). Cyclical processes in psychopathology. *Journal of Abnormal Psychology, 103,* 51–54.

Wachtel, P. L. (1995). The contextual self. In C. Strozier & M. Flynn (Eds.), *Trauma and self* (pp. 45–56). London: Rowman & Littlefield.

Wachtel, P. L. (1997). *Psychoanalysis, behavior therapy, and the relational world.* Washington, DC: American Psychological Association.

Wachtel, P. L. (1999). *Race in the mind of America: Breaking the vicious circles between blacks and whites.* New York: Routledge.

Wachtel, P. L. (2002). EMDR and psychoanalysis. In F. Shapiro (Ed.), *EMDR as an integrative psychotherapy approach: Experts of diverse orientations explore the paradigm prism* (pp. 123–150). Washington, DC: American Psychological Association.

Wachtel, P. L. (2003a). The surface and the depths: The metaphor of depth in psychoanalysis and the ways in which it can mislead. *Contemporary Psychoanalysis, 39,* 5–26.

Wachtel, P. L. (2003b). Full pockets, empty lives: A psychoanalytic exploration of the contemporary culture of greed. *American Journal of Psychoanalysis, 63,* 101–120.

Wachtel, P. L. (2005a). Implications of the two-configurations model. for the analysis of social and political phenomena. In J. Auerbach, K. Levy, & C. Schaffer (Eds.), *Relatedness, self-definition and mental representation: Essays in honor of Sidney J. Blatt* (pp. 241–254). London: Brunner-Routledge.

Wachtel, P. L. (2005b). Anxiety, consciousness, and self-acceptance: Placing the idea of making the unconscious conscious in an integrative framework. *Journal of Psychotherapy Integration, 14,* 243–253.

Wachtel, P. L. (2006). Psychoanalysis, science, and hermeneutics: The vicious circles of adversarial discourse. *Journal of European Psychoanalysis, 22,* 25–46.

Wachtel, P. L., & DeMichele, A. (1998). Unconscious plans, or unconscious conflicts? *Psychoanalytic Dialogues, 8,* 429–442.

Waelder, P. (1960). *Basic theory of psychoanalysis.* New York: International Universities Press.

Wallerstein, R., and Richards, A. (1984). The relation between psychoanalytic theory and psychoanalytic technique. *Journal of the American Psychoanalytic Association, 32,* 587–602.

Wallerstein, R. S. (1988). Psychoanalysis and psychotherapy. *Annual of Psychoanalysis, 16,* 129–151.

Wallerstein, R. S. (1989). The psychotherapy research project of the Menninger Foundation: An overview. *Journal of Consulting and Clinical Psychology, 57,* 195–205.

Wampold, B. E. (2001). *The great the debate: Models, methods, and findings.* Mahwah, NJ: Erlbaum.

Weeks, G. R. (Ed.). (1991). *Promoting change through paradoxical therapy* (rev. ed.). Philadelphia: Brunner/Mazel.

Weiss, J. (1998). Patients' unconscious plans for solving their problems. *Psychoanalytic Dialogues, 8,* 411–428.

Weiss, J., Sampson, H., & the Mt. Zion Psychotherapy Research Group. (1986). *The psychoanalytic process.* New York: Guilford Press.

Werman, D. A. (1984). *The practice of supportive psychotherapy.* New York: Brunner/Mazel.

Westen, D. (1989). Are "primitive" object relations really preoedipal? *American Journal of Orthopsychiatry, 59,* 331–345.

Westen, D. (1990). Toward a revised theory of borderline object relations: Contributions of empirical research. *International Journal of Psycho-Analysis, 71,* 661–693

Westen, D. (1991). Social cognition and object relations. *Psychological Bulletin, 109,* 429–455.

Westen, D. (1992a). Social cognition and social affect in psychoanalysis and cognitive psychology: From regression analysis to analysis of regression. In J. W. Barron, M. N. Eagle, & D. L. Wolitzky (Eds.). *Interface of psychoanalysis and psychology* (pp. 375–388). Washington, DC: American Psychological Association.

Westen, D. (1992b). The cognitive self and the psychoanalytic self: Can we put our selves together? *Psychological Inquiry, 3,* 1–13.

Westen, D. (2002). The language of psychoanalytic discourse. *Psychoanalytic Dialogues, 12,* 857–898.

Westen, D., & Gabbard, G. O. (2002a). Developments in cognitive neuroscience: I. Conflict, compromise, and connectionism. *Journal of the American Psychoanalytic Association, 50,* 53–98.

Westen, D., & Gabbard, G. O. (2002b). Developments in cognitive neuroscience: II. Implications for theories of transference. *Journal of the American Psychoanalytic Association, 50,* 99–134.

White, M., & Epston, D. (1990). *Narrative means to therapeutic ends.* New York: Norton.

Wile, D. (1984). Kohut, Kernberg, and accusatory interpretations. *Psychotherapy: Theory, Research, and Practice, 21,* 353–364.

Winnicott, D. W. (1953). Transitional objects and transitional phenomena: A study of the first not-me possession. *International Journal of Psycho-Analysis, 34,* 89–97.

Winnicott, D. W. (1955) Metapsychological and clinical aspects of regression within the psycho-analytical set-up. *International Journal of Psycho-Analysis, 36,* 16–26.

Winnicott, D. W. (1956). On transference. *International Journal of Psycho-Analysis, 37,* 386–388.

Winnicott, D. W. (1960). Ego distortion in terms of true and false self. *The maturational processes and the facilitating environment* (pp. 140–152). New York: International Universities Press.

Winnicott, D. W. (1965). The maturational processes and the facilitating environment. *International Psycho-Analysis Lib., 64,* 1–276.

Winnicott, D. W. (1968). Playing: Its theoretical status in the clinical situation. *International Journal of Psycho-Analysis, 49,* 591–599.

Winnicott, D. W. (1971). *Playing and reality.* New York: Basic Books.

Winnicott, D. W. (1975). *Through paediatrics to psycho-analysis.* New York: Basic Books.

Wolff, P. H. (2001, June). *Why psychoanalysis is still interesting.* Paper presented at the annual meeting of the Rapaport-Klein Study Group, Stockbridge, MA.

Zeanah, C. H., Anders, T. F., Seifer, R., & Stern, D. N. (1989). Implications of research on infant development for psychodynamic theory and practice. *Journal of the American Academy of Child and Adolescent Psychiatry, 28,* 657–668.

Zeig, J. K. (Ed.). (1985). *Ericksonian psychotherapy.* New York: Brunner/Mazel.

Zinbarg, R. E., Barlow, D. H., Brown, T. A., & Hertz, R. M. (1992). Cognitive-behavioral approaches to the nature and treatment of anxiety disorders. *Annual Review of Psychology, 43,* 235–267.

Author Index

Subject Index